THE **COMPACT CLINICAL**
Series Editor: Yvonne D'Arcy,

DISCARDED

Liza Marmo, MSN, RN-BC, CCRN, is currently a Education Specialist–Early Response Team Leader and a Clinical Adjunct Professor at the University of Dentistry and Medicine of New Jersey in Newark, New Jersey. Liza has worked in a variety of roles at the Morristown Medical Center in Morristown, New Jersey, for 20 years, including nurse manager at the Morristown Medical Center Pain Management Center. She has been Co-Chair of the Pain Steering Committee and Chair of Pain Resource Nurses. While in this role, she also maintained responsibility for HCAHPS in which the hospital met the national average. Ms. Marmo taught pain management in hospital orientation and provided education to staff nurses on pain management at Morristown Medical Center. Ms Marmo was the Principal Investigator for a research study on "Pain Assessment Tool in the Critically Ill CPACU Patient." She has had the opportunity to share her research efforts and her expertise in pain and critical care through publications and presentations, locally and nationally. Ms. Marmo currently holds certifications in AACN Critical Care and ANCC Pain Management

Yvonne D'Arcy, MS, CRNP, CNS, is the Pain and Palliative Care Nurse Practitioner at Suburban Hospital-Johns Hopkins Medical Center in Bethesda, Maryland. She has served on the board of directors for the American Society of Pain Management Nurses and has played an integral role in the formulation of several guidelines on the management of acute and chronic pain. She is a Principal Investigator at Suburban Hospital for Dissemination and Implementation of Evidence-Based Methods to Measure and Improve Pain Outcomes. Ms. D'Arcy is also the recipient of the Nursing Spectrum Nursing Excellence Award in the Washington, DC, Maryland, and Virginia districts for Advancing and Leading the Profession. She has contributed to numerous books and journals throughout her career. Books include *Pain Management: Evidence-Based Tools and Techniques for Nursing Professionals, Compact Clinical Guide to Chronic Pain, Compact Clinical Guide to Acute Pain, and Compact Clinical Guide to Cancer Pain* co-authored with Pamela Davies. Her book, *How to Manage Pain in the Elderly* is an *American Journal of Nursing* Book of the Year for 2010. Her book, *Compact Clinical to Women's Pain,* is scheduled for 2013 publication. Ms. D'Arcy lectures and presents nationally and internationally on such topics as chronic pain, difficult-to-treat neuropathic pain syndromes, and all aspects of acute pain management. Articles she has published can be found in an extensive number of journals, including but not limited to *American Nurse Today, Nursing 2011, Pain Management Nursing, PT Insider,* and *Nurse Practitioner Journal.*

Compact Clinical Guide to

CRITICAL CARE, TRAUMA AND EMERGENCY PAIN MANAGEMENT

An Evidence-Based Approach for Nurses

Liza Marmo, MSN, RN-BC, CCRN
Yvonne D'Arcy, MS, CRNP, CNS

SERIES EDITOR
Yvonne D'Arcy, MS, CRNP, CNS

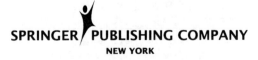

SPRINGER PUBLISHING COMPANY
NEW YORK

LIBRARY
CALDWELL COMMUNITY COLLEGE
HUDSON, NC

Copyright © 2013 Springer Publishing Company, LLC

All rights reserved. 13-MBT46.64

No part of this publication may be reproduced, stored in a retrieval system, or transmitted in any form or by any means, electronic, mechanical, photocopying, recording, or otherwise, without the prior permission of Springer Publishing Company, LLC, or authorization through payment of the appropriate fees to the Copyright Clearance Center, Inc., 222 Rosewood Drive, Danvers, MA 01923, 978-750-8400, fax 978-646-8600, info@copyright.com or on the web at www.copyright.com.

Springer Publishing Company, LLC
11 West 42nd Street
New York, NY 10036
www.springerpub.com

Acquisitions Editor: Margaret Zuccarini
Composition: S4Carlisle Publishing Services

ISBN: 978-0-8261-0807-4
E-book ISBN: 978-0-8261-0808-1

13 14 15 16 / 5 4 3 2 1

The author and the publisher of this Work have made every effort to use sources believed to be reliable to provide information that is accurate and compatible with the standards generally accepted at the time of publication. Because medical science is continually advancing, our knowledge base continues to expand. Therefore, as new information becomes available, changes in procedures become necessary. We recommend that the reader always consult current research, current drug information, and specific institutional policies before performing any clinical procedure or administering any drug. The author and publisher shall not be liable for any special, consequential, or exemplary damages resulting, in whole or in part, from the readers' use of, or reliance on, the information contained in this book. The publisher has no responsibility for the persistence or accuracy of URLs for external or third-party Internet Web sites referred to in this publication and does not guarantee that any content on such Web sites is, or will remain, accurate or appropriate.

Library of Congress Cataloging-in-Publication Data
Marmo, Liza.
 Compact clinical guide to critical care, trauma, and emergency pain management : an evidence-based approach for nurses / author, Liza Marmo ; contributing author and series editor, Yvonne M. D'Arcy.
   p. ; cm. — (Compact clinical guide)
 Includes bibliographical references and index.
 ISBN 978-0-8261-0807-4 — ISBN 0-8261-0807-5 — ISBN 978-0-8261-0808-1 (e-book)
 I. D'Arcy, Yvonne M. II. Title. III. Series: Compact clinical guide series.
 [DNLM: 1. Pain Management—nursing. 2. Critical Care. 3. Emergencies—nursing.
 4. Evidence-Based Nursing. 5. Wounds and Injuries—nursing. WY 160.5]
 616'.0472—dc23
                                        2012023435

Special discounts on bulk quantities of our books are available to corporations, professional associations, pharmaceutical companies, health care organizations, and other qualifying groups.

If you are interested in a custom book, including chapters from more than one of our titles, we can provide that service as well.

For details, please contact:
Special Sales Department, Springer Publishing Company, LLC
11 West 42nd Street, 15th Floor, New York, NY 10036-8002
Phone: 877-687-7476 or 212-431-4370; Fax: 212-941-7842
Email: sales@springerpub.com

Printed in the United States of America by Gasch Printing.

I dedicate this book to my husband Gary and children, Ashlie, Vincent, and Daniel who unconditionally love and support me through all my professional endeavors.

LIZA MARMO

Contents

Preface

Pain is one of the most common symptoms experienced by patients. Critically ill patients, particularly those not able to communicate, are at high risk for experiencing unrelieved pain. This population is often unable to speak for themselves and rely on their caregivers to be their voices. Many of us had limited education on pain while in school—my pain education was limited to just one lecture. We did the best that we could with the knowledge we had.

Each of us has gotten caught up in the common misconceptions surrounding pain. Comments such as "You can't give the patient anything for pain because you might drop their blood pressure" or "That patient is drug seeking because he calls for his pain medication like clockwork" and "Sleeping patients can't be experiencing pain" continue to exist today.

In the late 1990s the Joint Commission was buzzing about making pain a priority and mandating that each patient be assessed. I was asked to attend a day-long conference on pain management where Chris Pasero was the speaker. It was one of the best conferences I attended. Chris spoke so passionately about the plight of patients who experience pain—it was the day I changed how I render care to my patients. I took my new knowledge back to my department and began trying to make a difference.

As a nurse, I am in charge of each of my patients and often I am their voice. It is the responsibility of health care professionals to ensure the comfort of each of their patients and to minimize the untoward sequelae of unrelieved pain. We must ensure that those patients that can communicate are heard, and use our critical thinking and advanced assessment skills for those patients that cannot alert us if they are experiencing pain.

As Jo Eland, President of American Society of Pain Management Nurses, says "Nurses own pain." Pain is the one thing that nurses really own and have the ability to make a difference to our patients. It is imperative that all health care professionals understand pain and have a basic understanding of pain mechanisms, both physiologically and psychologically.

This knowledge is essential in attempting to alleviate the pain and the suffering that is associated with it.

This book in the Compact Clinical Guide series is for the health care professional who cares for patients in various settings that may be experiencing pain. The book provides some basic concepts on pain and pain medications, and then focuses on specific types of pain such as abdominal pain and chest pain. Each chapter contains short case studies that focus on the concepts of the chapter. All information is based upon evidence-based guidelines and evidence-based practice.

A critical care nurse for more than 10 years and with 10 years practicing in pain management, I hope that you find this book a helpful resource in managing your patients' pain and help in improving their outcomes.

Liza Marmo, MSN, RN-BC, CCRN

Acknowledgments

This book could not have been written without Yvonne D'Arcy, who not only served as the series editor, but also encouraged and challenged me throughout this endeavor. Without her mentoring, guidance, and support this book would not have come to fruition. I am forever and truly grateful.

1

The Problem of Pain in the Critically Ill

"Pain is a major health care problem. Although acute pain may reasonably be considered a symptom of disease or injury, chronic and recurrent pain is a specific healthcare problem, a disease in its own right." (IASP, 2011; EFIC, 2011)

Admission to a critical care setting is usually a threat to the life and well-being of the patient. Critical care nurses often see the intensive care unit as a place where fragile lives are carefully analyzed and cared for. Patients and their families often see admission to critical care as a sign of imminent death. Understanding what the critical care setting signifies to patients may help health care professionals care for their patients. However, communication with a critically ill patient is often challenging and frustrating due to the barriers that exist related to the patient's physiological condition, or the presence of endotracheal tubes which inhibit communication, or mind altering medications, or other conditions that affect cognitive function.

Researchers have long studied the patient experience related to an ICU stay. Many patients recall negative feelings related to fear, anxiety, sleep disturbance, cognitive impairment, and pain or discomfort. Many patients mistakenly believe that pain is to be expected and endured or they fear opioid use will result in addiction. Health care professionals are often unaware of a patient's discomfort or do not understand the physiological effects of uncontrolled/unrelieved pain. Despite the advances that have been made overall, unrelieved pain is still a major problem.

Pain is a stressor for the critically ill patient and provides significant challenges for the health care professional. Critically ill patients may suffer excessive pain from their life-threatening illnesses, injuries, or nursing care

1

and/or procedures (turning, endotracheal suctioning, removal of a chest tube). The critically ill often are unable to effectively communicate to their caregivers, making it difficult to assess and manage their pain effectively. In an effort to solve this ongoing problem, health care professionals must be able to recognize pain particularly in the critically ill. One must assume that all critically ill patients are in pain or are at high risk for pain.

The health care team must work together with the patient to establish common pain treatment goals. In order to select the most appropriate treatment, thorough pain assessment and in-depth understanding of pain physiology are needed. An understanding of how pain is processed at each stage allows the treatment plan to be tailored for each individual patient.

In most instances, the goal of the treatment strategy may be to achieve the maximal analgesia but when that is not possible, the goal shifts to reducing pain to a level that the patient finds tolerable and that allows for the performance of activities of daily living. Once that goal has been established the next step is to develop a plan to meet that goal.

PREVALENCE OF PAIN

Pain can significantly impact a patient's recovery. The exact prevalence is unknown although we know that it is high and can come from many different sources. Pain can occur as a result of surgery, procedures, illness, or trauma, and pain for most patients does not resolve until healing has occurred.

Apfelbaum, Chen, Mehta, and Gann (2003) conducted a randomized qualitative study of 250 patients who had recently undergone surgery. The study found that approximately 80% of patient's experienced acute pain after surgery. Of these patients, 86% had moderate, severe, or extreme pain, with more patients experiencing pain after discharge than before discharge. Almost 25% of patients who received pain medications experienced adverse effects, although almost 90% of them were satisfied with their pain medications. This study identified a need for additional efforts in order to improve pain suppression.

The American Association of Critical Care Nurses (AACN) supported the Thunder Project II, a large research study in which pain perception and responses to tracheal suctioning, as well as five other procedures, were evaluated (Puntillo et al., 2004, 2001). Thunder Project II was a comprehensive, descriptive study of pain perceptions and responses of patients to these six common procedures: turning, removal of wound drains, tracheal suctioning, removal of femoral catheters, insertion of central venous catheters, and non-burn wound dressing change. Data were obtained from

6,201 patients aged 4 to 97 years, 5,957 of which were adults. Numeric rating scales were used to measure pain intensity and procedural distress and word lists were used to measure pain quality. Mean pain intensity scores for turning and tracheal suctioning were 2.80 and 3.00, respectively (scale, 0–5). In adults, mean pain intensity scores for all procedures were 2.65 to 4.93 (scale, 0–10); mean procedural distress scores were 1.89 to 3.47 (scale, 0–10). The most painful and distressing procedure for adults was turning. Less than 20% of patients received opiates before procedures.

A study by Gélinas (2007) described the pain experience of cardiac surgery ICU patients. After the patients were transferred to the surgical unit, 93 patients were interviewed about their pain experience while they were in the ICU. Sixty-one patients (65.6%) recalled being ventilated and 72 patients (77.4%) recalled having pain. Turning was the most frequent source of pain experienced by these patients. A large proportion of the patients (47.3%) identified the thorax as the location of their pain. All patients had a sternal incision. Pain was mild for 16 patients, moderate for 21, and severe for 25 of them. While ventilated, head nodding and movements of the upper limbs were the most frequent means of communication used by the patients.

These findings are disturbing, and revealed that pain still exists and many the patients still experience moderate and severe pain despite all of the advances that have been made in pain management.

THEORIES OF PAIN

Pain has been experienced by everyone regardless of age, gender, or economic status. Pain is usually described as an unfavorable experience that has a lasting emotional and disabling influence on the individual. Theories that explain and assist in understanding what pain is, how it originates, and why we feel it are the Specificity Theory, Pattern Theory, and Gate Theory.

Since the beginning of time, the many theories regarding the cause, nature, and purpose of pain have been debated. Most early theories were based on the assumption that pain was a form of punishment. The word "pain" is derived from the Latin word "poena" meaning fine, penalty, or punishment. The ancient Greeks believed that pain was associated with pleasure because the relief of pain was both pleasurable and emotional. Aristotle reassessed the theory of pain and declared that the soul was the center of the sensory processes and the pain system was located in the heart. The Romans came closer to contemporary thought, viewing pain as something that accompanied inflammation.

In the second century, Galen offered the Romans his works on the concepts of the nervous system. In the fourth century, successors of Aristotle discovered anatomic proof that the brain was connected to the nervous system. Aristotle's belief prevailed until the 19th century, when German scientists provided unquestionable evidence that the brain is involved with sensory and motor function.

Specificity Theory

In the 17th century, Descartes described pain in physical terms. Pain was a physical occurrence traveling along a specific path suggesting that pain is caused by injury or damage to body tissue. The damaged nerve fibers in our bodies send direct messages through specific pain receptors and fibers to the pain center, which causes the individual to feel pain (Adams & Bromley, 1998). The amount of pain experienced by an individual is related to the severity of the injury.

The Specificity Theory was the most widely accepted theory of pain transmission through the end of the 19th century. The theory supports the idea that the body's neurons and pathways for transmission are as specific and unique as those for other body senses such as touch and taste. The free nerve endings in the skin act as pain receptors, accepting sensory input and transmitting this input along highly specific nerve fibers. These fibers synapse in the dorsal horns of the spinal cord, and cross over to the anterior and lateral spinothalmic tracts. The pain impulses then ascend to the thalamus and cerebral cortex, where painful sensations are perceived. The theory does not explain the difference in pain perception among individuals, nor does it satisfactorily account for the effect of physiologic variables, the effect of previous experience with pain, phantom limb pain, or peripheral neuralgias.

Pattern Theory

The Pattern Theory was introduced in the early 1900s. It identifies two major types of pain fibers, rapidly and slowly conducting fibers (A-delta and C fibers, respectively). The stimulation of these fibers forms a pattern. The theory also introduced the concept of central summation. Peripheral impulses from many fibers of both types are combined at the level of the spinal cord, and from there a summation of these impulses ascends to the brain for interpretation. The theory does not account for individual perceptual differences and psychological factors. The Pattern Theory claims that pain is felt as a consequence to the amount of tissue damaged (McCance & Huether, 1990).

Gate Control Theory

In 1962, Ronald Melzack and Patrick Wall proposed the Gate Control Theory. This theory explains how an individual's emotions and thinking can affect one's own perception of pain. It was hypothesized that there is a mechanism in the brain that acts as a gate to either increase or decrease the flow of nerve impulses from the peripheral nerve fibers to the central nervous system. If the gate is open it allows the flow of nerve impulses and as a result the brain perceives pain. If the gate is closed the nerve impulses do not let the brain perceive pain or decrease it.

Gate Control Theory is the first and the only theory to take into account psychological factors of pain experiences. Experiences of pain are influenced by many physical and psychological factors such as beliefs, prior experience, motivation, emotional aspects, anxiety, and depression, all of which can increase pain by affecting the central control system in the brain.

Neuromatrix Theory

In 1999, Melzack and Wall came up with a newer theory of pain, the Neuromatrix Theory (Melzack, 1999). The theory suggests that every human being has their own intrinsic network of neurons that is affected by all aspects of the person's physical, psychological, and cognitive traits, and their experience. Pain sensations are processed by a neural network in the brain. It integrates various inputs to produce the output pattern perceived as pain.

FACTORS AFFECTING PATIENTS' RESPONSES TO PAIN

Everyone has the same pain threshold; everyone perceives pain stimuli at the same stimulus intensity. What varies then is the patient's perception of and reaction to pain.

Age: The older adult with normal age-related changes in neurophysiology may have decreased perception of sensory stimuli and a higher pain threshold.

Sociocultural influences: People's response to pain is strongly influenced by the family, community, and culture. Sociocultural influences affect the way in which a patient tolerates pain, interprets the meaning of pain, and reacts verbally and nonverbally. Cultural influences teach an individual how much pain to tolerate, what types of pain to report and to whom to report the pain, and what kind of pain treatment to seek.

Emotional status: The sensation of pain may be blocked by intense concentration or may be increased by anxiety or fear. Pain often is increased when it occurs in conjunction with other illnesses or physiological discomforts such as nausea and vomiting.

Past experiences with pain: If the patient's childhood experiences with pain were responded to appropriately by supportive adults, as an adult they will usually have a healthy attitude.

Source and meaning: If the patient perceives the pain as deserved, the patient may actually feel relief that the punishment has commenced.

Knowledge deficit: If the patient has a clear and accurate perception of pain, it is far easier for health care professionals to increase the patient's knowledge of both the significance of pain and the strategies the patient can use to diminish discomfort.

REFERENCES

Adams, B., & Bromley, B. (1998). *Psychology for health care: Key terms and concepts.* New York, NY: Macmillan.

Apfelbaum, J. L., Chen, C., Mehta, S. S., & Gann, T. J. (2003). Postoperative pain experience: Results from a national survey suggest postoperative pain continues to be undermanaged. *Anesthesia and Analgesia, 97*(2), 534–540.

Gélinas, C. (2007). Management of pain in cardiac surgery ICU patients: Have we improved over time? *Intensive and Critical Care Nursing, 23*(5), 298–303.

McCance, K. L., & Huether, S. E. (1990). *Pathophysiology: The biologic basis for disease in adults and children.* St. Louis, MO: Mosby.

Melzack, R. (1999). From the gate to the neuromatrix. *Pain,* (Suppl. 6), S121–S126.

Puntillo, K. A., Morris, A. B., Thompson, C. L., Stanik-Hutt, J., White, C. A., & Wild, L. R. (2004). Pain behaviors observed during six common procedures: Results from Thunder Project II. *Critical Care Medicine, 32*, 421–427.

Puntillo, K. A., White, C., Morris, A. B., Perdue, S. T., Stanik-Hutt, J., Thompson, C. L., & Wild, L. R. (2001). Patients' perceptions and responses to procedural pain: Results from Thunder Project II. *American Journal of Critical Care, 10*, 238–251.

Weiner, K. (2003). *Pain issues: Pain is an epidemic.* Retrieved from http://www.aapainman age.org

2

Physiologic and Metabolic Responses to Pain

Pain is defined by the International Association for the Study of Pain (IASP) as "an unpleasant sensory and emotional experience associated with actual or potential tissue damage, or described in terms of such damage" (Merskey & Bogduk, 1994). From this definition, it would seem reasonable to think that pain is a pretty simple concept to understand; however, understanding pain pathophysiology is very complicated. Let's say you are preparing dinner in your kitchen, cutting up vegetables when the knife you are using slips and you feel this incredible painful sensation on your finger. You quickly drop the knife and pull your hand away. There is blood running from your finger and you feel a throbbing pain. Some people even feel light headed and nauseous. This entire process—the painful sensation of cutting your finger—was a very complex phenomenon. Pain serves as one of the body's defense mechanisms warning the brain that there may be potential tissue damage about to occur, although pain may be triggered without any physical damage to the body's tissues.

Our nervous system is associated with everything our body does in order to function—from regulating your breathing, to controlling your muscles, to sensing pain. The nervous system is divided into the peripheral nervous system and the central nervous system and both are involved in the pathophysiology of pain. The central nervous system consists of the brain, spinal cord, and optic nerves; the peripheral nervous system consists of sensory and motor nerves. The sensory nerves carry information from external stimuli to the spinal cord, brain, and motor nerves, then carry the information from the brain and spinal cord to organs, muscles, and glands. Motor nerves can be subdivided into the somatic nervous system and the autonomic nervous system.

The somatic nervous system controls skeletal muscle as well as external sensory organs such as the skin. The autonomic nervous system controls involuntary muscles, such as smooth and cardiac muscles. This system can be further divided into the parasympathetic and sympathetic branches.

The parasympathetic system is concerned with conserving energy, "rest and digest." The sympathetic system is activated during exercise, excitement, and emergencies—"flight, fight, or fright response."

SYSTEMIC EFFECTS
OF PHYSIOLOGICAL CHANGES

Physiological changes can have a serious impact on the cardiovascular, gastrointestinal, respiratory, genitourinary, musculoskeletal, and immune systems. Pain can increase the cardiac and respiratory rates, which increase the oxygen demand. Other physiological changes that take place can induce vomiting and potentially can pre-empt chronic pain conditions.

Cardiovascular System

The stress of unrelieved pain on the cardiovascular system increases the sympathetic nervous system activity, which increases heart rate, blood pressure, and peripheral vascular resistance. As the workload and stress of the heart increase, contributing to hypertension and tachycardia, the oxygen consumption of the myocardium also increases. As oxygen consumption decreases the supply available, myocardial ischemia and, possibly, myocardial infarction can occur. The oxygen supply may be further compromised by the presence of any pre-existing cardiac or respiratory disease or by hypoxemia due to impaired respiratory function (Macintyre & Ready, 2001).

Hypercoagulability occurs when there is a reduction in fibrinolysis compounded with an increased cardiac rate, workload, and blood pressure. This increases the risk of deep vein thrombosis (DVT) and pulmonary embolism (Wood, 2003).

Gastrointestinal System

Increased sympathetic nervous system activity can lead to temporary impaired gastrointestinal function resulting in gastric emptying and reduced bowel motility with the potential development of a paralytic ileus (Macintyre & Ready, 2001).

Respiratory System

Unrelieved pain can result in limited movement of the thoracic and abdominal muscles in an effort to reduce pain. This can cause some degree of respiratory abnormality with secretions and sputum being retained due to the patient being reluctant to cough. Atelectasis and pneumonia may ensue (Macintyre & Ready, 2001). Pulmonary dysfunction, caused by painful movement of the diaphragmatic muscles, is associated with a reduction in vital lung capacity, increased inspiratory and expiratory pressures, and reduced alveolar ventilation. This results in hypoxia, which can cause cardiac complications, disorientation, confusion, and delayed wound healing (Wood, 2003).

Genitourinary System

Unrelieved pain can increase the release of hormones and enzymes, such as catecholamines, aldosterone, ADH, cortisol, angiotensin II, and prostaglandins, which help to regulate urinary output and fluid and electrolyte balance, as well as blood volume and pressure (Pasero & McCaffery, 2010). This results in the retention of sodium and water, causing urinary retention. Increased excretion of potassium causes hypokalemia (Park et al., 2002). A decrease in extracellular fluid occurs as fluid moves into the intracellular compartments, causing fluid overload, increased cardiac workload, and hypertension (Pasero & McCaffery, 2010).

Musculoskeletal System

Involuntary responses to noxious stimuli can result in muscle spasm at the site of tissue damage (Pasero & McCaffery, 2010). Impaired muscle function and muscle fatigue can also lead to immobility, causing venous stasis, increased coagulability, and an increased risk of developing DVT (Park et al., 2002).

Pain can limit thoracic and abdominal muscle movement in an attempt to reduce muscle pain, also known as "splinting." The lack of respiratory muscle excursion can potentially lead to reduced respiratory function (Pasero & McCaffery, 2010).

Immune System

Depression of the immune system can occur as a result of unrelieved pain. This may predispose the patient to wound and chest infection, pneumonia, and, potentially, sepsis (Wood, 2003).

Nausea and Vomiting

When pain receptors in the central nervous system are stimulated, the center of the brain that is responsible for vomiting is activated causing vomiting to occur. Disturbance of the gastrointestinal tract can activate the release of neurotransmitters that can also cause vomiting. These neurotransmitters travel via the circulatory system to the chemoreceptor trigger zone in the brainstem and then on to the area of the brain that is responsible for vomiting, causing the patient to vomit (Jolley, 2001).

Chronic Pain

Poorly controlled acute pain can lead to debilitating chronic pain syndromes. Appropriate aggressive acute pain management is essential to prevent this from occurring (Pasero & McCaffery, 2010). Further discussion is given in the following sections.

PAIN BY DURATION

Acute Pain

Acute pain serves as a warning that illness or injury has occurred. The pain is usually confined to the affected area and is limited in duration to 3 to 6 months or until healing has occurred. Acute pain stimulates the sympathetic nervous system, resulting in increased heart and respiratory rates, sweating, dilated pupils, restlessness, and anxiety. Acute pain can be classified by mechanism: somatic, visceral, and referred. If acute pain is untreated it can become chronic pain (Kehlet, 2006).

Chronic Pain

Chronic pain, also called persistent pain, continues usually more than 3 to 6 months after the expected normal healing period. The pain may be continuous or intermittent. It may or may not be associated with a disease state. Chronic pain is poorly understood, complex, and often difficult to manage. Patients with chronic pain may not exhibit the behaviors associated with acute pain because the body has adapted to persistent pain impulses (Table 2.1).

PAIN BY MECHANISM

Somatic Pain

Somatic pain is caused by the activation of pain receptors in the skin, muscle, joints, or bone as a result of tissue damage. Somatic pain originates from specific nerve ending receptors, making it typically well localized with constant pain that can be described as sharp, aching, throbbing, or gnawing in character. Its cause is usually apparent and usually related to traumatic injury such as lacerations, sprains, fractures, and dislocations.

Table 2.1 ▪ *Acute Versus Chronic Pain*

Acute Pain	Chronic Pain
• Usually obvious tissue damage • Sudden onset • Short duration, resolves with healing • Somatic, visceral, referred • Physiological responses to acute pain include increased RR, HR, BP and reduction in gastric motility—sympathetic response • Associated anxiety • Serves a protective function • Effective therapy available	• Multiple causes (malignancy, benign) • Persistent, usually lasting more than 3 months beyond healing • Can be a symptom or diagnosis • Physiological responses are less obvious especially with adaptation • Psychological responses may include depression • Serves no adaptive purpose • May be refractory to treatment

Visceral Pain

Visceral pain nociceptors are those found in the internal organs of the main body cavities: thorax, abdomen, and pelvis. The causes of visceral pain may result from ischemia, inflammation, stretching, smooth muscle spasm, and distension of a hollow viscous or organ capsule. When visceral receptors are stimulated, poorly localized, diffuse, or vague complaints such as ache, pressure, cramping, throbbing are reported. These complaints may be felt at sites distant from the primary injury also known as referred pain. Visceral pain receptors travel along autonomic nerve fibers resulting in autonomic symptoms such as nausea/vomiting, hypotension, bradycardia, and sweating. Common types of visceral pain are gallbladder, appendicitis, and angina.

Neuropathic Pain

The Assessment Committee of the Neuropathic Pain Special Interest Group (NeuPSIG) of the International Association for the Study of Pain (IASP) recently revised the guidelines on neuropathic pain assessment, including the definition. Neuropathic pain has now been redefined as "pain arising as a direct consequence of a lesion or disease affecting the somatosensory system" (Haanpää et al., 2011).

One would think that injury to a nerve would deaden the sensation but the opposite sometimes occurs with neuropathic pain. Injury can cause numbness, pain with movement, or tenderness of a partially denervated body part. Pain is often described as electric, shocking, burning, shooting, and tingling. Abnormally amplified signals in the CNS due to wind-up result in central sensitization, which is an increased sensitivity of spinal neurons.

Neuropathic pain is commonly seen in patients with diabetes, shingles, herniated discs, and AIDS. It may also result from treatment with radiation or chemotherapy.

PHANTOM PAIN

Phantom pain occurs after amputation of a limb. The patient may experience painful sensations in the missing limb. As many as 70% of amputees report this phantom limb pain, usually within the first week after amputation. This type of sensation is generally intermittent and is often described as shooting, stabbing, pricking, squeezing, throbbing, and burning. Most patients report a decrease in pain over time. The exact etiology of phantom pain is unknown.

The origin of phantom pain is thought to be in the CNS and may be a somatosensory "memory" that involves complex neural interactions in the brain. Treatment for phantom pain is challenging and often unsuccessful.

CENTRAL PAIN

Central pain is a chronic neuropathic pain disorder that develops as a direct consequence of a lesion within the CNS (Gunnar, 2010). Most common causes include infarction, hemorrhage, abscess, tumors, and traumatic injury in the brain or spinal cord.

The term thalamic pain is used synonymously with central pain, although thalamic pain is caused by a lesion(s) in the thalamus. The intensity of pain ranges from mild to excruciating, but is constant, causing much suffering.

Patients with central pain often report burning, aching, and pricking. The location of the pain depends on the lesion involved; the pain may occur in an entire half of the body or in only a small area, such as a hand.

The specific mechanisms of central pain are poorly understood and no treatment is universally effective in treating the underlying cause along with symptomatic treatment.

NOCICEPTION

So just how do we feel pain? Though a person is not consciously aware of the process, the experience of pain involves a complex sequence of processes beginning with tissue damage. Nociceptive pain occurs as a result of the activation of the nociceptive system by noxious stimuli, inflammation, or disease (Woolf, 2004). The process of nociceptive pain is divided into four steps: (1) transduction, (2) transmission, (3) pain modulation, and (4) perception.

1. *Transduction:* Refers to mechanical, thermal, or chemical stimuli that result in tissue damage. Tissue damage releases chemical mediators,

such as histamine, substance P, serotonin (5HT), bradykinin, and prostaglandins. The nociceptors are activated and an action potential or nerve impulse is generated.

2. *Transmission:* The nerve impulse or action potential moves from the injury along the afferent nerve to the nociceptors in the spinal cord and brain.

3. *Perception:* The subjective conscious experience of pain is transmitted by neural activity.

4. *Pain modulation:* Neural activity via descending neural pathways from the brain influences pain transmission at the level of the spinal cord. The nociceptive message is subject to both enhancement and inhibition at all levels of the nervous system. This explains the variability of pain perception by people with the same pain experience.

PAIN PATHWAYS

Pain receptors, also known as nociceptors, are found in almost every tissue in the body. These nociceptors respond to thermal, chemical, and mechanical stimuli through a-delta, C, and a-beta fibers. The a-delta receptors contain small, myelinated fibers that rapidly transmit acute, sharp pain signals from the peripheral nerves to the spinal cord. C receptors have larger, unmyelinated fibers that transmit pain at a slower rate and are commonly associated with long-lasting, burning pain sensations. The a-beta receptors respond to nonpainful touch, such as a gentle rub or pressure.

Table 2.2 ■ *Nerves of Transmission*

A-Delta Fibers	C-Fibers
• Thinly myelinated, large	• Non-myelinated, small
• Fast (first) pain	• Slow (second) pain
• Associated with sharp, brief, pricking pain	• Associated with dull, burning, aching, prolonged pain
• Well localized	• More diffuse
• Elicited by mechanical or thermal stimuli	• Elicited mainly by chemical stimuli or persisting mechanical or thermal stimuli
• May be sensitized	• May be sensitized
• Resistant to local anesthetics but susceptible to pressure	• Susceptible to local anesthetics
• Responsible for I pain (early, sharp, brief pain)	• Responsible for II pain (dull, prolonged pain)

Table 2.3 ▣ *Nociceptors*

Nociceptors	Activated by	Type of Pain	Fibers
Mechanoreceptors	• Strong stimuli pinch • Sharp objects that penetrate • Squeeze • Pinch the skin • Sharp or pricking pain • Pressure • Abscess • Incision • Tumor growth	• Rapid • Sharp • Localized	• A-delta fibers
Thermal	• Burn • Scald • Strong mechanical stimuli		• A-delta fibers
Chemoreceptor	• Activated by chemicals • Ischemia • Infection	• Slow • Dull • Burning • Aching • Persistent pain	• C fibers

The peripheral and central nervous systems are involved with pain perception. The peripheral nerve fibers convey the painful stimuli to the spinal cord. Numerous ascending pathways transmit the stimuli through the dorsal root of a spinal nerve, ending in the dorsal horn of the spinal gray matter. In the substantia gelatinosa, located in the dorsal horn, the stimuli are directed to various parts of the spinal cord. Long nerve fibers, spinothalamic axons and spinoreticular axons, cross over to the opposite side of the spinal cord and ascend to the brain in the anterolateral column of the spinal white matter (Helms & Barone, 2008).

When tissue damage occurs from noxious stimuli, pain-producing substances are released into the extracellular fluid surrounding the pain fibers. These substances include bradykinin, cholecystokinin, serotonin, histamine, potassium ions, norepinephrine, prostaglandins, leukotrienes, and substance P (Helms & Barone, 2008). The brain and spinal cord also produce pain-relieving substances, endorphins and enkephalins. These chemicals attach to endogenous receptors in the brain, spinal cord, and peripheral tissues, activating the descending inhibitory system.

CHRONIC PAIN

Chronic pain can be a major problem for some people and affect their quality of life. It can be caused by alterations in nociception, injury, or disease and may result from current or past damage to the PNS, CNS, or may have no organic cause (Calvino and Grilo, 2006).

Pathophysiology of Chronic Pain

The exact mechanisms involved in the pathophysiology of chronic pain are complex and remain unclear. It is believed that following injury, rapid and long-term changes occur in parts of the CNS that are involved in the transmission and modulation of pain (nociceptive information) (Ko & Zhuo, 2004).

A central mechanism in the spinal cord, called wind-up, also referred to as hypersensitivity or hyperexcitability, may occur. Wind-up occurs when repeated, prolonged, noxious stimulation causes the dorsal horn neurones to transmit progressively increasing numbers of pain impulses.

The patient can feel intense pain in response to a stimulus that is not usually associated with pain, for example, touch. This is called allodynia.

This abnormal processing of pain within the PNS and CNS may become independent of the original painful event. In some cases, for example, amputation, the original injury may have occurred in the peripheral nerves, but the mechanisms that underlie the phantom pain are generated in both the PNS and the CNS.

REFERENCES

Haanpää, M., Attal, N., Backonja, M., Baron, R., Bennett, M., Bouhassira, D., . . . Treede, R. D. (2011). NeuPSIG guidelines on neuropathic pain assessment. *Pain*, *152*(1), 14–27.

Helms, J. E., & Barone, C. P. (2008). Physiology and treatment of pain. *Critical Care Nurse*, *28*(6), 38–49.

Woolf, C. J. (2004). Pain: Moving from symptom control toward mechanism-specific pharmacologic management. *Annals of Internal Medicine*, *140*(6), 441–451.

Additional Readings

Adams, B., & Bromley, B. (1998). *Psychology for health care: Key terms and concepts.* New York, NY: Macmillan.

Barber, J., & Adrian, C. (1982). *Psychological approaches to the management of pain.* New York, NY: Brunner/Mazel.

Brannon, L., & Feist, J. (2000). *Health psychology: An introduction to behaviour and health* (4th ed.). Belmont, CA: Brooks/Cole.

Bond, M. (1984). *Pain: Its nature, analysis and treatment* (2nd ed.). New York, NY: Churchill Livingstone.

Goleman, D., & Gurin, J. (1993). *Mind, body, medicine: How to use your mind for better health.* New York, NY: Consumer Report Books.

McCaffery, M., & Beebe, A. (1994). *Pain: Clinical manual for nursing practice.* Aylesbury, England: Mosby.

McCance, K., & Huether, S. (1990). *Pathophysiology: The biological basis for diseases in adults and children.* St Louis, MO: Mosby.

Plotnik, R. (1999). *Introduction to psychology* (5th ed.). Belmont, CA: Wadsworth.

Sheppard, J. (1981). *Advances in behavioural medicine* (Vol. 1). Sydney, Australia: Cumberland Collage of Health Science.

3

The Art and Science of Pain Assessment

Pain assessment is an essential part of good pain management. Assessment in general is a multifaceted process requiring understanding of pain management, assessment techniques, and advanced communication skills. Nurses play a central role in the management of patients' pain, which highlights the need for nurses to demonstrate excellence in every area of pain management to appropriately and effectively manage patients' pain.

Every patient has the right to have a report of pain acknowledged and promptly treated. Pain has a profound impact on the patient's quality of life and, as well, has physical, psychological, and social consequences. Brennan et al. (2007) has made a convincing case for pain management as a fundamental human right. Making pain management an essential component of health care is a challenge. Major changes need to occur to effectively address the needs of patients in pain.

One of the major factors that lead to inadequate pain management is the lack of regular pain assessment and reassessment. The failure of clinicians to assess pain can lead to undertreated pain and serious medical complications in the acute pain patient. Unrelieved pain after surgery increases heart rate, systemic vascular resistance, and circulating catecholamines, placing patients at risk of myocardial ischemia, stroke, bleeding, and other complications (Brennan et al., 2007).

Pain is one of the top reasons patients seek medical care in the emergency department (ED). Recent studies show that we currently do not address pain adequately or in a timely manner in the ED, although new ideas about pain management and patient satisfaction are evolving. Patients appear to have preferences and expectations for pain management in the ED that can be easily met.

Since the implementation of the 2000 Joint Commission (JC) standards for pain assessment and management, there have been significant improvements. reviewed medical records of 1,454 older patients who presented to the ED with broken hips. Within the study period, an average of

96% of patients with broken hips had pain documented in their medical records. Via use of a standard numeric rating scale (NRS), pain relief in the ED rose from 16.5% to 54.4%. This indicated an improvement in ED pain assessment, but also showed that still more can be done.

Conducted a study to investigate the outcome of nursing assessment, pain assessment, and nurse-initiated IV opioid analgesic compared to standard procedure for patients seeking emergency care for abdominal pain. There were 200 patients in this three-phase study. The nursing assessment and the nurse-initiated IV opioid analgesic resulted in a significant improvement in the frequency and reduction in time to receiving an analgesic. Patients perceived lower pain intensity and improved quality of care in pain management.

EDs should be able to assess and treat pain in triage. When a triage pain assessment is included, patients received pain medication more reliably and more quickly. Triage protocols that allow nurses to administer pain medication show even better performance on length of time to pain management. Pain treatment need not always involve medications but other adjuncts as well, including ice packs, splints, warm blankets, etc. Timeliness of these treatments is critical in the ED, and positively affects patient satisfaction.

The rate of uncontrolled pain in the critically ill remains high, with the majority of patients reporting moderate to severe levels of pain while in the intensive care unit (ICU). A systematic assessment of pain should routinely be done, and self-report by the patient should be the standard for pain assessment whenever possible. The routine assessment of pain with a validated pain assessment tool has been shown to decrease length of stay, decrease the duration of mechanical ventilation, and increase patient, family, and provider satisfaction.

The mandate for the proper assessment of pain has been required by the Agency for Healthcare Research and Quality (AHRQ) and JC. Many professional organizations, including the American Association of Critical Care Nurses (AACN), the American College of Chest Physicians (ACCP), the Society for Critical Care Medicine (SCCM) and the American Society for Pain Management (ASPM), have advocated for implementation of standardized pain assessment tools that include behavioral indicators in patients who are unable to self-report or in those whose self-report may be unreliable. Implementation of routine assessment of pain in the critically ill has demonstrated increased patient satisfaction.

Studies have shown that appropriate treatment of pain and anxiety is associated with decreased length of mechanical ventilation and a decreased rate of nosocomial infections. As well, systematic pain assessment in the critically ill has been shown to decrease ICU length of stay. The first step in providing adequate pain relief for patients is a systematic and consistent assessment and documentation of pain. Many patients in ICUs are unable to self-report pain due to the presence of mechanical ventilation, sedation, or critical illness. Even for patients capable of reporting their pain, the use of self-report as a method of pain assessment has limitations. In the absence of patient self-report, which is still considered the gold standard of pain assessment, the distress associated with pain can generate a broad range of observable behaviors that indicate the presence of pain, such as facial expression, physical movement, or autonomic responses. Many times, these behaviors are used by clinicians to signify the need for analgesia. When nurses are used as proxy reporters, the correlation between the nurse's assessment of pain and the patient's pain rating by self-report is low. Family members do poorly at identifying pain in the patient as well, reporting the presence of pain only 53% of the time.

In recent years, with the focus placed by regulatory agencies on the identification and treatment of pain, there has been a push toward the development of behavior-based pain scales to assess pain in those patient incapable of self-report. The tools are based on the identification of behaviors, such as facial expressions, vocalizations, withdrawal reflexes, and other motor movements that are associated with the existence of pain.

In 2001, the JC implemented pain management and assessment standards in an effort to improve pain management. The standards require that all hospitalized patients have the right to appropriate assessment and management of pain, with regular assessment and reassessment (JC, 2010). If a patient has increased pain, the health care provider uses his or her clinical judgment, consistent with the standards of good clinical practice, and increases the frequency of assessment accordingly (Herr & Garand, 2001). For either acute or persistent pain, a comprehensive ongoing assessment of pain and documentation of response to treatment are vital to effective pain management. The assessment should include both subjective and objective information and include the patient and/or the caretaker if the patient is unable to self-report pain intensity. It is essential that pain management is tailored to the individual needs of the patient and not be a cookie-cutter plan. If the patient is experiencing untoward side effects or the intensity of the patient's pain is not improving, then the patient needs to be reassessed and the treatment plan re-evaluated.

Many factors can influence a person's perception and reaction to pain. These may include (Arnstein, 2010):

▪ **Personal, ethnic, and cultural values and beliefs.** Cultural beliefs and values affect the way people respond to pain. Children learn what is acceptable and what is not when responding to pain. The meaning of pain itself may be significantly different in different cultures. In some, any expression of pain may be considered weak and shameful, while in others, loud demonstrations of pain are considered acceptable. Some cultures see pain as a punishment for wrongdoing. If a family of origin believes that males should not cry and must tolerate pain stoically, the male often will appear withdrawn and will refuse pain medications. Regardless of one's own culture and beliefs, health care providers must respect every person and strive to alleviate pain and suffering.

▪ **Emotional traits.** The association between pain and fear is complex. Fear often increases the person's perception of pain, and pain then increases feelings of fear and anxiety. The connection occurs in the brain because painful stimuli activate portions of the limbic system that control emotional responses. People who are critically ill often experience pain and elevated levels of anxiety due to their feelings of vulnerability. Practitioners need to address both pain and anxiety and need to use all appropriate measures to relieve patients' suffering.

▪ **Developmental traits.** Age affects the way people respond to pain. It influences both the development and the aging of the nervous system. Aging affects the whole body, causing painful degenerative disorders, increased frequency of injuries such as fractures and resultant common surgical procedures. The older adult with normal age-related changes in neurophysiology may have a decreased perception of sensory stimuli and a higher pain threshold.

▪ **Previous experiences associated with pain.** Memory of painful experiences, such as those that occurred as a young child, may increase sensitivity and decrease tolerance to pain. For example, a young child may remember the pain of an injection at the doctor's office and then may be afraid to visit the doctor again.

Pain does not discriminate among individuals and usually serves an important purpose. Although pain is unpredictable, decades of research have helped to gain an understanding of the pain experience. Everyone has the same pain threshold; everyone perceives pain stimuli at the same stimulus intensity. What varies is the patient's perception of and reaction to pain.

BASIC TERMINOLOGY

Understanding basic pain terminology will assist with assessing and appropriately identifying the type of pain and establishing appropriate treatment. Acute pain is usually a necessary ally that alerts the body that something is wrong and that immediate attention is needed. When pain is no longer a warning sign, it becomes a real concern. Pain can be classified in several different ways: acute, chronic, neuropathic, or combinations of several different pain types (Table 3.1).

Acute pain is pain that results from tissue damage or noxious stimuli that is time limited and resolves during the healing period. Acute pain is a warning that something is wrong. It results in a sympathetic nervous system response; increased blood pressure, pulse, and respirations; pupil dilation; muscle tension and rigidity; pallor; and diaphoresis. People may also demonstrate pain behaviors such as grimacing, moaning, groaning, and muscle guarding.

Table 3.1 ▦ *Types of Acute Pain*

Types	Receptors	Pain Characteristics	Causes
Somatic (Nociceptive)	• Activation of pain receptors in the skin and deep tissues	• Constant and well localized • Aching, throbbing, gnawing, dull, sore	• Bone metastases • Musculoskeletal injury
Visceral (Nociceptive)	• Activation of pain receptors resulting from stretching, distension, or inflammation of viscous tissue	• Pain is vague in quality • Deep, dull, aching, squeezing, cramping, pressure • Referred pain • Poorly localized	• Bowel obstruction • Biliary colic • Myocardial infarction • Tumors occupying the liver, pancreas, spleen
Neuropathic	• Injury to peripheral and/or central nervous system	• Radiating, shooting, burning, tingling, numbness • Pain with normal touch	• Spinal cord injury • Shingles • Peripheral nerve injury

Persistent pain or chronic pain is very different from acute pain in that the pain does not serve a useful purpose. Persistent pain is defined as pain that lasts beyond the normal healing periods; i.e., lasting longer than 3 months. Although persistent pain/chronic pain is not life threatening, it adversely affects the patient's life including emotional, behavioral, and psychological difficulties (Munafo & Trim, 2000, p. 10). Persistent pain/chronic pain may be limited, intermittent, or constant. Stress may worsen many types of persistent pain such as fibromyalgia or chronic regional pain syndrome. With persistent pain, the body adapts to the presence of pain and does not elicit a sympathetic response. The absence of a sympathetic response to pain behaviors does not negate the absence of pain. Vital signs are usually unchanged in persistent pain or chronic pain, but research has not shown that vital signs are reliable indicators of pain (Arbour & Gélinas, 2010; Herr et al., 2006). People with severe, persistent pain may not demonstrate the behaviors expected of a person with acute pain. They may have a flat expression even though experiencing significant pain

Clinical Pearl	Behaviors typically seen in persons with acute pain such as moaning or changes in heart rate or blood pressure cannot be used to evaluate the presence or intensity of persistent pain since these patients have adapted to pain.

ASSESSMENT

When assessing a patient, it is crucial to gather the key elements of a pain assessment to allow for the best treatment. There is no single approach that fits all patients or settings. The structure for assessment and assessment requirements are developed by each institution to meet the needs of their patients (Wells, Pasero, & McCaffery, 2008, p. 3). The institution should select a pain intensity rating that will elicit a full assessment to help formulate the plan of care. Since research suggests that pain at a level of 4 out of 10 is the point at which pain significantly interferes with function, most institutions choose that a full assessment be completed for pain levels of 4 or greater.

The pain management standards address the assessment and management of pain. The standards require organizations to:

■ Recognize the right of patients to appropriate assessment and management of pain

- Screen patients for pain during their initial assessment and, when clinically required, during ongoing, periodic re-assessments
- Educate patients suffering from pain and their families about pain management

The standards warrant that patients are asked about pain, depending upon the service the organization is providing. There are some services that do not require a pain assessment. For example, if a patient is having a MRI and is experiencing pain during the procedure, appropriate care should be made available to address the patient's pain. If screening indicates that pain does exist, the organization may assess and treat the pain; assess the pain and refer the patient for treatment; or refer the patient for further assessment. Patients are encouraged to report pain and to cooperate with the prescribed treatment.

When interviewing the patient, allow for an environment that encourages verbalizing a report of pain. The health care provider needs to ask open-ended questions and allow ample time for the patient to respond in his or her own words (Table 3.2).

At the initial patient encounter the patient is asked a screening question, "Are you experiencing pain or discomfort?" Some people may not respond to the word "pain," so by using a variety of qualifiers such as "aching," "hurting," or "discomfort" may help to illicit the best response. If the patient responds yes, the health care provider should then ask the patient to rate pain intensity on a scale of 0 to 10 with 10 being the worse pain and 0 being no pain at all.

Each institution determines an intensity level of the patient's self-report of pain to trigger a comprehensive pain assessment. Most hospitals or clinics perform a comprehensive pain assessment at the first visit or on admission. The health care provider should include at least these main characteristics of pain: location, intensity, quality, onset (pattern), duration (frequency), and aggravating and alleviating factors, pain goal, and functional impact of pain (Table 3.3).

Location. Ask the patient to point to the area that is painful. Is there more than one site? If the patient is unable to point, a figure drawing maybe used. The patient is asked to mark the location of the pain on a drawing (Figure 3.1). For multiple locations, the sites can be distinguished utilizing the letters to differentiate the sites.

Descriptors/characteristics. What does the pain feel like (e.g., aching, burning, sharp)? Document the patient's description in the patient's own words. Do not attempt to provide the patient with words. These

Table 3.2

PAIN ASSESSMENT GUIDE

TELL ME ABOUT YOUR PAIN

Words to describe pain

aching	throbbing	shooting
stabbing	gnawing	sharp
tender	burning	exhausting
tiring	penetrating	nagging
numb	miserable	unbearable
dull	radiating	squeezing
crampy	deep	pressure

Pain in other languages

itami	Japanese	dolor	Spanish
tong	Chinese	douleur	French
dau	Vietnamese	bolno	Russian

Intensity (0-10)
If 0 is no pain and 10 is the worst pain imaginable, what is your pain now? ... in the last 24 hours?

Location
Where is your pain?

Duration
Is the pain always there?
Does the pain come and go? (Breakthrough Pain)
Do you have both types of pain?

Aggravating and Alleviating Factors
What makes the pain better?
What makes the pain worse?

How does pain affect

sleep	energy	relationships
appetite	activity	mood

Are you experiencing only other symptoms?

nausea/vomiting	itching	urinary retention
constipation	sleepiness/confusion	weakness

Things to check
vital signs, past medication history, knowledge of pain, and use of noninvasive techniques

---

From Puntillo, K., Neighbor, M., O'Neil, N., & Nixon, R. (2010). Pain management nursing: Accuracy of emergency nurses in assessment of patients' pain. *Topics in Emergency Medicine, Volume 27*, 284.

Table 3.3 ▨ *PQRST Pain Assessment Acronym*

P – PROVOKES
- What are the aggravating factors, alleviating factors?
- What caused the current condition?
- What were you doing when it began?
- Does anything make it better or worse?
  (i.e., deep inspiration, movement etc.)

Q – Quality
- What does it feel like?
- Ask the patient to describe in his/her own words what the discomfort is like (sharp, stabbing, burning, crushing).
- Does anything change the pain (i.e., deep inspiration, cough, movement)?

R – Radiation/Region
- Where is it located?
- Does it go anywhere else?
- Ask the patient to point to where the pain is at its worst.

S – Severity
- How bad is the current condition?
- Severity of an individual's condition is difficult to assess and is subjective to the patient.
- Ask patient to rate any pain on a scale of 0 (no pain) to 10 (unbearable pain).
- If the patient has had pain before, determine if it is of greater or lesser severity than usual.

T – Time: Onset/ Duration
- Do you have any discomfort now?
- When did this episode of pain start?
- How long did it last?
- Is it constant or does it come and go?
- Did it come on suddenly or gradually over a period of time?

descriptors are very helpful in determining the type of pain and may determine the treatment plan.

Intensity. The appropriate pain scale corresponding to the patient's cognitive and communication abilities (e.g., Visual Analogue Scale [VAS], Numeric Rating Scale [NRS 0–10], Faces Scale, or Verbal Scale) is identified (see Chapter 4). The same pain rating scale is to be used consistently with this patient by all health care providers and documented in the patient's medical record.

Again, the patient is asked to rate pain intensity on a scale of 0 to 10, with 0 indicating no pain and 10 indicating the worst pain possible. If the patient has identified multiple pain sites, each painful site is rated and documented.

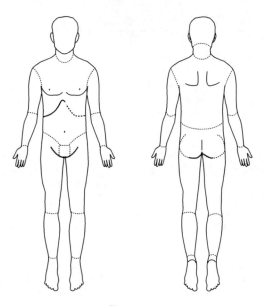

Figure 3.1

Onset/duration. How and when did the pain begin? Is it constant? Does it come and go?

Aggravating /alleviating factors. What factors make the pain worse? What makes the pain better? Include treatments and medications that are used to help. Questions related to alleviating features should include a thorough analgesic history and the effects of past treatments.

Functional impact of pain. This is an important question for patients who experience chronic pain or who are having recurrent episodes of acute pain. What effect is the pain having on your quality of life? The patient's response to previous or current pain treatments and the effect of pain on the patient's physical, mental (mood, sleep, appetite), social, and functional (work, activities of daily living) status are included.

COMFORT FUNCTION GOAL

A simple and effective method for building accountability for pain relief and improving patient outcomes is to establish and use comfort-function goals (Pasero & McCaffery, 2003). Comfort function goals require the collaboration of the health care practitioner and the patient to establish a plan that will result in the recovery of the patient and in pain control. The health care provider must clearly articulate the steps needed for the patient to recover (i.e., coughing, deep breathing, ambulation, etc.).

During the initial pain assessment of the patient, establishing the pain goal or comfort function goal is useful to set realistic expectations. Some patients may believe that they shouldn't experience any or little pain. The patient and care partner should be assured that every effort will be made to promote function and comfort, though there may be times when it may be unrealistic to eliminate all pain.

Patients are told that a pain rating from 1 to 3 generally recognizes that discomfort is present, but does not cause undue distress or interfere with activities. A pain rating greater than 3 may interfere with activities such as deep breathing, ambulating, or visiting, and will trigger a pain relief intervention. Pain studies have indicated that ratings of 4 or higher interfere with function (Pasero & McCaffery, 2003). To assess the comfort goal, ask the patient if he/she is satisfied with the level of pain control, and observe if the patient is able to perform the expected functional activity. The patient is asked if the comfort goal is achieved, and document the response with the pain assessment. The comfort function goal needs to be communicated to all who care for the patient and upon transfer to ensure that the patient's treatment plan is met.

Ongoing assessment and reassessment for the presence of pain are essential for effective pain management. Pain must be reassessed on a regular basis according to the type and intensity of the pain and the treatment plan. Pain is reassessed with each new report, increasing intensity, and if current pain treatment is no longer effective.

Throughout the literature, there is general agreement that patients should be involved in decisions about their medical care (Melnyk & Fineout-Overholt, 2011). Researchers have found that patients' involvement and participation in their health and treatment plans is essential to providing the highest quality of care. Patient participation contributes to positive patient outcomes such as satisfaction, autonomy, and perceived health-related quality of life. Promoting patient participation also enhances the patient's responsibility for treatment, psychological well-being, adherence to treatment, achievement of desired functional and clinical outcomes, cost effectiveness, and the development of a trusting relationship between the health care provider and the patient (Melnyk & Fineout-Overholt, 2011). Facilitating more patient participation in daily treatment decisions and care plans requires that health care practitioners and organizations provide for and encourage a more patient-centered approach to the provision of care.

Several studies of daily goal worksheets have been conducted over the last several years, with favorable outcomes and decreased lengths of stay.

In all of these studies, the daily goal worksheets were completed by inter-disciplinary teams and included little or no patient participation in goal formation.

However, five studies were found that evaluated the process of defining daily goals, and the incorporation of daily goals into patient care. Only the study by Potter and Mueller (2007) involved the input of patients and families in the development of daily goals.

In the study by Pronovost and colleagues (2003), a daily goals sheet was implemented in an adult intensive care setting in an attempt to improve communication among caregivers regarding patient goals and treatments. Results of the study included a 50% reduction in lengths of stay, improved perceptions of communication among caregivers, and improved commu-nication with family members using the goals form as a tool.

A similar study by Narasimhan (2006) also evaluated a daily goals worksheet in an intensive care setting. The worksheet was completed by the caregiver team during interdisciplinary rounds and posted at each patient's bedside. Researchers measured physicians' and nurses' understanding of the goals of care and length of stay in the intensive care unit. Use of the daily goal sheet resulted in improved understanding of care goals, improved communication between physicians and nurses, and decreased lengths of stay (Narasimhan, 2006).

Another study by the Joint Commission on Accreditation of Health-care Organizations (2007) examined the use of a multi-disciplinary goal sheet in an adult ICU. A standardized goal form was implemented for each patient, with documentation elicited from all caregivers. Results indicated an increase in nurses' and residents' understanding of daily therapy goals and a decreased patient mean length of stay of almost 50%.

REASSESSMENT FOLLOWING PAIN INTERVENTION

Reassessment of pain needs to be timed and performed in a manner that is comprehensive and appropriate to the patient's clinical situation to ensure safety and adequate pain relief. When an intervention such as medication is given, it is necessary to allow sufficient time for peak effect, such as 15 to 30 minutes after parenteral drug therapy or 1 hour after oral administration of an analgesic or nonpharmacologic intervention. Staff must be knowledgeable about the medication including the onset, peak, and duration of action being administered. Re-adjustments may include not only upward titration of treatment, but also tapering of the analgesics. Reassessment following each intervention should include the Four A's (Passik & Weinreb, 2000):

Analgesia: Reassess the patient's intensity after administration and determine if there is improvement.
■ Pain Intensity (0 to 10)

Activity: Determine the level of improvement in the patient's function.
■ Better able to move, follows therapeutic directions or sleep. Comfort function goal

Adverse effects: Note any untoward side effects of the intervention. The key is to give an effective dose of medication with the least amount of side effects.
■ Side effects, toxicity, sedation, constipation

Aberrant Drug-Taking Behaviors: Does the patient have any behaviors suggestive of drug abuse, such as "losing" multiple prescriptions or unauthorized dose escalation?

It may be unrealistic to eliminate all pain, but the patient must be assured that every effort will be made to promote function and comfort. Sequence of intervention and reassessment should continue until the patient reaches a satisfactory and/or functional pain level. If the patient's pain is not being relieved, a complete pain reassessment, re-evaluation, and modification of the current plan are needed. If a patient's pain and function level cannot be met despite the best efforts of the health care team, consultation by a Pain Specialist or Pain Team is generally recommended.

Pain is subjective; therefore, as health care practitioners, we must accept and respect the patient's self- report as the most reliable indicator of pain. Patients trust that their reports of pain will be believed and that they can openly report the information needed so that an adequate assessment is obtained and their pain can be appropriately treated.

Lack of accountability for health care practitioners assessing and providing pain-relieving interventions is one of the leading causes of the under-treatment of pain. With the implementation of the JC standards, there are now policies and procedures to address pain if patients continue to be under-treated.

A thorough pain assessment requires a skilled health care practitioner to ask the appropriate questions in a systematic and organized manner, which is a stepping stone toward effectively managing pain. An appropriate assessment will increase the likelihood that the patient's pain will be managed effectively. The goal of pain management is to achieve optimal comfort and function with minimal side effects from analgesic therapy.

Case Study

John Smith is a 55-year-old patient who presented to the emergency department at 5 p.m. after he fell while riding his bicycle in the afternoon. He is holding his left wrist and is reporting pain at 8/10, especially when he attempts to move his wrist. There is a visible deformity in the left wrist. He states the pain is excruciating and throbbing. John would like to get his pain to a 3/10 where he feels it will be tolerable. His wife had placed ice on his wrist, which he says has helped his pain a bit. He has not taken any medications for his pain. John is concerned how he will be able to work if his wrist is broken since he is an auto mechanic and sole provider for his family.

Questions to Consider

1. Perform a pain assessment using all the components discussed in this chapter.
2. What is John's comfort function goal? Is that a reasonable goal for his current medical condition?

REFERENCES

Arbour, C., & Gélinas, C. (2010). Are vital signs valid indicators for the assessment of pain in postoperative cardiac surgery ICU adults? *Intensive Critical Care Nursing, 26*(2), 83–90.

Arnstein, P. (2010). *Clinical coach for effective pain management.* Philadelphia, PA: F.A. Davis.

Brennan, F., Carr, D. B., & Cousins, M. (2007). Pain management: A fundamental human right. *Anesthesia & Analgesia, 105,* 205–221.

Herr, K., Coyne, P. J., Key, T., Manworren, R., McCaffery, M., Merkel, S., . . ., American Society for Pain Management Nursing. (2006). Pain assessment in the nonverbal patient: position statement with clinical practice recommendations. *Pain Management Nursing , 7*(2), 44–52.

Herr, K. A., & Garand, L. (2001). Assessment and measurement of pain in older adults. *Clinics in Geriatric Medicine , 17,* 457–478.

Joint Commission. (2010). *Joint Commission accreditation manual for hospitals: The official Handbook.* Oakbrook Terrace, IL: Author. Retrieved September 15, 2010, from http://amp.jcrinc.com/Frame.aspx

Joint Commission on Accreditation of Healthcare Organizations. (2007). Communicating through a daily goals form: Ensuring that physicians, nurses and pharmacists are on the same page. The Joint Commission Perspectives on Patient Safety, June 2007, *7*(6), 9–11.

Melnyk, B. M., & Fineout-Overholt, E. (Eds.). (2011). *Evidence-based practice in nursing and healthcare: A guide to best practice* (2nd ed.). Philadelphia, PA: Lippincott Williams & Wilkins.

Munafo, M., & Trim, J. (Eds.). (2000). *Chronic pain: A handbook for nurses.* London, UK: Butterworth-Heinemann.

Pasero, C., & McCaffery, M. (2003). Accountability for pain relief: Use of comfort-function goals. *Journal of PeriAnesthesia Nursing, 18*(1), 50–52.

Passik, S. D., & Weinreb, H. J. (2000). Managing chronic nonmalignant pain: Overcoming obstacles to the use of opioids. *Advances in Therapy, 17,* 70–83.

Potter, P., & Mueller, J. R. (2007). How well do you know your patients? *Nursing Management, 38*(2), 40–48.

Pronovost, P., Berenholtz, S., Dorman, T., Lipsett, P. A., Simmonds, T., & Haraden, C. (2003). Improving communication in the ICU using daily goals. *Journal of Critical Care, 18*(2), 71–75.

Puntillo, K., Neighbor, M., O'Neil, N., & Nixon, R. (2003). Accuracy of emergency nurses in assessment of patients' pain. *Pain Management Nursing, 4* (4), 171–175.

Wells, N., Pasero, C., & McCaffery, M. (2008). Improving the quality of care through pain assessment and management. In R. G. Hughes (Ed.), *Patient safety and quality: An evidence-based handbook for nurses* (chap. 17). Rockville, MD: Agency for Healthcare Research and Quality (US). Retrieved August 26, 2010, from http://www.ahrq.gov/qual/nurseshdbk/docs/WellsN_SMTEP.pdf

4

Assessment Tools

The definition of pain partly lies within the intricacy of its measurement. Pain is an individual and subjective experience influenced by various factors including physiological, psychological, and environmental factors. Most measures of pain are based on self-report, which is the gold standard. If done properly, these measures lead to sensitive and consistent results (Moore, Edwards, Barden, & McQuay, 2003). Self report measures may be influenced by mood, sleep disturbance, and medications (Scott & McDonald, 2008). Other measures when self-report is not possible because of cognitive impairment, and so on, will be discussed further in Chapter 5.

The most common approach to self-report is the patient's reporting of pain intensity or self-description of the pain. The health care professional must respect and believe the patient's self-report of pain. Pain assessment tools are useful in facilitating the collection of information during the initial and ongoing pain assessments. The critically ill trauma patient, and some patients in the emergency department (ED) are no exception in pain assessment, although sometimes these patients are a challenge—due to the seriousness of their condition they are at high risk for experiencing pain but are at times unable to communicate.

There are no objective measures of pain but other factors associated such as the stress response, behavioral responses, functional impairment, or physiological responses may provide additional information (Macintyre, Scott, Schug, Visser, & Walker, 2010). Regular, ongoing pain assessment and reassessment are done to ensure the efficacy of the pain management plan. The systematic use of formal pain measurement tools and documentation has been shown to improve the assessment and management of patients' pain (Lee, Hobden, Stiell, & Wells, 2003).

A number of scales are available that measure either pain intensity or pain relief following an intervention. There are a multitude of validated and reliable tools that are available to assist health care professionals in the measurement of pain. There is no one pain assessment tool that can objectively measure how much pain a patient experiences. Without accurate pain measurement, however, a patient's pain can be misinterpreted or underestimated, which often leads to the inadequate management of pain (Zwakhalen, Van Dongen, Hamers, & Abu-Saad, 2004). Even using a patient self-report or with pain behavioral observations, there is no reliable measurement as no two individuals experience pain the same.

Pain intensity can be defined as how much a person hurts or the magnitude of perceived pain (Turk & Melzack, 2001). Intensity is the most subjective item of the pain assessment. In order to achieve the most accurate pain assessment, the most appropriate pain rating scale should be selected. The tool should be appropriate for the patient's developmental, physical, emotional and cognitive status, as well as reliable, valid, and easy to use (Berry et al., 2001). The tool is used consistently each time unless the patient's condition warrants a change. Pain intensity should be measured at regular intervals, after intervention, and as needed. This will help the health care provider to determine the efficacy of the pain management plan.

In the clinical setting, pain intensity rating scales are most commonly used. These tools are one-dimensional, however, measuring only one aspect of the pain experience, that is, intensity. The ability to quantify the intensity of pain is an essential part of pain assessment but it fails to provide other information that is important to assessing pain and determining pain treatment (McCaffery & Pasero, 2010).

UNIDIMENSIONAL PAIN SCALES

Unidimensional scales assess a single dimension of patients' self-reports of pain—intensity. These types of scales are useful in acute pain such as trauma or postoperative pain and give quick feedback about the patient's pain intensity and response to treatment. Rating scales give patients a simple way to rate pain intensity but cannot be a substitute for a comprehensive pain assessment.

Since self-report is the most reliable indicator of pain, the health care provider must determine whether the patient is able to participate. The health care provider must give clear directions on use of the desired pain tool. It should not be assumed that the patient is incapable of self-report unless an attempt has been made (Pasero, 2009). Mild to moderate cognitively impaired patients have been shown to be able to report their pain using self-report tools if administered appropriately (Herr, Spratt, & Mobily, 2004).

Patients that are awake, alert, oriented, and on a ventilator may be able to communicate their self-report by pointing to the number on the pain tool; some may blink their eyes to indicate if they have pain (Pasero, 2002).

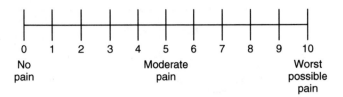

Figure 4.1 ■ Numerical Pain Rating Scale

Numerical Rating Scale

The Numerical Rating Scale (NRS; Figure 4.1) is the most commonly used scale. The NRS is a set of numbers (usually 0 to 10) represented along a horizontal or vertical line or on a pain thermometer. There may be a word at each end of the line; for example, 0 equals "no pain" and 10 equals the "worst pain imaginable." Patients are asked to point or draw around the number that best describes their pain intensity.

The scale is easy to use, providing consistency in interpretation of the patient's self-report of pain. If the patient cannot speak he or she may write the number on a piece of paper or respond by holding up the number of fingers that corresponds to the report of pain. Studies have shown that postoperative, critically ill, the visually impaired (if adapted), those with poor motor coordination, and older patients are able to use the NRS (Aubrun, Langeron, Quesnel, Coriat, & Riou, 2003; Ching & Burns, 2010; Piacentine et al., 2004).

Verbal Descriptor Scale

The Verbal Descriptor Scale (VDS) also assesses pain intensity by using graded words such as "no pain," "mild," "moderate," "severe," to "excruciating" to assess the patient's level of pain. The words are usually listed in order from the least intense to the most intense pain and the number of words used varies. The patient is asked to choose the word that best describes his or her intensity of pain. Some patients may prefer to use words to describe their pain rather than use a number (D'Arcy, 2007).

Studies have shown that these scales are of benefit for postoperative and critical care patients and patients with cognitive impairment, limited numerical skills, physical disabilities, or visual impairment, and older people (Ching & Burns, 2010; Kaasalainen & Crook, 2003).

Iowa Pain Thermometer

The Iowa Pain Thermometer (IPT; Figure 4.2) assesses pain by asking patients to indicate the intensity of their pain on a diagram of a thermometer. It is an adaptation of a verbal descriptor scale that visually represents

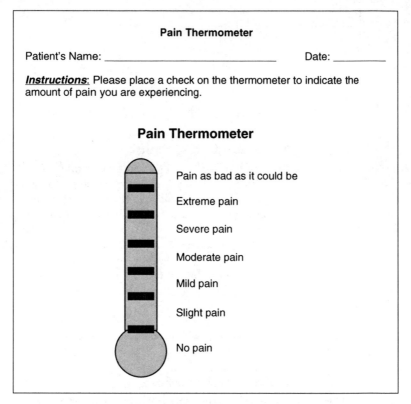

Figure 4.2 ■ Pain Thermometer (Heir & Mobily, 1993).

increasing degrees of pain along the thermometer. Words ranging from "no pain" to "pain as bad as it could be" correspond to different points on the diagram. This tool is appropriate for patients who have moderate to severe cognitive impairments, or who have difficulty communicating verbally.

Patients are shown the scale and asked to envision that, just as temperature rises in a thermometer, pain intensity increases as one moves to the top of the scale. The patient may place a check mark or point with the finger on the thermometer to indicate his/her current level of pain. Both the original and the revised IPT have been researched and found to be good tools for both younger and older patients (Herr et al., 2004). The combination of the thermometer and the verbal descriptors scale are recommended by national and international guidelines panels on pain in older persons (American Geriatrics Society, 2002; Hadjistavropoulos et al., 2007).

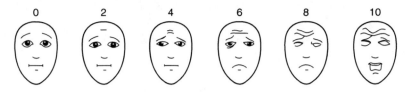

Figure 4.3 ■ FACES Pain Scale-Revised

FACES Pain Scale-Revised
(Bieri, Reeve, Champion, Addicoat, & Ziegler, 1990)

The FACES Pain Scale-Revised (FPS-R; Figure 4.3) was adapted from the FACES Pain Scale (Bieri et al., 1990). It does not contain smiling faces or tears, thus avoiding the confounding of affect and pain intensity (Hicks, Von Baeyer, Spafford, Van Korlaar, & Goodenough, 2001). The absence of smiles and tears in this faces scale may be useful for some patients. The FPS-R is recommended and preferred by older adults, those from ethnic minorities, and those with mild to moderate cognitive impairments.

The health care provider asks the patient to choose the face that best describes the pain they feel. The number that is associated with that face will be recorded by the provider.

Wong-Baker FACES Pain Rating Scale

The FACES scale (Figure 4.4) developed by Donna Wong was originally developed for the pediatric patient. The tool has been validated for use in adults and cognitively impaired populations. The scale has five cartoon-like faces that do not depict any gender or culture. The faces have expressions ranging from a broad smile to very sad and tearful, each face getting sadder (Wilson & Hockenberry, 2008); concern has been expressed regarding some of the expressions of the faces (crying face, smiling face, slight smile) and whether they could possibly alter the patient's pain report (Pasero & McCaffery, 2010). The scale has been translated into multiple languages.

Figure 4.4 ■ Wong-Baker FACES Scale. *Source:* From Hockenberry, M. J., & Wilson, D. (2009). *Wong's essentials of pediatric nursing* (8th ed.). St. Louis: Mosby.

> *Clinical Pearl*   When using the FACES scale, explain to the patient to select the face that describes how they hurt, not how their face looks.

The health care provider asks the patient to choose the face that best describes the pain they feel. The number that is associated with that face will be recorded by the provider.

MULTIDIMENSIONAL PAIN SCALES

Multidimensional tools are often used in assessing chronic or persistent acute pain. The most common multidimensional pain scales are the McGill Pain Questionnaire (MPQ) and the Brief Pain Inventory (BPI). Patients with chronic pain require a more comprehensive pain assessment with consideration of other aspects beyond the physical that include mood, behaviors, thoughts and beliefs, physiological effects and their interaction with others as this may impact the overall care of the patient. These tools take longer to administer than the one-dimensional scales and patients who are cognitively impaired or poorly educated may have difficulty completing these.

For patients admitted to the hospital that have an underlying chronic pain condition, a multidimensional pain scale may be more appropriate. Multidimensional tools, such as the MPQ and the Wisconsin Brief Pain Questionnaire (BPQ), measure pain intensity as well as the sensory, affective, and behavioral components of that pain, but take longer to administer and may not be practical for the ICU environment (Graf & Puntillo, 2003; Ho, Spence, & Murphy, 1996; Terai, Yukioka, & Asada, 1998). The MPQ and BPQ are reliable and valid tools but have not been tested or used in the ICU (Jacobi et al., 2002).

Brief Pain Inventory (BPI)

The BPI was originally developed to assess pain in cancer patients. It has been translated in over two dozen languages and is widely used in both clinical and research settings, including clinicians treating chronic nonmalignant pain. It assesses the patient's pain as well as the impact of the pain on daily function. BPI evaluates the patient's pain through a different number of scales. The patient is asked to mark on a drawing of a human body where he or she is experiencing the pain. The patient also reports medications and treatments in the past 24 hours. Patients also answer 11 NRS questions related to pain on their activities of daily living and function.

The Brief Pain Inventory-Short Form (BPI-SF) captures two broad pain domains: 1) the sensory intensity of pain, and 2) the degree to which pain interferes with different areas of life (Cleeland & Ryan, 1994). The 17-item scale also captures pain location, pain medication use, and response to treatments and can be completed in 5 minutes. The BPI-SF has been determined to be a reliable tool and has been validated in more than three dozen languages (Kalyadina et al., 2008; Keller et al., 2004; Klepstad et al., 2002; Mendoza et al., 2004; Mendoza, Mayne, Rublee, & Cleeland, 2006; Mystakidou et al., 2001; Yun et al., 2004). While this tool is shown to be excellent for monitoring the effects of pain and its treatment, the major disadvantage is that it takes time to complete (long version) and is unsuitable for those with cognitive impairment. Repeated use may be less desirable in the acute setting.

McGill Pain Questionnaire (MPQ)/ McGill Pain Questionnaire-Short Form (MPQ-SF)

The MPQ can be used to evaluate a person experiencing significant pain. It can be used to monitor the pain over time and to determine the effectiveness of any intervention. The MPQ has a long and short version that have been translated into several languages and used in the initial assessment and for research.

The MPQ is used to assess pain in three dimensions: sensory, affective, and evaluative using word descriptors from a patient's pain experience. The first section includes a drawing of the front and back of a human body on which patients can mark where they are experiencing pain. The second part is a six-word verbal descriptor scale (VDS) that patients use to record their pain intensity. The third section contains 78 adjectives divided into 20 sets that describe sensory, affective, and evaluative qualities of the patient's pain. The patient circles the words that best describe the pain experience. A score for each of the dimensions is generated, as well as a total score.

The MPQ is valid, reliable, and consistent in the ability to give seemingly appropriate description to a given pain experience (Correll, 2007).

The short form of the MPQ-SF contains 11 questions referring to the sensory terms of the pain experience and four related to the affective terms for a total of 15 descriptors (Melzack, 1987). Each descriptor is ranked on a four-point intensity scale (0 = none, 1 = mild, 2 = moderate, 3 = severe). The MPQ-SF also has a single VAS item for pain intensity and a VRS for rating the overall pain experience. The pain rating index of the standard MPQ is also included, as well as a VAS. The MPQ-SF has been validated and correlates well with the long form (Correll, 2007; Melzack, 1987). While this shortened version only takes approximately 5 minutes, it may still be too burdensome for the acute care setting. The MPQ-SF has been used in research studies in the ICU.

The foundation of pain assessment is the patient self-report. Pain assessment tools assist in providing a quantitative assessment of pain by measuring intensity used in conjunction with the other elements of pain assessment to provide an ongoing evaluation of the pain management plan.

There are times in which communication barriers exist, such as with cognitive impairment, a nonverbal or unconscious patient, where the patient is unable to self-report. The next chapter will discuss pain assessment in specialty population areas.

Case Study

Sandy is a 45-year-old female who was in a motor vehicle accident and is now admitted to the ICU after she underwent exploratory laparotomy. This is her first postoperative day. As you enter her room, she smiles at you and continues talking and joking with her visitor. Your assessment reveals the following information: BP = 120/80; HR = 80; R = 18; on a scale of 0 to 10 (0 = no pain/discomfort, 10 = worst/pain/discomfort).

She rates her pain as 8 using the Numeric Rating Scale.

Questions to Consider

1. On the patient's record what would you document that represents your assessment of Sandy's pain?
2. Does her pain rating scale match her report of pain?

REFERENCES

AGS Panel on Persistent Pain in Older Persons. (2002). The management of persistent pain in older persons. *Journal of American Geriatric Society, 50*(Suppl. 6), S205–S224.

Aubrun, F., Langeron, O., Quesnel, C., Coriat, P., & Riou, B. (2003). Relationship between measurement of pain using visual analog score and morphine requirements during postoperative intravenous morphine titration. *Anesthesiology, 98,* 415–1421.

Piacentine, L., Maloni, H., Mogensen, K., McNair, N., Hickey, A., & Oloomi, C. W. (2004). In M. K. Bader & L. R. Littlejohns (Eds.), *AANN core curriculum for neuroscience nursing* (4th ed.). Philadelphia, PA: Sanders.

Berry, P. H., Chapman, C. R., Covington, E., Dahl, J., Katz, J., Miaskowski, C., & McLean, M. J. (2001). *Pain: Current understanding of assessment, management, and treatments.* Reston, VA: National Pharmaceutical Council.

Bieri, D., Reeve, R., Champion, G. D., Addicoat, L., & Ziegler, J. (1990). The faces pain scale for the self-assessment of the severity of pain experienced by children: Development, initial validation and preliminary investigation for ratio scale properties. *Pain, 41,* 139–150.

Ching, J. M., & Burns, S. M. (2010). Pain, sedation, and neuromuscular blockade management. In M. Chulay & S. M. Burns (Eds.), *AACN essentials of critical care nursing* (2nd ed.). New York, NY: McGraw Hill Publishers.

Cleeland, C. S., & Ryan, K. M. (1994). Pain assessment: Global use of the brief pain inventory. *Annals Academy of Medicine Singapore, 19,* 129–138.

Correll, D. J. (2007). The measurement of pain: Objectifying the subjective. In S. D. Waldman (Ed.), *Pain management* (pp. 197–211). Philadelphia, PA: Elsevier.

D'Arcy, Y. (2007). *Pain management: Evidence-based tools and techniques for nursing professionals.* Marblehead, MA: HcPro.

Graf, C., & Puntillo, K. A. (2003). Pain in the older adult in the intensive care unit. *Critical Care Clinics, 19*(4), 749–770.

Hadjistavropoulos, T., Herr, K., Turk, D. C., Fine, P. G., Dworkin, R. H., Helme, R., . . . Williams, J. (2007). An interdisciplinary expert consensus statement on assessment of pain in older persons. *Clinical Journal of Pain, 23*(Suppl. 1), S1–S43.

Herr, K., Bjoro, K., & Decker, S. (2006). Tools for assessment of pain in nonverbal older adults with dementia: A state-of-the-science review. *Journal of Pain Symptom and Management, 31,* 170–192.

Herr, K., Coyne, P. J., Key, T., Manworren, R., McCaffery, M., Merkel, S., . . . Wild, L. (2006). Pain assessment in nonverbal patients: Position statement with clinical practice recommendations. *Pain Management Nursing, 7,* 44–52.

Herr, K., Spratt, K. F., Garand, L., & Li, L. (2007). Evaluation of the Iowa pain thermometer and other selected pain intensity scales in younger and older adult cohorts using controlled clinical pain: A preliminary study. *Pain Medicine, 8,* 585–600.

Herr, K. A., Spratt, K., & Mobily, P. R. (2004). Richardson G. Pain intensity assessment in older adults: use of experimental pain to compare psychometric properties and usability of selected pain scales with younger adults. *Clinical Journal of Pain, 20*(4), 207–219.

Hicks, C. L., Von Baeyer, C. L., Spafford, P. A., Van Korlaar, I., & Goodenough, B. (2001). The faces pain scale revised: toward a common metric in pediatric pain measure. *Pain, 93*(2), 173–183.

Ho, K., Spence, J., & Murphy, M. F. (1996). Review of pain management tools. *Annals Emergency Medicine, 27,* 427–432.

Jacobi, J., Fraser, G. L., Coursin, D. B., Riker, R. R., Fontaine, D., Wittbrodt, E. T., . . . Lumb, P. D. (2002). Clinical practice guidelines for the sustained use of sedative and analgesics in the critically ill adult. *Critical Care Medicine, 30*(1), 119–141.

Kalyadina, S. A., Ionova, T. I., Ivanova, M. O., Uspenskaya, O. S., Kishtovich, A. V., Mendoza, T. R., . . . Wang, X. S. (2008). Russian brief pain inventory: Validation and application in cancer pain. *Journal of Pain Symptom Management, 35*(1), 95–102.

Kaasalainen, S., & Crook, J. (2003). A comparison of pain-assessment tools for use with elderly long-term-care residents. *Canadian Journal of Nursing Research, 35*(4), 58–71.

Keller, S., Bann, C. M., Dodd, S. L., Schein, J., Mendoza, T. R., & Cleeland, C. S. (2004). Validity of the brief pain inventory for use in documenting the outcomes of patients with noncancer pain. *Clinical Journal of Pain, 20*(5), 309–318.

Klepstad, P., Loge, J. H., Borchgrevink, P. C., Mendoza, T. R., Cleeland, C. S., & Kaasa, S. (2002). The Norwegian brief pain inventory questionnaire: Translation and validation in cancer pain patients. *Journal of Pain Symptom Management, 24*(5), 517–525.

Lee, J. S., Hobden, E., Stiell, I. G., & Wells, G. A. (2003). Clinically important change in the visual analog scale after adequate pain control. *Academy of Emergency Medicine, 10*(10), 1128–1130.

Macintyre, P., Scott, D. A., Schug, S. A., Visser, E. J., & Walker, S. M. (Eds.). (2010). *Acute pain management: Scientific evidence* (3rd ed.). Melbourne, Australia: Australian and New Zealand College of Anaesthetists and Faculty of Pain Medicine. Retrieved from http://www.anzca.edu.au/resources/books-and-publications/Acute%20pain% 20management%20-%20scientific%20evidence%20-%20third%20edition.pdf

Melzack, R. (1987). The short-form McGill pain questionnaire. *Pain, 30,* 191–197.

Mendoza, T. R., Mayne, T., Rublee, D., & Cleeland, C. S. (2006) Reliability and validity of a modified brief pain inventory short form in patients with osteoarthritis. *European Journal of Pain, 10*(4), 353–361.

Mendoza, T. R., Chen, C., Brugger, A., Hubbard, R., Snabes, M., Palmer, S. N., . . . Cleeland, C. S. (2004). The utility and validity of the modified brief pain inventory in a multiple-dose postoperative analgesic trial. *Clinical Journal of Pain, 20*(5), 357–362.

Moore, A., Edwards, J., Barden, J., & McQuay, H. (2003). *Bandolier's little book of pain.* Oxford, England: Oxford University Press.

Mystakidou, K., Mendoza, T., Tsilika, E., Befon, S., Parpa, E., Bellos, G., . . . Cleeland, C. (2001). Greek brief pain inventory: Validation and utility in cancer pain. *Oncology. 60*(1), 35–42.

Pasero, C. (2002). The challenge of pain assessment in the PACU. *Journal of Perianesthesia Nursing, 17,* 348–350.

Pasero, C. (2009). Challenges in pain assessment. *Journal of Perianesthesia Nursing. 24,* 50–54.

Pasero, C., & McCaffery, M. (2010). *Pain assessment and pharmacological management.* St. Louis, MO: Mosby.

Scott, D. A., & McDonald, W. M. (2008). Assessment, measurement and history. In P. E. Macintyre, D. Rowbotham, & S. Walker (Eds.), *Textbook of clinical pain management* (2nd ed.).

Terai, T., Yukioka, H., & Asada, A. (1998). Pain evaluation in the intensive care unit: Observer reported faces scale compared with self reported visual analog scale. *Regional Anesthesia Pain Medicine, 23,* 147–151.

Turk, D. C., & Melzack, R. (Eds.). (2001). *Handbook of pain assessment* (2nd ed.). New York, NY: The Guilford Press.

Wilson, D., & Hockenberry, M. (Eds.). (2008). *Wong's clinical manual of pediatric nursing* (7th ed.). St. Louis, MO: Mosby.

Yun, Y. H., Mendoza, T. R., Heo, D. S., Yoo, T., Heo, B. Y., Park, H. A., . . . Cleeland, C. S. (2004). Development of a cancer pain assessment tool in Korea: A validation study of a Korean version of the brief pain inventory. *Oncology, 66*(6), 439–444.

Zwakhalen, S. M., Van Dongen, K. A., Hamers, J. P., & Abu-Saad, H. H. (2004). Pain assessment in intellectually disabled people: Non-verbal indicators. *Journal of Advanced Nursing, 45,* 236–245.

5

Assessing Pain in Specialty Populations

Since pain is a subjective experience, we simply measure it by the patient's self-report. Sounds simple? Unfortunately, patients who have cognitive/expressive deficits, are intubated or sedated, or unconscious may not be able to provide a self-report. So how does the health care professional know if the patient is experiencing pain? Think of how many times you have cared for an intubated patient, lying so still in the bed, looking comfortable, breathing so easily while on the ventilator. You gently call the patient's name and the patient does not respond. So is the patient in pain or not? What about the elderly woman with dementia who is admitted to the intensive care unit (ICU) from the nursing home with congestive heart failure. She is bed-ridden and moans all day and night. When she is asked if she is in pain, she only moans. Is she in pain or is it her dementia? Individuals who cannot communicate their pain remain a challenge and are at even greater risk for inadequate pain control. They may experience unnecessary painful treatments and procedures because the patient is unable to self-report and the health care professional is unable to determine if pain is present.

Patients that are unable to communicate are at increased risk for untreated pain because of various factors, including:

- Altered mental status
- Mechanical ventilation
- Sedating medications (Marmo & Fowler, 2010)

When patients cannot self-report, other methods must be utilized to assess for pain. Valid and reliable methods to assess pain in nonverbal patients are apparently needed. Behavioral pain assessment tools have been developed but most are in early stages and still being validated.

Critically ill and nonverbal patients have many challenges and pain assessment is included. Patients in this setting endure pain and discomfort from surgical procedures, posttrauma injuries, prolonged immobilization, invasive devices, and often just the routine care that the patient receives.

45

Patients may already have pain from chronic conditions, which also may be a barrier in assessing pain.

The Thunder Project II was a multisite research project with 6,201 patients sponsored by the American Association of Critical-Care Nurses (AACN). The study was designed to gather patients' pain perceptions and responses for certain procedures, such as chest tube insertion/removal and central line removal, during different phases of the procedure and compare the patients' pain perceptions and responses. Pain intensity increased at the time of all procedures, but more than 63% of patients received no analgesics and less than 20% received opioids (Puntillo et al., 2001). The most painful procedures found were turning and drain removal.

The research revealed information about the behavioral responses related to the specific procedures performed. A 30-item behavioral tool was used before and during the procedure to observe patient behaviors. Specific behaviors were identified in relation to procedural pain, such as:

- Grimacing
- Wincing
- Shutting of eyes
- Verbalizations
- Moaning
- Clenching of fists
- Rigidity (Puntillo et al., 2004)

The evidence is overwhelming, indicating that pain is problematic in all patient populations, particularly to the most vulnerable. In interviews conducted within 5 days after discharge from an ICU, 63% of surgical patients rated their ICU pain as being moderate to severe in intensity (Puntillo, 1990). The Study to Understand Prognoses and Preferences for Outcomes and Risks of Treatment (SUPPORT) included 9,105 patients and focused on treatment preferences and patterns of decision making among critically ill patients. Interviews regarding pain were obtained from 5,176 patients and pain was reported to occur in almost 50% of seriously ill patients and described as severe in 15% of patients (Desbians & Broste, 1996). This research suggests that pain is a serious issue that is not effectively managed or treated in sedated or mechanically ventilated patients in ICUs.

Subjective pain rating scales such as the verbal descriptor scale (VDS) or the numerical rating scale (NRS) are not appropriate in the unresponsive patient. Behavioral and physiological indicators may be the only information to utilize in order to develop a pain management plan of care (Chong & Burchett, 2003; Puntillo et al., 1997, 2002).

Clinical Pearl	Behavioral scales are not intensity scales. Behavior observation scores should be considered along with knowledge of existing painful conditions and reports from family members or a caregiver who knows the older adult and his or her behaviors. It is important to note that some older adults may not demonstrate obvious pain behaviors or cues.

Clinical Pearl	Behavioral scales are only used for patients who are cognitively impaired.

A 2006 published review and recommendations from the American Society for Pain Management Nursing (ASPMN) support a hierarchical approach for assessing pain in nonverbal patients (Herr, Bjoro, & Decker, 2006).

The ASPMN recommendations emphasize that a self-report should be elicited whenever possible (Herr et al., 2006). The following should be considered in assessing pain in patients who are not able to provide their own report:

- **Attempt a self-report of pain:** Have patients with mild to moderate cognitive impairment, delirium, low level of consciousness, or who are intubated, etc., make an attempt at self-report. Such patients may be able to provide a self-report of pain and attempts should be made.
- **Search for potential causes of pain:** Does the patient have a history of pain or a pain-related condition (e.g., osteoporosis, diabetic neuropathies, trauma, fractures, etc.)? Does the patient have any invasive tubes, wounds, or edema, etc.? Are you turning, positioning, suctioning, or transferring the patient? Is the patient having physical therapy?
- **Observe patient behaviors:** The American Geriatrics Society (AGS) identified pain indicators that may be exhibited in patients who are cognitively impaired older adult (American Geriatrics Society Panel on Persistent Pain in Older Persons [AGS], 2002). There are six categories:
  1. Facial expressions
  2. Verbalizations, vocalizations
  3. Body movement
  4. Changes in interpersonal interactions
  5. Changes in activity patterns or routines
  6. Mental status changes

It is important to understand that if a person does not exhibit any of these behaviors, it does not necessarily indicate that the patient is not experiencing pain.

■ **Surrogate reporting by family members or care-givers who know the patient**: Discussing with the family or caregivers those behaviors that the patient may exhibit when experiencing pain will assist the health care provider in identifying and treating the pain.

■ **Attempt an analgesic trial**: After going through all the previous steps, an analgesic trial can be given. Based upon the patient's response, a pain treatment plan can be developed if pain is determined with certain procedures or conditions that are likely to cause pain or when pain behaviors continue after attention to basic needs and comfort measures is given.

BEHAVIORAL PAIN ASSESSMENT TOOLS

A challenge to assessment of pain is the patient who is unable to self-report. Some patients are mistakenly believed to be pain free because they are unconscious, cognitively impaired, etc. Health care providers must suspect pain in all of these individuals. Behavioral assessment tools may assist the clinician to identify the presence of pain as well as to evaluate a decrease in pain behaviors following an intervention, but this should not be used in isolation. A patient who displays only a few behaviors may have as much pain as a patient with many more behaviors (Agency for Healthcare Research and Quality [AHRQ], 2008).

Until recently, the Face, Legs, Activity, Cry, Consolability (FLACC) Behavioral Pain Scale had been the only appropriate scale available for use in the ICU setting. The FLACC scale was designed to rate indicators of pain in children under the age of 7 years. In a recent study by Voepel-Lewis, Zanotti, Dammeyer, and Merkel (2010), the reliability and validity of the FLACC Behavioral Pain Scale in critically ill adults and children unable to self-report pain was evaluated. Twenty-nine critically ill adults and eight children were observed and scored for pain. Three nurses simultaneously but independently evaluated the patient before administration of an analgesic or during a painful procedure, and 15 to 30 minutes after the administration or procedure. There were a total of 73 observations. FLACC scores correlated highly with the other two scores ($p = 0.963$ and 0.84), supporting criterion validity. Significant decreases in FLACC scores after analgesia or at rest supported construct validity of the tool. The intraclass correlation coefficients (0.67 to 0.95) support excellent interrater reliability of the tool and internal consistency was excellent. The researchers have concluded that FLACC can be used across many populations of patients and multiple settings.

There are various tools that have been developed to assess pain in nonverbal patients. Tools developed to assess pain with mechanically ventilated and/or unconscious patients are few in number. The number of studies has increased over the recent years although more studies are required to establish the reliability, validity, and usefulness of the tools in a variety of clinical settings. Appropriateness of a pain assessment tool is based upon the patient's cognitive ability, among other factors, as well as research for reliability and validity in a similar clinical setting. When the appropriate tool is selected, the name of the tool is documented in the patient record so that it is used consistently among the health care providers. If there is a change in the patient's condition, a more appropriate tool is selected and the patient's medical record is updated. The scoring between the tools is not exchangeable because each tool utilizes different factors to reach the final score.

There are two types of behavioral assessment tools for the cognitively impaired: pain behavior scales and pain behavior checklists. Pain behavior scales are scored by identifying an observed behavior in a number of dimensions. In order for a particular pain behavior scale to be used, the patient needs to be able to respond in all of the dimensions of the tool. The cumulative pain score is not the same as a pain intensity score. Any positive score may indicate that pain is present and the score can be used to evaluate the intervention, but cannot be interpreted to mean pain intensity.

Behavior checklists differ from pain behavior scales in that they do not evaluate the degree of an observed behavior. These checklists are useful in identifying pain behaviors unique to that individual (AHRQ, 2008). Checklists can provide a base for determining what behaviors indicate pain, while the assessment tools use these behaviors to create assessment categories. A decrease or change in the total number of behaviors may be used to indicate more or less pain or used to evaluate a response to an intervention.

Clinical Pearl	Behaviors may not always be indicative of pain but could be in response to another distress.

REASSESS AND DOCUMENT

Just as with patients who self-report pain, reassessment of pain with nonverbal patients needs to occur after any intervention and regularly over time. Reassessment should occur utilizing the same initial behavioral pain assessment tool and observing for changes in those behaviors with effective treatment over time.

PAIN ASSESSMENT IN ADVANCED DEMENTIA (PAINAD) SCALE

The Pain Assessment in Advanced Dementia (PAINAD) scale is easy to use to assess pain in older adults who have advanced dementia. This patient population is at high risk for not having their pain assessed or treated. This pain behavior tool has been designed to assess pain by looking at five specific indicators (Table 5.1).

Table 5.1 ■ *Pain Assessment in Advanced Dementia (PAINAD) Scale*

Items	0	1	2	Score
Breathing independent of vocalization	Normal	Occasional labored breathing. Short period of hyperventilation.	Noisy labored breathing. Long period of hyperventilation. Cheyne-Stokes respirations.	
Negative vocalization	None	Occasional moan or groan. Low-level speech with a negative or disapproving quality.	Repeated troubled calling out. Loud moaning or groaning. Crying.	
Facial expression	Smiling or inexpressive	Sad. Frightened. Frown.	Facial grimacing.	
Body language	Relaxed Tense	Distressed pacing. Fidgeting.	Rigid. Fists clenched. Knees pulled up. Pulling or pushing away. Striking out.	
Consolability	No need to console	Distracted or reassured by voice or touch.	Unable to console, distract or reassure.	
Total				

A health care professional can use the scale with minimal observation time. The health care professional observes the older adult for 3–5 minutes during activity/with movement (such as bathing, turning, transferring). For each item included in the PAINAD, the provider selects the score (0, 1, 2) that reflects the current state of the behavior. The score for each item is then added to get a total score. Total scores range from 0 to 10 with a higher score suggesting more severe pain (0 equals "no pain"; 10 equals "severe pain"). After each use of the PAINAD scale, compare the total score to the previous score. A higher score suggests an increase in pain, while a lower score suggests pain is decreased.

Follow-up studies of the PAINAD demonstrate good internal consistency, interrater reliability, and test and retest reliability. No cutoff score was provided for the PAINAD, although lower total scores resulted when analgesia was provided (Lane et al., 2003). A recent review of pain scales for use in older adults with cognitive impairment or communication difficulties recommended the PAINAD scale as the most feasible scale for clinical practice of all currently available and validated scales (van Herk et al., 2007).

THE CHECKLIST OF NONVERBAL PAIN INDICATORS (CNPI)

The Checklist of Nonverbal Pain Indicators (CNPI) (Table 5.2) was developed from the University of Alabama Birmingham Pain Behavior Scale (UAW-PBS) to assess pain in cognitively impaired elders. The CNPI is known for its validity based on pain behaviors exhibited in cognitively impaired adults. Populations for use include patients who are unable to validate the presence of pain or quantify pain intensity by self-report methods. Initially developed for cognitively impaired older adults, it is has been used with other nonverbal populations.

The tool consists of six categories: 1) nonverbal vocalization, 2) facial grimacing or wincing, 3) bracing, 4) rubbing, 5) restlessness, and 6) vocal complaints. The frequency of the behaviors is collected when observing the patient at rest and during movement.

The number of behaviors present at the time of assessment is the pain score. Each item is scored (1 = present, 0 = not present), both at rest and on movement, for a possible range of scores from 0 to 6 points for each situation and a combined total of 12 points. Cognitively impaired older adults show fewer pain behaviors at rest, so patients with one or two pain behaviors at rest or with movement may warrant treatment.

A study was conducted comparing cognitively intact older adults with cognitively impaired older adults and the results showed no differences

Table 5.2 ▓ *Checklist of Nonverbal Pain Indicators (CNPI)*
Instructions: Observe the patient for the following behaviors both at rest and during movement.

	Behavior With	*Movement*	*At Rest*
1.	Vocal Complaints: Nonverbal (sighs, gasps, moans, groans, cries)		
2.	Facial: Grimaces/winces (furrowed brow, narrowed eyes, clenched teeth, tightened lips, jaw drop, distorted expressions)		
3.	Bracing: Clutching or holding onto furniture, equipment, or affected area during movement		
4.	Restlessness: Constant or intermittent shifting of position, rocking, intermittent or constant hand motions, inability to keep still		
5.	Rubbing: Massaging affected area		
6.	Vocal Complaints: Verbal (words expressing discomfort or pain [e.g., "ouch," "that hurts"]; cursing during movement; exclamations of protest [e.g., "stop," "that's enough"])		
Subtotal Scores			
Total Score			

Scoring: Score 0 if the behavior was not observed. Score 1 if the behavior occurred even briefly during activity or at rest. The total number of indicators is summed for the behaviors observed at rest, with movement, and overall. There are no clear cutoff scores to indicate severity of pain; instead, the presence of any of the behaviors may be indicative of pain, warranting further investigation, treatment, and monitoring by the practitioner.
Adapted from Feldt, K. S. (2000). The checklist of nonverbal pain indicators (CNPI). *Pain Management Nursing, 1*(1), 13– 21; Horgas, A. L. (2003). Assessing pain in persons with dementia. In M. Boltz (series ed.) *Try this: Best practices in nursing care for hospitalized older adults with dementia. Fall, 1*(2). The Hartford Institute for Geriatric Nursing.

between the two groups with observed pain behaviors (Feldt, 2000). The cognitively intact group showed less nonverbal indicators at rest and with movement than the impaired group, indicating that with rest both groups of patients appeared comfortable. Health care professionals should understand that even low scores may warrant pain treatment. There are two barriers with using this tool: There is no retest reliability, and there is a need for testing this tool in a larger patient population (Feldt, 2000). The CNPI has been shown to be a reliable and valid assessment tool in older adults with acute or chronic pain, in critical care units, and adults with dementia.

CRITICAL-CARE PAIN OBSERVATION TOOL (CPOT)

The Critical Care Pain Observation Tool (CPOT; Table 5.3) measures a patient's pain level by looking at four behavioral dimensions: 1) facial expression, 2) body movements, 3) muscle tension, and 4) ventilator compliance for intubated patients or vocalization for extubated patients or patients who were never intubated but who are nonverbal (Gelinas & Johnston, 2007). A maximum score of 8 is allowed by the CPOT (Gelinas et al., 2006). Patients are scored in each dimension between 0 and 2 giving an overall score of 0 (no pain) to 8 (maximum pain). Descriptions are given to explain the behaviors expected for each increment, enabling consistent scoring within each area. The tool also includes a picture of facial expressions and directions for use of the tool. The CPOT scale guidelines (Gelinas & Johnston, 2007; Gelinas, 2009) recommend providing nursing intervention for a pain score greater than or equal to 2.

The French and English versions of the CPOT were tested with cardiac surgery and ICU adults with various diagnoses (trauma, postoperative, and medical cases). It demonstrated moderate to high interrater reliability. Discriminant validity was supported with higher CPOT scores during a nociceptive procedure (turning) compared with rest or a non-nociceptive procedures (Gelinas et al., 2006). Based upon the results, the CPOT seems to be a beneficial tool for critically ill nonverbal patients, although further studies are needed in other populations.

The Gelinas et al. (2006) study also used patients' self-reports of pain, which is considered the gold standard to reporting pain; it showed that pain intensity correlated moderately with CPOT scores. No statistically significant correlation was found between a patient's self-report and the physiological indicators.

In the Gélinas and Johnston (2007) study, the results of the CPOT showed a marked increase in pain scores during turning but much less of an increase while taking a noninvasive blood pressure. A weak relationship between patients self-reports of pain and the physiological indicator was found and as a result Gélinas and Johnston (2007) do not advocate the use of physiological changes in pain assessment except as a cue to further assessment. Although there is some evidence that certain physiological changes, such as an increase in systolic blood pressure do correlate with an increase in

Table 5.3 ■ *Critical-Care Pain Observation Tool (CPOT)*

Indicator	Description	Score	
Facial Expression	No muscular tension observed.	Relaxed, neutral	0
	Presence of frowning, brow lowering, orbit tightening, and levator contractions.	Tense	1
	All of the above facial movements plus eyelid tightly closed.	Grimacing	2
Body Movements	Does not move at all, which does not mean the absence of pain.	Absence of movements	0
	Slow cautious movements, touching or rubbing the pain site, seeking attention through movements.	Protection	1
	Pulling tube, attempting to sit up, moving limbs/thrashing not following commands, striking at staff, trying to climb out of bed.	Restlessness	2
Muscle Tension	No resistance to passive movements.	Relaxed	0
	Resistance to passive movements.	Tense, rigid	1
	Strong resistance to passive movements, inability to complete them.	Very tense or rigid	2
Compliance with the ventilator (intubated patient)	Alarms not easily activated, easy ventilation. OR	Tolerating ventilator or movement	0
	Alarms stop spontaneously.	Coughing but tolerating	1
	Asynchrony; blocking ventilation, alarms frequently activated.	Fighting ventilator	2
Vocalization (extubated patients)	Talking in normal tone or no sound.	Talking in normal tone or no sound	0
	Sighing, moaning.	Sighing, moaning	1
	Crying out, sobbing.	Crying out, sobbing	2
		Total (0-8)	__

self-reported pain levels (Foster et al., 2003; Labus et al., 2003), most guidelines do not recommend relying on these changes as the main method of pain assessment (Herr et al., 2006). This is because physiological changes can usually be attributed to a wide range of factors, so it is very difficult to establish which change is pain related.

BEHAVIORAL PAIN SCALE (BPS)

The Behavioral Pain Scale (BPS) developed by Payen et al. (2001) was based on findings from the study of Puntillo et al. (1997). Puntillo found a correlation of certain behavioral indicators and patients' self-reports of pain. The BPS pain scale is used in patients who are sedated and mechanically ventilated and is based on a sum score of three dimensions: 1) facial expression, 2) movements of upper limbs, and 3) compliance with mechanical ventilation. Each pain indicator is scored from 1 (no response) to 4 (full response), with a maximum score of 12. A health care professional selects the descriptor in each dimension that best describes the behavior displayed by the patient. It has been shown using this tool that there is moderate to strong correlation with the number of observed behaviors to the patient's report of the intensity of pain. Initial validity and reliability was established during painful procedures (such as endotracheal suctioning) and nonpainful procedures (central venous catheter dressing change). Nociceptive stimulation resulted in higher BPS values than did nonnociceptive stimuli. Excellent interrater reliability was also found upon multiple testing. The BPS has been tested by Payen et al. (2001), Aissaoui et al. (2005), and Young et al. (2006). One limitation of BPS is that responsiveness (increase in score in response to noxious stimuli) decreases substantially with deepening levels of sedation and that it can only be used in the ventilated patient (Sessler, Grap, & Ramsay, 2008).

In a more recent study, Chanques et al. (2009) adapted the BPS for use in nonintubated ICU patients unable to self-report their pain because of the existence of delirium. The "vocalization" domain was inserted in place of the intubated dimension to create the BPS-nonintubated (BPS-NI) scale, ranging from 3 (no pain) to 12 (most pain). The BPS-NI was tested in a medical ICU. The results of the BPS-NI scores were higher during nociceptive procedures than at rest and there were no changes in BPS-NI scores during non-nociceptive procedures, establishing discriminative validity. The BPS-NI had good internal consistency and good interrater reliability. Chanques et al. (2009) concluded that for patients with dementia, pain level can be assessed with the BPS-NI scale since the instrument exhibited good psychometric properties.

ASSUME PAIN PRESENT (APP)

Patients who are chemically paralyzed and those with brain injury remain a challenging population in which to assess pain. There is no assessment tool available nor is there subjective data to utilize in order to determine pain. The health care provider must utilize a comprehensive clinical assessment based upon the following:

■ Patient's history and current condition
■ Behaviors if present
■ Pre-existing painful condition (chronic pain condition, arthritis, spinal stenosis, etc.)
■ Is there acute pain present (burns, trauma, or surgery)?
■ Does the potential for pain exist if the patient is receiving paralytics?
■ Invasive and noninvasive procedures
■ Extended stay in critical care

   Once the assessment is performed and if the circumstances suggest that pain is probable, then the practitioner may Assume Pain Present (APP). APP is not a substitute for a pain assessment, but a conclusion of the assessment because there is no behavioral assessment tool to quantify patient behaviors. The practitioner must document the criteria used to reach the conclusion of the APP assessment. The patient should be treated appropriately and reassessed regularly to determine effectiveness of treatment (Herr et al., 2006).

Case Study

Mr. Vincent is an 85-year-old male who has a history of mild dementia, atrial fibrillation, stroke, and cancer of the colon. He lives with his family. He was admitted to the medical ICU with a diagnosis of pneumonia 10 days ago. He had a tracheostomy tube placed 2 days ago because he has been unable to be weaned from the ventilator. His current vital signs are BP 156/82, P 88, R 20, T 99.4, O_2 sat 93%. He has a left subclavian central line and left radial arterial line. The thoracic surgeon placed a right chest tube yesterday because of a large pleural effusion. Mr. Vincent has been immobile and has lost a lot of movement in his limbs. His family is very supportive of his care.

Questions to Consider

1. Is Mr. Vincent at risk for pain?
2. What screening tools would you use to assess/monitor Mr. Vincent's pain?
3. Would the family play a role in the assessment process? If yes, what would be the role?
4. Name other factors that you may want to consider as part of the assessment process.

REFERENCES

American Geriatrics Society Panel on Persistent Pain in Older Persons. (2002). Clinical practice guidelines: The management of persistent pain in older persons. *JAGS, 50*, S205–S224. Retrieved from http://www.americangeriatrics.org/products/positionpapers/persistent_pain_ guide.shtml

Chanques, G., Payen, J. F., Mercier, G., de Lattre, S., Viel, E., Jung, B., . . . Jaber, S. (2009). Assessing pain in non-intubated critically ill patients unable to self-report: An adaptation of the behavioral pain scale. *Intensive Care Medicine, 35*, 2060–2067.

Chong, C., & Burchett, K. (2003). Pain management in critical care. *British Journal Anaesthesia CEPD Reviews, 3*(6), 183–186.

Feldt, K. (2000). The checklist of nonverbal pain indicators (CNPI). *Pain Management Nursing, 1*, 13–21.

Herr, K., Bjoro, K., & Decker, S. (2006). Tools for assessment of pain in nonverbal older adults with dementia: A state of the science review. *Journal of Pain and Symptom Management, 31*(2), 170–192.

Herr, K., Coyne, P. J., Manworren, R., McCaffery, M., Merkel, S., Pelosi-Kelly, J., & Wild, L. (2006). Pain assessment in the nonverbal patient: Position statement with clinical practice recommendations. *Pain Management Nursing, 7*(2), 44–52.

Kabes, A. M., Graves, J. K., & Norris, J. N. (2009). Further validation of the nonverbal pain scale in intensive care patients. *Critical Care Nurse, 29*(1), 59–66.

Payen, J. F., Bru, O., Bosson, J. L., Lagrasta A., Novel, E., Deschaux, I., . . . Jacquot, C. (2001). Assessing pain in critically ill sedated patients by using a behavioral pain scale. *Critical Care Medicine, 29*, 2258–2263.

Puntillo, K. A., Miaskowski, C., Kehrle, K., Stannard, D., Gleeson, S., & Nye, P. (1997). Relationship between behavioral and physiological indicators of pain, critical care patients' self-reports of pain, and opioid administration. *Critical Care Medicine, 25*(7), 1159–1166.

Puntillo, K. A., Stannard, D., Miaskowski, C., Kehrle, K., & Gleeson, S. (2002). Use of a pain assessment and intervention notation (P.A.I.N.) tool in critical care nursing practice: nurses' evaluations. *Heart and Lung, 31*(4), 303–314.

Sessler, C. N., Grap, M. J., & Ramsay, M. A. E. (2008). Evaluating and monitoring analgesia and sedation in the intensive care unit. *Critical Care, 12*(Suppl. 3), S2.

Stolee, P., Hillier, L. M., Esbaugh, J., Bol, N., McKellar, L., & Gauthier, N. (2005). Instruments for the assessment of pain in older persons with cognitive impairment. *Journal of the American Geriatrics Society, 53,* 319–326.

Van Herk, R., Van Dijk, M., Baar, F. P. M., Tibboel, D., & de Wit, R. (2007). Observation scales for pain assessment in older adults with cognitive impairments or communication difficulties. *Nursing Research, 56*(1), 34–43.

Voepel-Lewis, T., Zanotti, J., Dammeyer, J. A., & Merkel, S. (2010). Reliability and validity of the face, legs, activity, cry, consolability behavioral tool in assessing acute pain in critically ill patients. *American Journal of Critical Care, 19,* 55–61. doi: 10.4037/ajcc2010624

6

Medication Management With Nonopioid Medications

The mainstay for treating acute pain is medication management. Most patients with a pain complaint expect to receive a medication prescription when they see their health care provider. However, for some conditions, such as acute low back pain, the current recommendations are not pain medications; they are acetaminophen/nonsteroidal anti-inflammatory drugs (NSAIDs) and continued activity rather than opioids and bedrest (Chou et al., 2009). About 15% of the patients who have acute low back pain progress to chronic low back pain. Medication management for chronic low back pain is recommended, accompanied by a plan of care that includes medications along with other therapies, such as physical therapy and counseling (D'Arcy, 2009b). Opioids currently are, in most cases, reserved for severe pain that impairs functionality (Chou et al., 2009).

To treat acute pain with medications requires a pain assessment; history and physical examination; and a medication review that includes over-the-counter medications, herbal supplements, and vitamins (Bruckenthal, 2007). Most patients with pain have tried first to self-treat; they have tried pain medications in the past and know which work the best and which are less effective. When patients have information about medications that are effective for relieving their pain, consider this to be information that is similar to what a patient with diabetes provides about his or her daily insulin doses to a new health care provider. Just because a patient is familiar with medication names and doses does not make him or her a "drug seeker."

There are genetic factors that influence the effectiveness of pain medications specific to each individual, so when a patient says, "the only medication that works for me is morphine," it may really be a reflection of how his or her genetic makeup has reacted to medications tried in the past. The patient should never be penalized or negatively labeled for providing information on how specific medications have worked for him or her in the past.

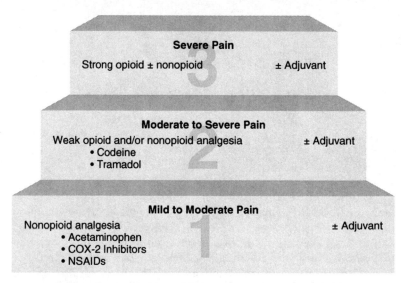

Figure 6.1 ▓ World Health Organization's analgesic ladder.

This section will provide information about using pain medications of various types—NSAIDs, opioids, and other coanalgesics, such as antidepressants. The information will be taken from current guidelines developed by the American Pain Society (APS), the American Geriatrics Society (AGS), the American Academy of Pain Medicine (AAPM), and other national organizations. Included will be an order set for pain management based on the World Health Organization (WHO) analgesic ladder and medication charts (Figure 6.1). The topics of addiction, dependency, and tolerance will be discussed in the last section of the book. Information on integrative therapies that can be combined with medication management will be provided at the end of this section.

GENERAL GUIDELINES

All patients have the right to have their pain treated, and most health care providers make honest efforts at getting patients' pain to a tolerable level (Brennan, Carr, & Cousins, 2007). Most patients with acute or surgical pain realize that "pain free" is not a reasonable goal to set and that a risk–benefit analysis is used to determine what type of medication management will provide the best outcome for the patient. However, pain has become an extremely common patient complaint that often requires the use of nonopioid medications, opioid analgesics, and coanalgesics.

Most prescribers have very little concern when opioids are needed for short-term pain management, but when opioid therapy is required for the long term, their concern increases, and fears of addicting the patient to the medication or fear of increased regulatory oversight can affect the prescriber's willingness to continue providing opioid medications to the patient with chronic pain (D'Arcy, 2009a). For acute pain, this issue is not as significant, but there are still some health care providers who feel that they are contributing to addiction when opioids are used in the acute care setting. This can lead the prescriber to consider the nonopioid medications as a first-line medication when an opioid may be indicated. Alternatively, the prescriber may try an opioid that he or she perceives has a lower potential for abuse or addiction, such as acetaminophen with codeine, even though the patient may be reporting severe pain. Selecting a medication that will be effective for the patient's pain complaint can be by trial and error until the right medication and dose are found.

Some patients who have acute pain will progress to chronic pain management. All patients who are being considered for chronic opioid therapy should be screened for risks that include opioid misuse, development of aberrant medication-taking behaviors, and addiction (Chou et al., 2009). The development of a comprehensive treatment plan that includes the use of various medications is extremely important to the success of pain management (Institute for Clinical Systems Improvement, 2008). If long-term opioids are being considered, an opioid agreement may be created that outlines when the medications will be refilled, the risks and benefits of the medications, the use of random urine screens, and the consequences of violating the agreement (Trescot et al., 2008). A sample opioid agreement can be obtained at the AAPM website. At the other end of the spectrum, the undertreatment of pain can produce a plethora of unwanted side effects, especially with older patients. Some of the significant consequences of undertreated pain include the following:

- Depression
- Impaired cognition
- Sleep disturbances
- Poorer clinical outcome
- Decreased functional ability
- Decreased quality of life
- Anxiety
- Decreased socialization
- Increased health care utilization and costs (American Geriatrics Society [AGS], 2002; Brennan et al., 2007; D'Arcy, 2007; Karani & Meier, 2004).

In a recent survey conducted by Stanford University, 40% of the respondents reported that pain interfered with enjoyment of life and pleasurable activities, and that chronic pain adversely affected their mood (Stanos, Fishbain, & Fishman, 2009). Although 63% of the survey respondents indicated that they had gone to their health care provider, only 31% of the patients reported that they had either complete or a great deal of pain relief. In addition, less than 50% reported a lot of control over their pain. What this tells us about acute pain that progresses to chronic pain and its management is that the problem is very big and the ability of health care providers to control the pain is limited.

Among pain specialists, there is currently a movement toward considering chronic pain as a disease in and of itself (Brennan et al., 2007). There is also evidence to support the idea that untreated or undertreated acute pain can lead to more difficult-to-treat chronic pain syndromes, such as complex regional pain syndromes. Becoming more aware of patients with acute pain who report high levels of pain for many clinic visits or return visits is important for providers working with these patients, because this can be the beginning of a chronic pain condition. The effect of chronic pain on the patient is so profound that it constitutes a major threat to health and wellness. Unrelieved chronic pain can have many different physiologic effects, such as the following:

- Reduced mobility
- Loss of strength
- Disturbed sleep
- Decreased immune function
- Increased susceptibility to disease
- Dependence on medications for pain relief
- Depression and anxiety (Brennan et al., 2007)

Because of the magnitude of the problem of pain and the impact on the individual patient's well-being, health care providers need to become proficient in prescribing and dosing medications for pain of all types. WHO developed an analgesic ladder (Figure 6.1) that provides guidance to prescribers about their choices of pain medications. Although the ladder was originally developed for cancer pain, it has been adapted for use in many areas of pain management to include acute pain.

WHO ANALGESIC LADDER

Level I Medications: Mild to Moderate Pain

Medications to treat mild to moderate pain, which are on the first step of the analgesic ladder, include acetaminophen; NSAIDs, both selective and nonselective; and adjuvant medications or coanalgesics. These medications can add to pain relief, although they are not primarily classed as pain medications. These medications include antidepressants, anticonvulsants, muscle relaxants, and topical medications.

Level II Medications: Moderate to Severe Pain

On the middle step of the analgesic ladder are the medications for moderate to severe pain, for example, a combination medication with an opioid, such as hydrocodone or oxycodone (OxyContin), and acetaminophen. In addition, tramadol (Ultram) and tapentadol (Nucynta), medications with combined mu agonist and selective serotonin reuptake inhibitor (SSRI) actions, are included in this level of medications for moderate pain. Adjuvant medications for this level could include the muscle relaxants and antidepressants of the lower level, but the acetaminophen or NSAIDs of the lower level could also be used at this point for additional pain relief.

Level III Medications: Severe Pain

Patients who are reporting severe pain require strong opioid medications for pain relief. Included in this group of medications are the opioids, such as morphine, fentanyl (Sublimaze), hydromorphone (Dilaudid), and methadone (Dolophine). As with the other steps, adjuvant medication should be continued here to help reduce opioid needs and provide additional pain relief (D'Arcy, 2007).

Clinical Pearl	Although the WHO analgesic ladder provides some guidance in the choice of medications, the overall assessment, history and physical comorbidities, and organ functions need to be considered when selecting a medication for pain.

It is important to remember that the patient's report of pain is more than a number. There are many pieces of the patient puzzle that need to fit together just right to find an effective method for pain relief. Although the severity ratings of the analgesic ladder are a guide to choosing the correct medication because there is a group of medications at each pain level, the practitioner can individualize the medication selection. The efficacy of the medication is an individualized response based on the patient's report of decreased pain or increased functionality (D'Arcy, 2007).

PHYSICIAN'S ORDERS
Pain Management Standard Order Set

ALLERGIES ➤

I HEREBY AUTHORIZE THE PHARMACY TO DISPENSE A GENERIC EQUIVALENT UNLESS THE PARTICULAR DRUG IS CIRCLED.

PATIENT PLATE

ORDERS ***PLEASE WRITE WITH BALLPOINT PEN***

Medications must be written with one dose and one time interval. Select only one medication from each section.

Mild Pain. Pain Intensity Rating 1-3
☐ Tylenol ☐ Tylenol #3 (Tylenol with codeine)
*No more than 4 grams of Tylenol per day
☐ Ibuprofen (starting dose 200 mgs twice a day)
☐ Celebrex (Starting dose 100 mg twice a day - no more than 400 mgs per day)
☐ PO ☐ PRN ☐ Scheduled
Dose ☐ One tablet ☐ Two tablets ☐ Other ____________
Interval-every ☐ 4 hours ☐ 6 hours ☐ 8 hours

Moderate Pain. Pain Intensity Rating 4-6 * Consider total daily intake of Tylenol
☐ Vicodin (Hydrocodone with Tylenol) ☐ Percocet (Oxycodone with Tylenol)
☐ Oxy IR (oxycodone) ☐ Oxycontin (extended release oxycodone)
*Suggested starting dose one tablet every 4 hours except for oxycontin which is given every 12 hours
☐ PO ☐ PRN ☐ Scheduled
Dose ☐ One tablet ☐ Two tablets ☐ Other ____________
Interval-every ☐ 4 hours ☐ 6 hours ☐ 8 hours ☐ 12 hours

Severe Pain. Pain Intensity Rating 7-10
☐ MSIR (oral morphine) ☐ MS Contin (Extended release morphine)
Suggested starting dose 15 milligrams every 4 hours except MS Contin which is given every 12 hours
☐ Dilaudid (hydromorphone) Suggested starting dose 2 milligrams every 4 hours
☐ PO ☐ PRN ☐ Scheduled
Dose ____________
Interval-every ☐ 4 hours ☐ 6 hours ☐ 8 hours ☐ 12 hours

Parenteral Pain Medications- For use as primary medication or for breakthrough pain
☐ Morphine (suggested 2 milligrams every hour) ☐ Dilaudid (suggested- 0.5 milligrams every 3 hours)
*Caution in elderly. May accumulate with decreased renal clearance
☐ Fentanyl - dosed in **MICROGRAMS** (suggested 25 **micrograms** every hour)
☐ Toradol * Five day maximum use * reduce dose in elderly * Creat > 1.2 or hx of GI bleed-do not use suggested 15 milligrams every 6 hours
☐ IV ☐ SQ ☐ IM ☐ PRN ☐ Scheduled
Dose ____________
Interval-every ☐ hour ☐ 2 hours ☐ 4 hours ☐ 6 hours ☐ 8 hours ☐ 12 hours

Fentanyl Patch
☐ Duragesic patch - not recommended for acute postoperative use, change every 72 hours
Start opioid naïve patients on 25 **microgram** patch. Takes 12 - 18 hours to begin relieving pain.
☐ 25 microgram ☐ 50 microgram ☐ 75 microgram ☐ 100 microgram ☐ 200 microgram

Laxative
☐ Senakot one tab ☐ Milk of Magnesia 30 ml ☐ Dulcolax one tab/Suppository ☐ Colace 100 mg
☐ Other ____________
☐ PO ☐ Rectal suppository ☐ PRN ☐ Scheduled
☐ every day ☐ twice per day

Antiemetic
☐ Phenergan ☐ Reglan ☐ Zofran ☐ Compazine ☐ Scopolamine patch 1.5 mg disk - change every 3 days
☐ PO ☐ Rectal ☐ IV ☐ PRN ☐ Scheduled
Dose ____________
Interval-every ☐ 4 hours ☐ 6 hours ☐ 8 hours ☐ 12 hours

PAIN DISTRESS/ INTENSITY SCALE

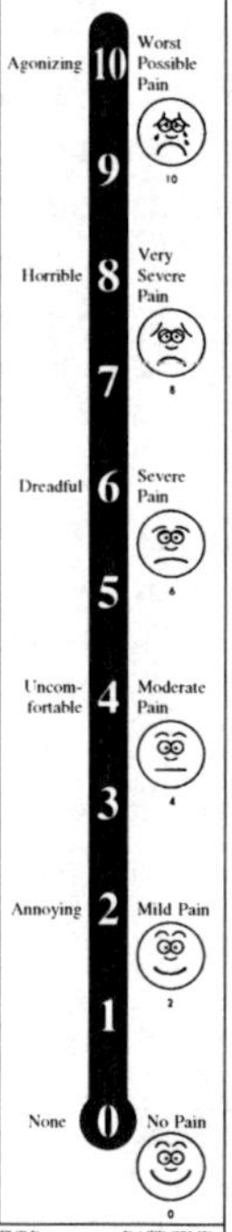

PLEASE WRITE WITH BALLPOINT PEN	UNIT SECRETARY DATE/TIME	RN SIGNATURE DATE/TIME	PHYSICIAN'S SIGNATURE DATE/TIME

MEDICAL RECORDS

Figure 6.2 ■ Pain management order set exemplar. *Source:* Courtesy of Suburban Hospital—Johns Hopkins Medical Center, Bethesda, MD.

For treating acute pain, a pain management order set that clarifies which medications are available to treat the stated level of pain is useful for general directions. A sample of an order set is provided in Figure 6.2.

Another use for this order set is education. It can help prescribers understand which medication is appropriate to treat the various levels of pain. This avoids the use of acetaminophen with codeine to treat severe pain and indicates which medications might be better choices.

NONOPIOID ANALGESICS FOR PAIN (ACETAMINOPHEN AND NSAIDs)

Although acetaminophen and NSAIDs are considered to be weaker medications for pain, they can provide a good baseline of relief that can help decrease the amount of opioid required to treat pain. Both acetaminophen and NSAIDs are seriously overlooked and underutilized as coanalgesics when higher intensity pain is reported. Multi-modal analgesia, which is recommended for complex pain needs and for postoperative pain relief, may consist of any combination of medications that may include the use of acetaminophen and NSAIDs. However, there are some important considerations when adding these medications into a pain regimen. These medications are not benign and have risk potential that should be considered prior to use in all patients. They also have maximum dose levels that create a ceiling for dose escalations.

Acetaminophen (APAP, Paracetamol)

Acetaminophen is used worldwide to treat pain. Known as paracetamol in Europe, it is associated with the Tylenol brand in the United States and is widely added to many over-the-counter pain relievers, such as Excedrin, Midol, and the various Tylenol products. The newest formulation is intravenous acetaminophen (Oremev). It is available as tablets, gel caps, and elixirs, and as pediatric formulations. Most homes have some type of acetaminophen compound that the family uses for relief of minor aches and pains. Because it is so popular and easy to obtain, some 24.6 billion doses were sold in 2008 (Pan, 2009).

Acetaminophen is classed as a para-acetaminophen derivative *(Nursing 2010 Drug Handbook,* 2009), and has a similar pain relief profile to aspirin without the potential to damage the gastric mucosa (APS, 2008). The pain relief efficacy of acetaminophen is superior to placebo but slightly less effective than NSAIDs (APS, 2008). The action of the medication is thought to be the inhibition of prostaglandins and other pain-producing substances *(Nursing 2010 Drug Handbook,* 2009). It is entirely metabolized in the liver and can cause blood pressure elevations (Buvanendran & Lipman, 2009).

Advantages of acetaminophen over NSAIDs include the following:
- Fewer gastrointestinal (GI) adverse effects
- Fewer GI complications

In general, acetaminophen is safe and effective when used according to the directions and labeling on the over-the-counter preparations and the prescription-strength medication information. There are serious concerns today about acetaminophen overdose, both intentional and unintentional.

The Food and Drug Administration (FDA) has been holding hearings and is considering reducing the recommendations for the daily total dose from 4,000 mg per day to a lower limit. The FDA is also considering making the 500-mg strength tablets available only by prescription and limiting the number of doses in each package (Alazraki, 2009).

The concerns underlying these fears are related to some very serious statistics about the increase in liver disease related to acetaminophen use. There is a clear connection with acetaminophen overuse and liver disease and failure. Total acetaminophen doses should not exceed 4,000 mg per day, including any combination medication taken by the patient that may include acetaminophen (Trescott et al., 2008). Even at this dose, there is an associated risk of hepatotoxicity (APS, 2008).

From 1998 to 2003, acetaminophen was the leading cause of acute liver failure in the United States (Alazraki, 2009). Between 1990 and 1998, there were 56,000 emergency department visits, 26,000 hospitalizations, and 458 deaths reportedly connected to acetaminophen overdoses (Alazraki, 2009). Many of these overdoses were unintentional and caused by a knowledge deficit about the "hidden" acetaminophen found in combination medications. Some of the most common prescription strength combinations with acetaminophen include the following:

- Tylenol #3
- Vicodin
- Percocet
- Ultracet

Other over-the-counter medications that can contain hidden acetaminophen include the following:

- Alka-Seltzer Plus
- Cough syrups, such as NyQuil/DayQuil Cold and Flu Relief
- Over-the-counter pain relievers, such as Pamprin and Midol Maximum-Strength Menstrual Formula

Care should be taken with older patients, patients with liver-impaired function, and any patient who uses alcohol regularly (American Geriatrics Society [AGS], 2009; APS, 2008). In these cases, acetaminophen doses should not exceed 2,000 mg per day or should not be used at all (AGS, 2009). The risk of liver failure is very real. It is imperative for all patients who are taking Tylenol to read and understand the medication administration guidelines and recommendations. Exceeding daily recommended doses of acetaminophen can have deadly consequences.

One little-known impact is the effect of acetaminophen on the anticoagulant warfarin (Coumadin). Careful monitoring of anticoagulation should take place when a patient is taking both acetaminophen and warfarin because acetaminophen is an underrecognized cause of over-anticoagulation when both medications are being used concomitantly (APS, 2008).

Aspirin

Aspirin is one of the oldest pain relievers known to humans. It is classed as a salicylate. Before the beginning of modern medicine, salicylate-rich willow bark was used as one of the earliest forms of pain relief. Many Americans use aspirin for minor aches and pains, and because of its action on platelet activity, it has been promoted for early in-the-field treatment for patients who are experiencing heart attack. It was traditionally used for pain relief of osteoarthritis, rheumatoid arthritis, and for other inflammatory conditions but has been replaced by newer NSAIDs (APS, 2008; *Nursing 2010 Drug Handbook*, 2009).

Aspirin is available in many different doses, but the most common dose is 500 to 1,000 mg every 4 or 6 hours with a maximum dose of 4,000 mg per day (APS, 2008). It is available in buffered, sustained-release, and chewable formulations.

Despite its easy availability and widespread use, there are some serious adverse effects connected with regular aspirin use. These include the following:

- GI distress
- GI ulceration and bleeding
- Prolonged bleeding times
- Reye syndrome
- Aspirin hypersensitivity

These reactions to aspirin are quite serious and, in some cases, life threatening. GI ulceration and bleeding can cause death. Aspirin is not recommended for children younger than the age of 12 because of the potential for Reye syndrome, which can develop when a child has a viral illness and aspirin is given for pain relief (APS, 2008). Aspirin hypersensitivity reactions can be minor or very severe. A minor reaction presents as a respiratory reaction with rhinitis, asthma, or nasal polyps. A smaller group of patients can get more serious reactions that include the following:

- Urticaria
- Wheals
- Angioneurotic edema
- Hypotension
- Shock and syncope (APS, 2008)

Although aspirin seems like a very simple analgesic, care should be taken with any aspirin use.

THE NSAID DEBATE

NSAIDs of all types are commonly used for pain that is mild to moderate in intensity. They can be used for pain that is inflammatory and as an analgesic for low-level pain or as a coanalgesic. They are available in different combinations in both prescription strength and over-the-counter preparations. They do have a maximum dose that limits dose escalation beyond the maximum dose ceiling.

NSAIDs have two different types of actions: selective and nonselective.

▪ *Nonselective NSAIDs* affect all types of prostaglandins found in the stomach, kidneys, heart, and other organs of the body.
▪ *Selective NSAIDs* protect the prostaglandins that coat the stomach lining but do affect the other types of prostaglandins found elsewhere in the body.

The most common use of NSAIDs is to treat pain that is caused by inflammation, such as arthritis or common musculoskeletal injuries (APS, 2008; D'Arcy, 2007).

NSAIDs have long been a standard for pain relief in older patients. Relatively cheap, they are easily accessible at most supermarkets or drugstores. They are available as over-the-counter formulations and in prescription strength as well. The most common uses are for arthritis pain, headaches, and minor sprains and strains.

Based on the differences in actions, the NSAIDs are clearly divided into two classes: *nonselective* and *COX-2 selective*. The nonselective NSAIDs include ibuprofen (Motrin, Advil), naproxen (Naprosyn), and ketoprofen (Orudis). They affect production of the prostaglandins that coat and protect the lining of the stomach and those that are found in other organs of the body, including the kidneys and the heart. The only COX-2 selective NSAID medication available at this time is celecoxib (Celebrex). Celecoxib spares the stomach prostaglandins and does not affect platelet aggregation, so blood clotting is not affected. Mechanisms for both types of NSAIDs can be found at http://www.fda.gov.

Newer research from the FDA indicates that all NSAIDs, not only the COX-2 selective medications such as Celebrex, have the potential for increased cardiovascular risk, renovascular risk, stroke, and myocardial infarction (Bennett et al., 2005; D'Arcy, 2007). GI bleeding with NSAIDs continues to be a risk; for those patients who are taking aspirin as a cardiac prophylaxis, the risk increases several fold with concomitant NSAID and aspirin use (D'Arcy, 2007; Exhibit 6.1).

Exhibit 6.1

Medication Guide for Nonsteroidal Anti-inflammatory Drugs (NSAIDs)
(*See the end of this Medication Guide for a list of prescription NSAID medicines.*)

What is the most important information I should know about medicines called nonsteroidal anti-inflammatory drugs (NSAIDs)?
NSAID medicines may increase the chance of a heart attack or stroke that can lead to death. This chance increases:
- with longer use of NSAID medicines
- in people who have heart disease

NSAID medicines should never be used right before or after a heart surgery called a "coronary artery bypass graft (CABG)."
NSAID medicines can cause ulcers and bleeding in the stomach and intestines at any time during treatment. Ulcers and bleeding:
- can happen without warning symptoms
- may cause death

The chance of a person getting an ulcer or bleeding increases with:
- taking medicines called "corticosteroids" and "anticoagulants"
- longer use
- smoking
- drinking alcohol
- older age
- having poor health

NSAID medicines should only be used:
- exactly as prescribed
- at the lowest dose possible for your treatment
- for the shortest time needed

What are nonsteroidal anti-inflammatory drugs (NSAIDs)?
NSAID medicines are used to treat pain and redness, swelling, and heat (inflammation) from medical conditions such as:
- different types of arthritis
- menstrual cramps and other types of short-term pain

Get emergency help right away if you have any of the following symptoms:
- shortness of breath or trouble breathing
- chest pain

(*continued*)

- weakness in one part or side of your body
- slurred speech
- swelling of the face or throat

Stop your NSAID medicine and call your health care provider right away if you have any of the following symptoms:

- nausea
- more tired or weaker than usual
- itching
- your skin or eyes look yellow
- stomach pain
- flu-like symptoms
- vomit blood
- there is blood in your bowel movement or it is black and sticky like tar
- skin rash or blisters with fever
- unusual weight gain
- swelling of the arms and legs, hands, and feet

These are not all the side effects with NSAID medicines. Talk to your health care provider or pharmacist for more information about NSAID medicines.

Other information about nonsteroidal anti-inflammatory drugs (NSAIDs):

Aspirin is an NSAID medicine but it does not increase the chance of a heart attack. Aspirin can cause bleeding in the brain, stomach, and intestines. Aspirin can also cause ulcers in the stomach and intestines. Some of these NSAID medicines are sold in lower doses without a prescription (over-the-counter). Talk to your health care provider before using over-the-counter (OTC) NSAIDs for more than 10 days.

Who should not take a nonsteroidal anti-inflammatory drug (NSAID)?

Do not take an NSAID medicine:

- if you had an asthma attack, hives, or other allergic reaction with aspirin or any other NSAID medicine
- for pain right before or after heart bypass surgery

Tell your health care provider:

- about all of your medical conditions.
- about all of the medicines you take. NSAIDs and some other medicines can interact with each other and cause serious side effects.

(continued)

- keep a list of your medicines to show to your health care provider and pharmacist.
- if you are pregnant. NSAID medicines should not be used by pregnant women late in their pregnancy.
- if you are breastfeeding. Talk to your doctor.

What are the possible side effects of nonsteroidal anti-inflammatory drugs (NSAIDs)?
Serious side effects include:
- heart attack
- stroke
- high blood pressure
- heart failure from body swelling (fluid retention)
- kidney problems including kidney failure
- bleeding and ulcers in the stomach and intestine
- low red blood cells (anemia)
- life-threatening skin reactions
- life-threatening allergic reactions
- liver problems including liver failure
- asthma attacks in people who have asthma
Other side effects include:
- stomach pain
- constipation
- diarrhea
- gas
- heartburn
- nausea
- vomiting
- dizziness

NSAID Medicines That Need a Prescription:

Generic Name	Trade Name
celecoxib	Celebrex
diclofenac	Cataflam, Voltaren, Arthrotec combined with misoprostol
diflunisal	Dolobid
etodolac	Lodine, Lodine XL

(*continued*)

Generic Name	Trade Name
fenoprofen	Nalfon, Nalfon 200
flurbiprofen	Ansaid
ibuprofen with combunox	Motrin, Tab-Profen, Vicoprofen* (combined with hydrocodone), (combined with oxycodone)
indomethacin	Indocin, Indocin SR, Indo-Lemmon, Indomethagan
ketoprofen	Oruvail
ketorolac	Toradol
mefenamic acid	Ponstel
meloxicam	Mobic
nabumetone	Relafen
naproxen	Naprosyn, Anaprox, Anaprox DS, ECNaprosyn, Naprelan, PREVACID NapraPAC (copackaged with lansoprazole)
oxaprozin	Daypro
piroxicam	Feldene
sulindac	Clinoril
tolmetin	Tolectin, Tolectin DS, Tolectin 600

*Vicoprofen contains the same dose of ibuprofen as OTC NSAIDs, and is usually used for less than 10 days to treat pain. The OTC NSAID label warns that long term continuous use may increase the risk of heart attack or stroke.

Note: *This Medication Guide has been approved by the U.S. Food and Drug Administration.*

GI Risks With NSAIDs

One of the major risks with nonselective NSAIDs is gastric ulceration. Gastric ulcers develop within a week in about 30% of patients started on nonselective NSAIDs (Wallace & Staats, 2005). Most patients with these ulcers are asymptomatic and only seek medical care when the bleeding becomes obvious with tarry stools or hematemesis.

Some practitioners prescribe proton pump inhibitors (PPI), such as omeprazole (Prilosec), which only provides protection for the upper GI system. Patient compliance with PPI for protection is also suspect. A recent study found that by the time the patients received three prescriptions for a PPI as NSAID prophylaxis, the nonadherence rate for patients with PPIs was as high as 60.8% (D'Arcy, 2010; Sturkenboom et al., 2003).

Some older patients are also using an aspirin a day for cardioprotective effect; adding the incidence of ulcer formation with aspirin to the NSAID risk only increases the potential for GI bleeding. Patients who use higher doses and are older have an increased occurrence rate of GI side effects (Perez-Gutthann, Garcia Rodriguez, & Raiford, 1997). Additionally, chronic alcohol use with NSAIDs increases the risk of GI bleeding and ulceration. Deciding if NSAIDs are an appropriate treatment option for the patient depends largely on the individual patient's history and medical situation.

Cardiovascular Risks With NSAIDs

For patients who have had recent heart bypass surgery, patients with heart disease, and patients who have had transient ischemic attacks or strokes, NSAID use presents a higher risk for cardiovascular events and their use is not recommended (Bennett et al., 2005). For these patients, an alternate form of analgesic is recommended.

When trying to determine if NSAIDs are a good treatment option, consider that naproxen interferes with the inhibitory effect of aspirin (Capone et al., 2005) and that similar effects may be seen with concomitant use of ibuprofen (Advil, Motrin), acetaminophen (Tylenol), and diclofenac (Cataflam, Voltaren; Catella-Lawson et al., 2001). Weighing the risks and benefits of using NSAIDs for a patient who is using aspirin for cardiac prophylaxis should include consideration of an increased risk of GI events and that the aspirin effectiveness may be decreased.

Overall, the recommendations for using NSAIDs for pain relief indicate that the medication should be used at the lowest dose for the shortest time (Bennett et al., 2005). For older patients this means that long-term use of NSAIDs for chronic conditions such as arthritis can lead to serious and even life-threatening events.

New Developments With NSAIDs

Newer forms of NSAIDs have come to market recently. These types of NSAIDs are called targeted topical medications and are applied directly to the site of pain. Some of the medications are applied as liquids, whereas others have been made into patches. The newest formulation is a liquid made of diclofenac sodium, a topical solution called Pennsaid. The liquid can be applied directly to the knees for patients with osteoarthritis.

Diclofenac also comes as a 1% gel formulation that is rapidly absorbed and is recommended for use on joints with osteoarthritis. The patient will need to apply the solution or gel to the affected joint four times per day for maximum pain relief.

A patch containing 1% of diclofenac epolamine (Flector) has been used successfully for minor orthopedic injuries, such as strains and sprains. The patch should be applied directly to the site of the injury. Despite the topical application, each medication has recommendations to use the smallest dose possible for the shortest time, and GI side effects, although rare, cannot be excluded.

Case Study

Lawrence is a 45-year-old thoracotomy patient. He has had chest surgery yesterday for lung cancer and is complaining of pain that is not relieved with his epidural. He complains of shoulder pain and incisional discomfort. Additionally, he has a history of gastro-esophageal reflux disease (GERD) and is currently taking nothing by mouth. What can you add to improve his pain control?

Questions to Consider

1. What kind of non-opioid medication can you add to help improve the patient's pain control? Would you consider Oremev (acetaminophen given intravenously) or ketoralac (Toradol)?
2. Does the fact that Lawrence has GERD limit your ability to give him an NSAID like Toradol?
3. For his shoulder pain, what would you consider adding in a topical medication: NSAID cream or liquid, a topical NSAID patch, or a lidocaine patch (Lidoderm)?
4. How should you educate Lawrence about using NSAIDs. Can you offer him options for added pain relief that take his GERD into consideration?

REFERENCES

Alazraki, M. (2009). *Raw risk of over-the-counter meds: How many Tylenols have you taken today?* Retrieved from http://www.dailyfinance.com/

American Geriatrics Society (AGS). (2002). Panel on persistent pain in older persons. *Journal of the American Geriatrics Society, 50*(6), 1–20.

American Geriatrics Society (AGS). (2009). Pharmacological management of persistent pain in older persons. *Journal of the American Geriatrics Society, 57*(8), 1331–1346.

Bennett, J. S., Daugherty, A., Herrington, D., Greenland, P., Roberts, H., & Taubert, K. A. (2005). The use of nonsteroidal anti-inflammatory drugs (NSAIDs): A science advisory from the American Heart Association. *Circulation, 111*(13), 1713–1716.

Brennan, F., Carr, D. B., & Cousins, M. (2007). Pain management: A fundamental human right. *Anesthesia & Analgesia, 105*(1), 205–221.

Bruckenthal, P. (2007). Controlled substances: Principles of safe prescribing. *The Nurse Practitioner, 32*(5), 7–11.

Buvanendran, A., & Lipman, A. (2009). Nonsteroidal anti-inflammatory drugs and acetaminophen. In J. Ballantyne, S. Fishman, & J. Rathmell (Eds.), *Bonica's management of pain* (4th ed., pp. 1157–1171). Philadelphia, PA: Lippincott Williams and Wilkins.

Capone, M. L., Sciulli, M. G., Tacconelli, S., Grana, M., Ricciotti, M., Renda, G., . . . Patrignani, P. (2005). Pharmacodynamic interaction of naproxen with low-dose aspirin in healthy subjects. *Journal of the College of Cardiology, 45*(8), 1295–1301.

Catella-Lawson, F., Reilly, M., Kapoor, S., Cucchiara, A., DeMarco, S., Tournier, B., . . . FitzGerald, G. (2001). Cyclooxygenase inhibitors and the antiplatelet effects of aspirin. *New England Journal of Medicine, 345*(25), 1809–1817.

Chou, R., Fanciullo, G. J., Fine, P. G., Adler, J. A., Ballantyne, J. C., Davies, P., . . . Miaskowski, C. (2009). Clinical guidelines for the use of chronic opioid therapy in chronic noncancer pain. *The Journal of Pain, 10*(2), 113–130.

D'Arcy, Y. (2007). *Pain management: Evidence based tools and techniques for nursing professionals.* Marblehead, MA: HCPro.

D'Arcy, Y. (2009a). Be in the know about pain management. *The Nurse Practitioner, 34*(4), 43–47.

D'Arcy, Y. (2009b). Treating low back pain with evidence-based options. *The Nurse Practitioner.*

Institute for Clinical Systems Improvement. (2008). *Assessment and management of chronic pain.* Bloomington, MN: Author.

Karani, R., & Meier, D. (2004). Systematic pharmacologic postoperative pain management in the geriatric orthopaedic patient. *Clinical Orthopaedics and Related Research, 425,* 26–34.

Nursing 2010 Drug Handbook. (2012). Philadelphia, PA: Wolters Kluwer/Lippincott Williams and Wilkins.

Pan, G. J. D. (2009). *Acetaminophen: Background and overview.* Retrieved from www.fda.gov.

Perez-Gutthann, S., Garcia Rodriguez, L., & Raiford, D. S. (1997). Individual nonsteroidal anti-inflammatory drugs and other risk factors for upper gastrointestinal bleeding and perforation. *Epidemiology, 8,* 18–24.

Stanos, S. P., Fishbain, D. A., & Fishman, S. M. (2009). Pain management with opioid analgesics: Balancing risk and benefit. *Physical Medicine & Rehabilitation, 88*(3, Suppl. 2), S69–S99.

Sturkenboom, M. C., Burke, T. A., Tangelder, M. J., Dieleman, J. P., Walton, S., & Goldstein, J. L. (2003). Adherence to proton pump inhibitors or H2-receptor antagonists during the use of non-steroidal anti-inflammatory drugs. *Alimentary Pharmacology and Therapeutics,* 18(11–12), 1137–1147.

Trescot, A. M., Helm, S., Hansen, H., Benyamin, R., Glaser, S. E., Adlaka, R., . . . Manchikanti, L. (2008). Opioids in the management of chronic non-cancer pain: An update of American Society of Interventional Pain Physicians' (ASIPP) guidelines. *Pain Physician, 11*(Suppl. 2), S5–S62.

Wallace, M., & Staats, P. (2005). *Pain medicine and management.* New York, NY: McGraw-Hill.

Additional Resources

Chu, L. F., Clark, D. J., & Angst, M. S. (2006). Opioid tolerance and hyper-algesia in chronic pain patients after one month of oral morphine therapy: A preliminary prospective study. *The Journal of Pain, 7*(1), 43–48.

Dworkin, R. H., O'Connor, A. B., Backonja, M., Farrar, J. T., Finnerup, N. B., Jensen, T. S., . . . Wallace, M. S. (2007). Pharmacologic management of neuropathic pain: Evidence-based recommendations. *Pain, 132*(3), 237–251.

Fine, P., & Portnoy, R. (2007). *A clinical guide to opioid analgesia.* New York, NY: Vendome Group Health Care.

Veterans Health Administration, Department of Defense. (2003). *VA/DoD clinical practice guideline for the management of opioids therapy for chronic pain.* Washington, DC: Author.

7

Opioid Analgesics

OVERVIEW OF OPIOID MEDICATIONS

Opioids are medications that are derived from the opium poppy, *Papaver somniferum*. They have a long history of pain relief and have been used in various forms since the time of the Sumerians, such as elixirs and potions, and also smoked; in the Sumerian culture, the poppy was depicted in art as "the plant of joy" (Osler, cited in Fine & Portnoy, 2007). Reports from early Greek, Egyptian, and Roman societies described the fact that many of the leaders and everyday citizens used opium for pain relief. In the 16th century, the use of laudanum, an opium-derived elixir, was common for various pain complaints. It was during this time that dependence and tolerance were first observed to be occurring in laudanum users. In the early days of the United States, cocaine-containing elixirs and tonics for pain relief were sold by peddlers. Laudanum was a major pain reliever for households in the Civil War era of the 1860s.

The term *opioid* or *opiate* denotes a class of medications that are derived from the latex sap of the opium poppy or created as analogs to these natural substances. Opium has a two-sided history: one as a potent analgesic and the other as a recreational drug. For example, it was smoked for its euphoric effect in the opium dens of China and also used for pain relief. Early herbalists recognized the analgesic potential of opium and used it to treat many different types of pain in their patients.

During the 19th century, China's trade with the British consisted of large amounts of opium. The supply was high and demand for the product was just as great, leading to wars and infighting over the use of opium to balance trade. Morphine was first isolated in 1895 in Germany, where the medication was thought to be useful as a cure for opium addiction (McCoy, cited in Fine & Portnoy, 2007). The development of the hypodermic syringe in the mid-19th century gave medical practitioners another route for delivering opioid medications injected directly into the site of the pain.

By the 20th century, opioid use not only was seen as beneficial for treating pain but also had become problematic as opioid abuse increased. The United States passed the first two acts for controlling the use of opioids: the Pure Food and Drug Act (1906) and the Harrison Narcotics Act (1914). As late as 1970, the Federal Controlled Substances Act provided standards for the monitoring, manufacturing, prescribing, and dispensing of opioids and created the five-level classification of controlled substances that we use today.

In general, opioids are some of the best medications we have to control pain. They come in various formulations and have few adverse side effects when compared with other medication types.

Natural derivatives of opium include morphine, codeine, and heroin. Synthetic analogues, such as fentanyl (Sublimaze) and meperidine (Demerol), were developed much later as attempts to perfect compounds for better pain relief. All of the opioid compounds share certain features.

▪ Opioids work by binding sites in the body called mu receptors to produce analgesia. Mu receptors are found in many places in the body, including the brain and spinal column neurons.

▪ Their main action is analgesia.

▪ Side effects, such as sedation, constipation, and nausea, are common.

▪ They all are potentially addicting. Analgesia is the goal of opioid administration. The cytocrome P450 system, located in the liver, transforms some opioids into usable metabolites (Fine & Portnoy, 2007). The rate that opioids are metabolized varies from person to person, with the range being ultraslow to ultrarapid. Additionally, 5% to 10% of Caucasians lack the ability or have poor ability to convert codeine to morphine (Løvlie et al., 2001). In some older individuals, changes in proteins may limit the binding ability of opioid medications (Zurakowski, 2009).

The Various Forms of Opioids

Some opioids are used in the natural form, such as morphine and heroin. Other natural opium alkaloids include codeine, noscapine, papaverine, and thebaine. These alkaloids can be further reduced into more common analgesic compounds. The alkaloid thebaine is used to produce semisynthetic opioid morphine analogues, such as oxycodone (Percocet, Percodan), hydromorphone (Dilaudid), hydrocodone (Vicodin/Lortab), and etorphine (Immobilon). Other classes of morphine analogues include the 4-diphenylpiperidines: meperidine (Demerol), diphenylpropylamines, and methadone (Dolophine). Each of these compounds was developed to either increase analgesic effect or reduce the potential for addiction.

Although all of the opioid substances can be classed as pain relievers, their potency varies. Etorphine is one of the most potent of the analogue compounds, with very small amounts providing a great effect. All members of the morphine group have one chemical similarity in common—a piperidine ring or a greater part of the ring must be chemically present to be classified as a morphine.

The main binding sites for opioids, the mu receptors (Holden, Jeong, & Forrest, 2005), are found in the following areas:

- Brain cortex
- Thalamus
- Periaqueductal gray matter
- Spinal cord substantia gelatinosa (Fine & Portnoy, 2007)

Other secondary binding sites include the kappa and delta sites. Kappa sites are found in the brain's hypothalamus, periaqueductal gray matter, claustrum, and spinal cord substantia gelatinosa. The delta receptors are located in the pontine nucleus, amygdala, olfactory bulbs, and the deep cortex of the brain. Recently, an opioid receptor-like site was discovered and named opioid receptor-like 1 (Figure 7.1). The activity at this site is thought to be related to central modulation of pain but does not appear to have an effect on respiratory depression (Fine & Portnoy, 2007).

When an opioid is introduced into a patient's body, it looks for the binding site that conforms to a specific protein pattern, which will allow

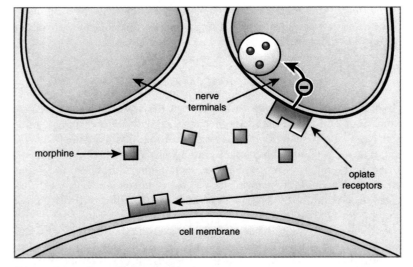

Figure 7.1 ▥ Opioid receptor-like 1 site.

the opioid to bind to the receptor site and create analgesia, an agonist action. At one time, the binding action for opioids was believed to be a simple lock-and-key effect: Introduce the medication, find the binding site, and bind, thus creating analgesia. Today, we know that the process is much more specific and is more sophisticated than a simple lock-and-key model.

Once the opioid molecule approaches the cell, it looks for a way to bind. On the exterior of each cell are ligands, or cellular channel mechanisms,connecting the exterior of the cell with the interior and conveying the opioidmolecule into the cell. The ligands are affiliated with the exterior receptor sites and can contain various G proteins. These G proteins couple with the opioid molecule and mediate the action of the receptor (Fine & Portnoy, 2007). "One opioid receptor can regulate several G proteins, and multiple receptors can activate a single G protein" (Fine & Portnoy, 2007, p. 11). As efforts progress to better identify the process, more than 40 variations in binding site composition have been identified (Pasternak, 2005). These differences explain some of the variation in patient response to opioid medications.

The body also has natural pain-facilitating and pain-inhibiting substances. These include the following:

- *Facilitating:* substance P, bradykinin, and glutamate
- *Inhibiting:* serotonin, natural or synthetic opioids, norepinephrine, gamma-aminobutyric acid (GABA)

When these substances are activated or blocked, pain can be relieved or increased. These more complex mechanisms are difficult to tease out, and trying to link them to analgesia and opioid effect can be misguided. More information on pain-facilitating and pain-inhibiting substances can be found in Chapter 1.

TYPES OF OPIOID MEDICATIONS

Opioid medications are very versatile in that they can be given as a stand-alone medication, such as codeine, or combined with another type of nonopioid medication, such as a nonsteroidal anti-inflammatory drug (NSAID; e.g., ibuprofen [Combunox] or acetaminophen [Tylenol #3 or Percocet]). Some of the medications have elixirs, such as morphine (Roxanol), and others have a suppository form, such as hydromorphone (Dilaudid). Because the elixir form can be very bitter, adding a flavoring available at most pharmacies can help the patient tolerate the taste of the medication.

The duration of the oral short-acting preparations is usually listed as 4 to 6 hours, but each patient has an individual response and ability to metabolize medications. Most of the combination medications are considered short acting, and the combination of another type of medication such as acetaminophen limits the amount of medication that can be taken in a 24-hour period. Preparations in which opioids are combined with acetaminophen follow the recommended dose for daily acetaminophen use to 4,000 mg/day maximum (American Pain Society [APS], 2008).

Other medications, especially those on the third level of the World Health Organization (WHO) analgesic ladder, have extended-release (ER) formulations. These formulations not only make the medication a pure opioid agonist but also, when ER formulations are used, they extend the dosing time to 12 to 24 hours, as with ER morphines (MS Contin, Avinza, Kadian) or ER oxycodone (Oxycontin). These ER medications are particularly helpful for patients in whom pain is present throughout the day, such as patients with chronic pain and patients with cancer. These ER medications are not designed to be used in patients with acute pain who are opioid naïve (patients who have not been taking opioid medications), but for those who have been taking the short-acting medications regularly to control their pain.

Some long-acting opioid medications, such as the fentanyl patch (Duragesic), have specific short-acting medication requirements before they can be used (e.g., before using Duragesic 25 mg, the patient must have been using the opioid equivalent of Dilaudid 8 mg by mouth per day for 2 weeks prior to patch application). Every patient who uses an ER opioid medication for pain should have a short-acting medication to use for breakthrough pain that occurs with increased activity or for end-of-dose failure that allows pain levels to increase (APS, 2008).

No matter what type or form of opioid medication is being considered for use, the health care provider should be aware of the risks and benefits of each medication and weigh the options carefully. A full history and physical and risk assessment for opioid therapy should be performed.

SHORT-ACTING COMBINATION MEDICATIONS

Short-acting pain medications come in a wide variety of types. Some are combined with acetaminophen or other nonopioid medications, and others are opioid medications, such as oxycodone, that only last for several hours at the recommended doses. For most patients with an acute injury, such as surgery, a short-acting medication is appropriate, and the patient will use it intermittently throughout the period of recovery. Once the surgical pain resolves, the patient no longer needs to take the opioid medication and should stop medication use. Patients with chronic pain require a more complex medication regimen to control their pain effectively, especially if the chronic pain is an underlying condition to an acute pain presentation.

Most short-acting medications are oral formulations, given as either pills or elixirs. For surgical pain, a short-acting medication may be needed in the immediate postoperative period, and these are given as intermittent intravenous (IV) doses or through patient-controlled analgesia (PCA). One route of administration that is no longer recommended is the intramuscular (IM) injection. Because the administration of medication via the IM route allows for irregular absorption of the medication and tissue sclerosis, most national guidelines and pain specialists have eliminated the IM route from their recommendations (American Society of Pain Management Nursing [ASPMN], 2010; APS, 2008).

Conversely, for patients with chronic pain, the pain will continue with no end point and therefore medication use will continue. For these patients, a careful assessment of pain patterns and intensities throughout the day will help determine when and how the opioid medication will be prescribed. If the pain is only episodic or present at certain times of day, a short-acting medication may provide all the pain relief that is needed. However, most patients with chronic pain have pain that is continuous, so adding an ER medication is common.

Most short-acting opioid medications are designed for moderate to severe pain intensities. Onset of action is usually 10 to 60 minutes with a short duration of action of 2 to 4 hours (Katz, McCarberg, & Reisner, 2007). Overall advantages to short-acting medications include a synergistic effect with the combination of medications that can improve pain relief and provide a better outcome.

MEDICATIONS

Short-Acting Combination Medications: Intermittent Pain, Breakthrough Pain

▓ *Codeine-Containing Medications: Codeine, Tylenol #3 (Codeine 30 mg Combined With Acetaminophen 325 mg)*
Used to treat mild to moderate pain, codeine[1] is noted to have a "number needed to treat" of 11. That means the first analgesic effect would be seen in the 12th patient who was given the medication for pain relief.

---

[1]Codeine should be used with caution in breastfeeding women who may inadvertently give their infants a morphine overdose if they are ultrarapid codeine metabolizers (*Nursing 2010 Drug Handbook*, 2009).

About 10% of people lack the enzyme needed to activate codeine (APS, 2008). Codeine has a high profile for side effects, such as constipation, and gastrointestinal (GI) disturbances, such as nausea and vomiting (APS, 2008). It is often used as a component in cough syrups as a cough suppressant (*Nursing 2010 Drug Handbook*, 2009). The medication can also be given in an elixir form, which is convenient for patients who have difficulty swallowing or for use with enteral feeding tubes.

■ *Hydrocodone-Containing Medications: Vicodin, Lortab, Norco, and Lortab Elixir*

Hydrocodone-containing medications are designed to be used for moderate pain. They usually contain 5 to 10 mg of hydrocodone with 325 mg or 500 mg of acetaminophen. Many patients tolerate the medication very well for intermittent pain or for breakthrough pain. It is available in an elixir form that is very effective and can be used with patients who have difficulty swallowing pills or for use with enteral feeding tubes. Norco has a higher dose of hydrocodone per tablet.

■ *Oxycodone-Containing Medications: Oxycodone, Percocet, Roxicet, Percodan, and Oxfast*

Medications with oxycodone are designed for treating moderate-level pain. They are commonly used for postoperative pain in the acute care setting and for patients with chronic pain. Percocet is a combination medication with 5 mg of oxycodone and 325 mg of acetaminophen. Percodan is a combination of oxycodone and aspirin. If the patient requires a higher dose of medication for pain control, combining an oxycodone 5 mg tablet with a combined form such as Roxicet will provide additional pain relief but still maintain the acetaminophen dose at 325 mg. To help patients tolerate the medication without nausea, giving the medication with milk or after meals is recommended (*Nursing 2010 Drug Handbook*, 2009).

■ *Oxymorphone-Containing Medications: Opana*

Opana is a medication designed to treat moderate to severe pain. It has a more extended half-life than other medications of the same class, resulting in a decreased need for breakthrough medications (Adams et al., 2005; Adams & Abdieh, 2004). Opana should be taken 1 hour before or 2 hours after a meal (*Nursing 2010 Drug Handbook*, 2009). It is also available in an injectable form for use during labor (*Nursing 2010 Drug Handbook*, 2009).

■ *Tramadol: Ultram and Ultracet*

Tramadol is a unique medication that combines a mu agonist, an opioid-like medication, and a selective serotonin reuptake inhibitor–type medication. It is designed for use with moderate pain. Doses should be reduced for older patients and in patients with increased creatinine levels or cirrhosis. Tramadol may increase the risk of seizures and serotonin syndrome (*Nursing 2010 Drug Handbook*, 2009). Patients should be instructed to taper off the medication gradually when discontinuing it. It should not be stopped suddenly (*Nursing 2010 Drug Handbook*, 2009). Tapentadol (Nucynta) is a medication similar to tramadol. It has a dual action of mu agonism but it also has a selective serotonin and norepinephrine reuptake inhibitor action with a lessened serotonin effect when compared to tramadol. It is indicated for acute pain and may have some activity for neuropathic pain. Dose adjustment should be made for elderly patients and patients with renal or hepatic dysfunction.

■ *Hydromorphone: Dilaudid*
Dilaudid is an extremely potent analgesic and it is designed for use with severe level pain. In the oral form, it comes in 2 mg and 4 mg tablets. In the IV form, 0.2 mg of Dilaudid is equal to 1 mg of IV morphine. Dilaudid is a medication that is commonly used only after the other medications for pain (e.g., Vicodin and Percocet) are trialed unsuccessfully.
Because of the strength of this medication, it is possible to get good pain relief with small amounts and to potentially have fewer side effects. See Chapter 12 for PCA use.

■ *Morphine: Immediate-Release Morphine (MSIR) and Roxanol (Elixir)*
Morphine is the gold standard for severe level pain relief. It is the standard for equianalgesic conversions and has a long history of use for pain control. It is available in many different forms: pills, elixir, IV, and suppository. The biggest drawback to morphine is the side effect profile; constipation, nausea and vomiting, delirium, and hallucinations are some of the most commonly reported adverse effects.

■ *Fentanyl Transmucosal (Sublimaze): Actiq, Fentora, and Onsolis*
There is no oral pill formulation possible for fentanyl. The route of administration is either transdermal or buccal. When used buccally for breakthrough or incident pain in opioid-tolerant patients (patients who take opioid medications regularly), the transmucosal medications can be rubbed across the buccal membrane and absorbed directly into the cardiac circulation. Fentanyl's fast absorption rate makes this medication a risk for oversedation, so the indication is only for breakthrough pain in opioid-tolerant cancer patients or patients with chronic pain who take opioid medications on a daily basis.
     If the entire dose of an Actiq oralet is not used, it should be placed in a childproof container until the remainder is needed. This medication in patch or oral form is not intended for use for acute or postoperative pain (*Nursing*

2010 Drug Handbook, 2009). It is not meant to be used in opioid-naïve patients because serious oversedation can occur (Fine & Portnoy, 2007). If a patient with chronic pain or cancer pain is having surgery or has another acute pain complaint and he or she is using buccal fentanyl for pain control, care must be taken in providing IV pain medications to avoid oversedation.

ER MEDICATIONS: AROUND-THE-CLOCK PAIN RELIEF

For opioid-tolerant patients or patients with chronic pain, ER medications can give a consistent blood level of medication, providing a steady comfort level. This may increase functionality and improve quality of life, enhance sleep, and let the patient participate in meaningful daily activities. ER medications have a slower onset of action from 30 to 90 minutes, with a relatively long duration of action of up to 72 hours (Katz et al., 2007).

When a patient has pain that lasts throughout the day and the patient is taking short-acting medications and has reached the maximum dose limitations of the nonopioid medication, the prescriber should consider switching the patient to an ER or long-acting medication. Candidates for this type of therapy in acute care are trauma patients with extensive orthopedic injuries who will require long-term rehabilitation and will need to have tolerable pain to participate in their recovery.

Some of the short-acting medications have an ER formulation, including Vicodin ER, Opana ER, Ultram ER, Oxycontin, Exalgo, Kadian, Avinza, and MS Contin. Most are pure mu agonist medications, such as morphine, with an ER action that allows the medication to dissolve slowly in the GI tract. Some ER medications are encapsulated into beads that allow gastric secretions to enter the bead and force the medications out. Other ER formulations have a coating around an ER plasticized compound that keeps the medication from dissolving too quickly. Most ER medications either have or are developing a formula that makes them more tamper resistant to avoid improper use. When ER medication is being started with a patient, the patient should be instructed on the important aspects of the medications, which includes the following:

- ER medications of all types should never be broken, chewed, or degraded in any way to enhance the absorption of the medications. To do so risks all the medication being given at one time, and there is then a high risk of potentially fatal oversedation.
- Most ER medications should not be taken with alcohol. To do so degrades the ER mechanism and allows for a faster absorption of the medication, which can cause potentially fatal oversedation.

Table 7.1 ■ *Equianalgesic Table for Opioid Conversion*

Analgesics	Generic	Brand Name	Oral	Parenteral	
Immediate release	morphine	Roxanol, MSIR	30 mg	10 mg	Relative potency 1:6 with acute dosing and 1:2 to 1:3 with chronic dosing
	oxycodone	Roxicodone, Oxy IR	20 mg	NA	
	hydromorphone	Dilaudid	7.5 mg	1.5 mg	
	oxymorphone	Opana, Numorphan	10 mg	1 mg	Extended half-life with short-acting oral form
	hydrocodone	Vicodin, Lortab	30 mg	NA	
	fentanyl	Sublimaze	NA	100 mcg	
	methadone	Dolophine	5–10 mg	10 mg	Use with caution: Half-life of 12–150 hr accumulates with repeated dosing
	meperidine	Demerol	NR	NR	Use with caution. Toxic metabolite normeperidine can cause seizures
Not recommended for opioid-naïve patients	morphine	MSContin, Avinza, Kadian	20–30 mg	NA	
	oxycodone	Oxycontin	20–30 mg	NA	
	fentanyl transdermal	Duragesic	NA	25 mcg	

Basic IV conversion: Morphine 1 mg = Dilaudid 0.2 mg = Fentanyl 10 mcg.

NR = not recommended.

When switching from one opioid to another, reduce the dose by 25%–50% with adequate breakthrough medication.

When switching to methadone, reduce the equianalgesic dose by 75%–90%.

Breakthrough medication should be available when controlled-release medications are being used.

All opioid medications should be carefully dosed and titrated with consideration for the individual patient and medical condition of the patient.

Sources: American Pain Society (2008), Fine Portnoy (2007); Inturrisi & Lipman (2010); Smith & McCleane (2009).

■ ER medications are not meant to be injected.

■ ER medications should not be crushed and inserted into enteral feeding tubes.

■ ER medications are not meant to be used on an as-needed basis, but rather as scheduled daily doses.

■ If the patient experiences end-of-dose failure several hours before the next dose of medication is due, the interval should be shortened or, more commonly, the dose should be increased (APS, 2008).

When converting a patient from short-acting medications, the rules of thumb are as follows:

■ If the medication is the same (e.g., Percocet to Oxycontin), equivalent doses of the medication can be prescribed.

■ If the medication is a different drug (e.g., Percocet to MS Contin), the daily dose should be calculated using the equianalgesic conversion table (see Table 7.1) and reduced usually by 30%. To ensure that adequate pain relief is maintained, additional doses of breakthrough medication should be prescribed about 5% to 15% of the total daily dose to be taken every 2 hours as needed (APS, 2008).

■ ***Methadone: Dolophine and Methadose***

Methadone is considered to be a long-acting medication because it has an extended half-life of 15 to 60 hours (APS, 2008). Pain relief for the oral form, however, is less extended at 4 to 6 hours (*Nursing 2010 Drug Handbook*, 2009). Therein lies the danger. Given that the half-life is very long and the pain relief is shorter, dosing must be done very carefully to avoid oversedation, which may become apparent only a day or two after the doses are given. Dose escalation should be done no more frequently than every 3 to 7 days (APS, 2008).

Methadone can be prescribed legally by general practitioners in primary care and acute care for pain relief. It is also used for methadone maintenance to control addiction in heroin addicts. To prescribe methadone for these patients requires a special licensure. The addiction program has no connection to prescribing methadone for pain management. However, because there is such a risk with methadone, the current recommendation of the APS is that only pain management practitioners or those skilled and knowledgeable about the medication prescribe the drug (APS, 2008).

An additional risk factor for methadone is the potential for QT corrected interval prolongation and, at higher doses, for torsades de pointes (APS, 2008). Primary care providers are advised to obtain a baseline electrocardiogram (ECG) for patients who are on daily methadone and continue to obtain regular ECGs as the doses escalate more than 200 mg/day (APS, 2008).

Fentanyl Patches: Duragesic

Fentanyl patches can provide a high level of pain relief and are used for various chronic pain conditions. Patches are the only transdermal opioid application available for use. The Duragesic patch is a delivery system that contains a specified dose of fentanyl in a gel formulation. It is designed for use with opioid-tolerant patients and should never be used for acute pain or with opioid-naïve patients.

The patch is applied to clean intact skin and delivers the specified amount of medication over a period of 72 hours (e.g., 25 mcg/hr). The medication effect begins as the medication depot develops in the subcutaneous fat, and it can take from 12 to 18 hours for pain relief to begin (D'Arcy, 2007, 2009a). It can also take up to 48 hours for steady-state blood levels to develop; therefore, when the patch is being started, the patient will need additional breakthrough pain medication (D'Arcy, 2009a).

There are some safety concerns with the Duragesic patch. More than 100 patients have died related to fentanyl patch use and misuse. When a patch is prescribed for pain relief, patient education should include the following points:

- Do not cut the patch. To do so will result in a dose-dumping effect where all the medication is released at one time, resulting in an overdose.
- Do not apply heat over the patch. To do so may result in accelerated medication delivery, also resulting in potential overdose.
- Dispose of the patch in a closed container, flush it down a toilet, or seal it in a sealable bag with kitty litter or used coffee grounds. Because there is medication left in the patch, safe disposal is necessary to avoid diversion and minimize contamination.
- Do not place the patch in a regular wastebasket when discarding. There is about 16% of the dose remaining in the patch after use and a small animal or child could remove the patch and chew or come in contact with it.

Before a 25 mcg fentanyl patch is placed, the patient should be taking one of the following: 30 mg of oxycodone per day for 2 weeks, 8 mg of hydromorphone per day for 2 weeks, or 60 mg of oral morphine per day for 2 weeks (Janssen prescribing information available at www.Janssen. com).

MEDICATIONS THAT ARE NO LONGER RECOMMENDED

There are two pain medications that are no longer recommended for use related to toxic metabolites, high acetaminophen doses, or high profile for side effects.

■ *Propoxyphene With Acetaminophen: Darvocet*

Darvocet is a medication that has fallen out of favor and is being considered for withdrawal by the U.S. Food and Drug Administration because of the high levels of acetaminophen. It is designed to treat mild level pain, but its analgesic action is created primarily by the high dose of acetaminophen it contains. Each tablet contains 650 mg of acetaminophen and 50 or 100 mg of propoxyphene. It is very easy to reach daily maximum doses of acetaminophen with just a few tablets of Darvocet. Additionally, there is a toxic metabolite called norpropoxyphene that can build up with use and can cause seizures (APS, 2008). For these reasons, it is not used very often by pain specialists for pain control, and it is not recommended for patients with renal impairment or in older adults (APS, 2008). As of December 2010 this medication has been removed from the market by the FDA.

■ *Meperidine: Demerol*

Meperidine (Demerol) has also fallen out of favor. It is no longer considered a first-line pain medication (APS, 2008; D'Arcy, 2007). Meperidine has a toxic metabolite called normeperidine that accumulates with repetitive dosing (APS, 2008). This metabolite can cause tremors and seizures. Other drawbacks include the need to use high doses to achieve an analgesic effect that is accompanied by sedation and nausea (D'Arcy, 2007). If Demerol is going to be used, there are certain recommendations that include the following:

■ Demerol should never be used in children and infants.
■ It should never be used in patients with renal impairment (e.g., older patients or patients with sickle cell disease).
■ Hyperpyrexic syndrome with delirium can occur if Demerol is used in patients who are taking monoamine oxidase inhibitors, which can be potentially fatal.
■ If used, it should never be administered for more than 1 to 2 days at doses not to exceed 600 mg/24 hr (APS, 2008).

Table 7.2 ■ *Common Opioid Medications*

		Common Opioid Medications–Short Acting	
Generic Name	*Trade Name/ Combination Name*	*Usual Starting Dose–Adults*	*Maximum dose*
codeine	Tylenol #3	30 to 60 mg by mouth every 4–6 hr	12 tablets in a 24-hr period Limited by acetaminophen*; available as an elixir
hydrocodone	Lortab Vicodin	5–10 mg by mouth every 4–6 hr 5–10 mg by mouth every 6 hr	Limited by acetaminophen dose*
oxycodone	Percocet	5 mg every 6 hr	Limited by acetaminophen dose*
tramadol	Ultram Ultracet	25 mg by mouth in AM	Maximum 400 mg per day Limited by acetaminophen dose*
tapentadol	Nucynta	50, 75, or 100 mg every 4–6 hr	No more than 700 mg on day 1 and thereafter 600 mg maximum
oxymorphone	Opana	10–20 mg by mouth every 4–6 hr	
hydromorphone	Dilaudid	2–4 mg by mouth every 4–6 hr	Limited only by adverse side effects such as respiratory depression, sedation, nausea
morphine	Morphine Immediate Release- MSIR Roxanol	5–15 mg by mouth every 4 hr 5–30 mg by mouth every 4 hr	Limited by adverse side effects such as respiratory depression, sedation, nausea
methadone	Dolophine	2.5–10 mg by mouth every 3–4 hr	Extreme care with dosing and medication initiation Half-life ranges from 12–150 hr

(continued)

morphine	Oramorph SR/Kadian Avinza MsContin	20 mg every 12 hr or 40 mg once daily 20–30 mg by mouth daily 15 or 30 mg every 12 hr	
oxycodone	Oxycontin	10 mg every 12 hr	
oxymorphone	Opana ER**	5 mg every 12 hr	
tramadol	Ultram ER**	100 mg once daily	300 mg per day
dilaudid	Exalgo	8–64 mg daily converted from current opioid doses using Exalgo conversion equivalents—give 50% of converted daily dose	
morphine sulfate with naltrexone	Embeda	Convert the patient's total daily dose of current opioid and rescue dose by 50% when initiating therapy—dose every 12 hours	

*Acetaminophen dose should be limited to 4,000 mg per day.

Medication information taken from *Nursing 2010 Drug Handbook*; opioid analgesia from Fine & Portnoy (2007) and APS (2008).

**Not intended to be crushed, chewed, or used when alcohol is being ingested. For use with opioid tolerant patients on a schedule basis—not prn. Medication information taken from *Nursing 2010 Drug Handbook* and opioid analgesia from Fine & Portnoy (2007); APS (2008); and PI forExalgo, Embeda, and Nucynta.

Note: In order to be considered opioid tolerant, the patient should be taking at least 60 mg of oral morphine per day or 25 mcg of fentanyl patch per hr, 30 mg of oxycodone per day, 8 mg of oral hydromorphone per day, 25 mg of oral oxymorphone per day for a week or longer.

Source: D'Arcy & Bruckenthal (2011)

MIXED AGONISTS/ANTAGONIST MEDICATIONS

There is a group of medications that have both agonist and antagonist actions at the various binding sites throughout the body. These medications are called *mixed agonist/antagonist medications* and include the following:

- Nubain
- Talwin
- Buprenex

These medications act further down on the spinal cord at the kappa receptor sites, so there is less potential for respiratory depression. Because these medications have both agonist and antagonist actions, they have the potential for reversing the opioid effect of pure opioid agonists, such as morphine. If a patient is taking morphine, giving a mixed agonist/antagonist medication will reverse the analgesic effect of the morphine and pain relief is lessened. This group of medications also has a high profile for adverse side effects, such as confusion and hallucinations, and has dose ceilings that limit dose escalations (APS, 2008).

SELECTING AN OPIOID

Selecting an opioid for an individual patient may be a trial-and-error process. Each individual has a genetic preference for one or more types of opioids; therefore, the practitioner must determine which opioid works best for the patient. For most patients who are hospitalized and have severe pain, the analgesic will need to be administered by the IV route. For other patients with acute injuries, a short-acting oral medication may be enough to control the pain (Table 7.2).

Many patients with pain have tried opioids before. They may know which opioid works best and which ones do not work at all. If the patient can provide information on the efficacy of pain medications, it should not be considered as drug seeking or potential addiction. If a patient has used a medication successfully, starting with one that was effective will, in many cases, provide the best outcome.

Conversely, if a patient says he or she has tried a medication but it did not work, get more information about when, for what indication, and what doses were tried. In many cases, patients with chronic pain have been underdosed with medications, and they then believe the medications are "not working" or are ineffective. If the correct dose of medication had been provided, the medication could have provided good pain relief. It is always wise to revisit the use of a medication that has been underdosed by using appropriate doses for treating pain unless there are side effects that would contraindicate the use of the drug (Figure 7. 2).

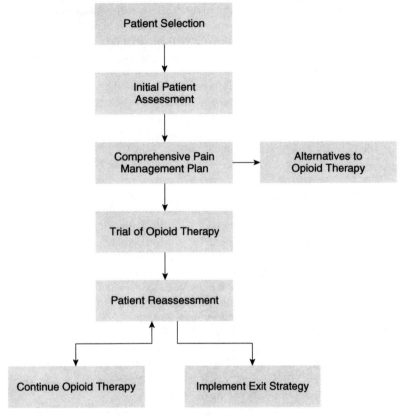

Figure 7.2 ■ Algorithm for opioid treatment of chronic pain.

OPIOIDS IN THE OLDER PATIENT

Older patients have a large number of conditions, such as osteoarthritis and other painful comorbidities. Choosing a medication to treat acute pain in these patients is more of a challenge. The myth that older patients do not tolerate pain medications is just that, a myth. Older patients can even use opioid medication with good results if careful dosing and titration takes place.

The American Geriatrics Society (AGS) has released a new set of pain management guidelines for persistent pain in older patients (2009). These new guidelines indicate that opioids are an option for the older patient when moderate to severe pain is present.

For older patients, pain is experienced in the same way, but aging can change the way the nervous system perceives the pain and transmission may be altered (Huffman & Kunik, 2000; McLennon, 2005). Aging can also change the way the older patient's body processes pain medications and can increase the potential for adverse effects. Some of the reasons an older patient may experience adverse effects include the following:

- Muscle-to-fat ratios change as patients age, causing the body fat composition to be altered.
- Poor nutrition can decrease protein stores, which in turn can decrease the binding ability of some medications.
- Because of the changes in the protein-binding mechanisms, drugs may need to compete for binding sites, making one or more of the patient's medications ineffective.
- Aging affects the physiologic functions of metabolism, absorption, medication clearance (including a slowed GI motility), decreased cardiac output, and decreased glomerular filtration rate.
- Baseline changes in sensory and cognitive perception, such as sedation or confusion, can be an increased risk for some patients.
- Drug excretion and elimination are reduced by 10% for each decade after 40 years of age because of decreased renal function (Bruckenthal & D'Arcy, 2007; D'Arcy, 2009b; Horgas, 2003).

The old adage of starting low and going slow still applies to starting opioid therapy in older adults. Older patients are not all the same and bodies age in different ways. Using conservative doses and monitoring the patient carefully for side effects can help ensure that opioids are providing optimal pain relief while also being used safely.

TIPS FOR STARTING ANALGESIC MEDICATION IN THE OLDER PATIENT

Because the older patient has pain needs and requires more monitoring of dosing and adverse effects, starting new medications can be somewhat complicated. Recommendations for pain medications for the older adult (AGS, 2002, 2009) include the following:

- Decrease acetaminophen dose if the patient has a history of alcohol use/abuse or liver or renal impairment. The maximum daily dose should be decreased from 4 g per day by 50% to 75% or not used at all.
- Reduce beginning opioid doses by 25% to 50% to decrease the potential for oversedation.
- Scheduling medication may provide better pain relief and reduce the likelihood of needing increased doses for uncontrolled pain.

■ Monitor older adults being started on opioid therapy daily if not more frequently because organ impairment may decrease the elimination of the medication.

■ Avoid the use of the following medications because of unwanted side effects and/or toxic metabolites: meperidine, propoxyphene, pentazocine, indomethacin, and amitriptyline (McLennon, 2005).

TREATING THE SIDE EFFECTS OF OPIOID TREATMENT

All opioids have the potential for side effects. There is no magic opioid or pain medication that does not have the potential for constipation, sedation, or pruritus. Opioids can be used in the presence of side effects, but treatment options to control the unwanted effects or dose reductions to minimize the side effects should be used. One important concept to remember here is that adding a medication that is sedating, such as promethazine, can potentiate sedation from an opioid. Before deciding that an opioid is too sedating, look at all sedating medications that are being used concomitantly and try to minimize the use of additional sedating agents.

Constipation

Constipation is a common side effect of opioid use. It is the one effect to which the patient will not become tolerant. Every patient who is prescribed an opioid should have a laxative of some type. Stool softeners are also used to ease bowel movements. Stimulant laxatives are used to counteract the constipation. Combination stool softener/laxatives are available over the counter in most drugstores. Recommended types of laxatives include the following:

■ Senna or Senna with stool softener—increases bowel motility
■ bisacodyl—increases bowel motility
■ lactulose-osmotic laxative sorbitol—osmotic laxative; easily found in Sorbee candies
■ methylnaltrexone (Relistor)—approved for opioid-induced constipation for patients with advanced illness or palliative care; SC injectable (APS, 2008)

Sedation

Patients may become sedated when opioids are first started, but most become tolerant to the effect within a period of 2 weeks or less. If sedation persists or reaches high levels, dose adjustments should be made so that serious oversedation does not occur. Sedation occurs most commonly at the beginning of opioid therapy (D'Arcy, 2007). Patients should be monitored for sedating effects of the opioid and additive sedating effects from medications such as antiemetics, sedatives, antihistamines, muscle relaxants, sleeping medications, benzodiazepines, and so forth.

To counteract sedation, stimulants such as caffeine, dextroamphetamine, methylphenidate, or modafinil can be used. The sedating medications listed previously are most commonly used for patients with chronic cancer pain. Most patients adjust to the sedating effects of opioids within a few weeks at the longest, but the use of caffeine can be recommended for almost any patient.

In acute care, oxygen monitoring or capnography can be used to monitor sedation that could lead to respiratory depression. When giving opioids to postoperative patients, it is wise to monitor the use of other sedating medications with patients who are using opioids for postoperative pain control.

Pruritus (Itching)

Some patients started on opioids or taking high doses of opioids may develop pruritus, commonly known as itching. It was thought to be the result of a histamine release, and is not an indication of a true allergy. Current thinking indicates that it may have its source in an unknown cerebral function. The most common way to counteract the itching is to use an antihistamine such as diphenhydramine (Benadryl). If the itching persists, changing to another opioid may reduce or eliminate this effect. For postoperative patients on PCA and epidurals, the use of small doses of Nubain 2.5 mg IV, a mixed agonist/antagonist medication, is an *off-label* use for treating pruritus.

Delirium/Confusion

Delirium can be caused by opioids, and it is usually a temporary state. Many patients, especially older ones, become confused when they are moved from their usual living situation and put into a new situation or have surgery and start opioids. For patients with chronic pain, the incidence of confusion or delirium should be much less. If the patient becomes delirious, changing the opioid, reducing the dose, or stopping the opioid may provide the needed intervention. Some opioids, such as morphine, have a higher profile for confusion. Changing to another medication, such as low-dose Dilaudid, may provide adequate pain relief and lessen the potential for confusion.

Nausea and Vomiting

Opioids have a high profile for nausea and vomiting. For most opioids, taking the medication with a small amount of food or milk will help reduce the effect. If the nausea and vomiting do not resolve, using an antiemetic regularly until the effect abates is the best option. Because all antiemetics are sedating, there will be an additive sedating effect when the medications are combined. Recommended antiemetics include the following:

- ondansetron
- Phenergan[2]
- Reglan
- meclizine or cyclizine, for motion-induced nausea
- scopolamine patches, for severe cases (APS, 2008)

> ### Case Study
>
> Sharon P., 32 years old, is admitted after a fall from a ladder. She has a broken femur, two broken ribs, and a pelvic fracture. There is a suspicion that she has two compression fractures in her lumbar spine, but she has refused to go for an MRI. She complains of pain repeatedly. She will not move for the physical therapist and complains that the pain is too severe to do anything but stay in one position in bed. She has been told about the need for moving once the surgery was done to repair her femur. She says she can't use the incentive spirometer, and she just feels the pain is too much to bear. She always rates it at 10/10. She has been using a Dilaudid PCA and has 250 attempts and 61 injections, and her dose has not been increased since the PCA was first set up 3 days ago.
>
> How can you impress on Sharon that even though she has pain, she will need to move? How will you improve her pain control?

---

[2] Phenergan should be used with caution with IV administration. This medication can cause tissue necrosis.

Questions to Consider

1. What can you add to the medication regimen that will improve the pain relief: NSAIDs, acetaminophen, coanalgesics, or will you change the opioid?
2. Does Sharon have realistic expectations for pain relief?
3. If Sharon has a chronic pain condition, will it color the way she reacts when she has acute pain?
4. Can you start Sharon on an ER pain medication?
5. What types of interventional pain options could you use to improve Sharon's pain?

REFERENCES

Adams, M., & Abdieh, H. (2004). Pharmokinetics and dose-proportionality of oxymorphone extended release and its metabolites: Results of a randomized crossover study. *Pharmacotherapy, 24*(4), 468–476.

Adams, M., Pienazek, H., Gammatoni, A., & Abdieh, H. (2005). Oxy morphone extended release does not affect CVP2C9 or CYP3A4 metabolite pathways. *Journal of Clinical Pharmacology, 45*, 337–345.

American Geriatrics Society. (2002). Persistent pain in the older patient. *Journal of the American Geriatrics Society, 50*, S205–S224.

American Geriatrics Society. (2009). Persistent pain in the older patient. *Journal of the American Geriatrics Society, 57*, 1331–1346.

American Pain Society. (2008). *Principles of analgesic use in the treatment of acute pain and cancer pain.* Glenview, IL: Author.

American Society of Pain Management Nursing. (2010). *Core curriculum for pain management nursing.* Dubuque, IA: Kendall Hunt Publishing

Bruckenthal, P., & D'Arcy, Y. (2007). Assessment and management of pain in older adults: A review of the basics. *Topics in Advanced Practice Journal, 7*(1). Retrieved Jul. 13, 2009, from http://www.medscape.com/viewarticle

D'Arcy, Y. (2007). *Pain management: Evidence-based tools and techniques for nursing professionals.* Marblehead, MA: HCPro.

D'Arcy, Y. (2009a). Avoid the dangers of opioid therapy. *American Nurse Today, 4*(5), 18–22.

D'Arcy, Y. (2009b). *Pain in the older adult.* Indianapolis, IN: Sigma Theta Tau.

D'Arcy, Y., & Bruckenthal, P. (2011). *Safe opioid prescribing for nurse practitioners.* New York: Oxford University Press.

Fine, P., & Portnoy, R. (2007). *A clinical guide to opioid analgesia.* New York: Vendome Group Health Care.

Holden, J. E., Jeong, Y., & Forrest, J. M. (2005). The endogenous opioid system and clinical pain management. *AACN Clinical Issues, 16*(3), 291–301.

Horgas, A. (2003). Pain management in elderly adults. *Journal of Infusion Nursing, 26*(3), 161–165.

Huffman, J., & Kunik, M. (2000). Assessment and understanding of pain in patients with dementia. *The Gerontologist, 40*(5), 574–581.

Inturrisi, C., & Lipman, A. (2010). Opioid analgesics. In S. M. Fishman, J. C. Ballantyne, & J. P. Rathmell (Eds.), *Bonica's management of pain* (pp. 1174-1175). Baltimore, MD: Lippincott Williams & Wilkins

Katz, N., McCarberg, B., & Reisner, L. (2007). *Managing chronic pain with opioids in primary care.* Newton, MA: Inflexxion.

Løvlie, R., et al. (2001). Polymorphisms in CYP2D6 duplication-negative individuals with the ultrarapid metabolizer phenotype: A role for the CYP2D6*35 allele in ultrarapid metabolism? *Pharmacogenetics, 11*(1), 45–55.

McLennon, S. M. (2005). Persistent pain management. *National Guidelines Clearinghouse.* Retrieved from www.guideline.gov

Nursing 2013 Drug Handbook. (2012). Philadelphia: Lippincott Williams & Wilkins.

Smith, H., & McCleane, G. (2009). Opioids issues. In H. Smith (Ed.), *Current therapy in pain* (pp. 408-420). Philadelphia, PA: Saunders Elsevier

Additional Resources

Chou, R., Fanciullo, G., Fine, P., Adler, J., Ballantyne, J., Davies, P., . . . Miaskowski, C. (2009). Opioid treatment guidelines: Clinical guide lines for the use of chronic opioid therapy in chronic noncancer pain. *The Journal of Pain, 10*(2), 113–130.

McCoy, A. W. (n.d.). *Opium: Opium history up to 1858 A.D.* Retrieved from http://opioids.com/opium/history/index.html

Osler, W. (n.d.). *The plant of joy.* Retrieved from http://www.opiates.net/

8

Coanalgesics for Additive Pain Relief

COANALGESICS FOR ACUTE PAIN

Coanalgesics are a varied group of medications that can provide additive pain relief when they are added to nonsteroidal anti-inflammatory drugs (NSAIDs) or opioids (American Pain Society [APS], 2008). They can have independent analgesic activity for some painful complaints, and can counteract select adverse effects of analgesics (APS, 2008). This group of medications was developed to treat a wide variety of conditions, such as seizures or muscle spasms, and were originally intended for symptom control of the various conditions. However, in many cases, patients reported pain relief when these medications were prescribed for them, leading health care providers to consider their additional application for pain relief.

Although some classes of these medications are not used for acute pain, there are some that can be used effectively, such as muscle relaxants. Some of these medications are being used to treat pain on an *off-label* basis. If pain has been determined to have a neuropathic source, antidepressants, antiseizure medications, or topical medications, such as lidoderm patches, can be trialed to see if there is any definitive benefit for relieving the pain. An example of this type of pain is in a patient who has a large amount of tissue damage from surgery or swelling where nerves are being compressed, causing additional pain.

Medications that are considered to be coanalgesics for pain management include the following:

- Antidepressants
- Anticonvulsants
- Muscle relaxants
- Topical agents
- Cannabinoids
- *N*-methyl-d-aspartate (NMDA) receptor blockers
- Alpha 2-adrenergic agonists
- Benzodiazepines

▦ Antispasmodic agents
▦ Stimulants (APS, 2008)

Although these medications were not developed for pain control, they have been used for adjunct pain relief and are found to be effective. For some medications, such as gabapentin (Neurontin), pregabalin (Lyrica), and duloxetine (Cymbalta), the pain application became so prevalent that the manufacturers sought and received Food and Drug Administration (FDA) approval for pain management. Many patients with neuropathic pain benefit greatly from the addition of one or more of these agents to help decrease pain. Because many patients with chronic pain are depressed, the use of antidepressants has improved the quality of pain relief and enhanced sleep for many of these patients.

When the World Health Organization (WHO) ladder was developed with medication choices for pain management (see Chapter 6), the focus was on dividing different types of opioid medications. However, the ladder also includes adjuvant medications, or coanalgesics, on each step of the ladder. Only broad classes of these medications and no specific medications are listed, so the choice of coanalgesic is patient dependent (Dalton & Youngblood, 2000).

Trying to group these medications into a single class of coanalgesics is difficult. They all have such different mechanisms of action and applications. These medications can enhance the effect of opioids or other medications that are being used for pain relief, or they can stand alone as single-agent pain relievers (APS, 2008). Some of the benefits of using these medications include the following:

▦ Enhance pain relief
▦ Allow lower doses of opioids (opioid-sparing effect)
▦ Manage refractory pain
▦ Reduce side effects of opioids related to opioid sparing (APS, 2008)

Commonly used coanalgesics include the following:

▦ Acetaminophen (Tylenol)
▦ Ibuprofen (Advil, Nuprin), naproxen (Naprosyn), or naproxen sodium (Aleve)
▦ Celecoxib (Celebrex)
▦ Gabapentin (Neurontin) and pregabalin (Lyrica)
▦ Duloxetine hydrochloride (Cymbalta)
▦ Topical lidocaine (Lidoderm) and capsaicin 8% patch (Qutenza)
▦ Cyclobenzaprine hydrochloride (Flexeril), carisoprodol (Soma), or metaxalone (Skelaxin)
▦ Diazepam (Valium) or alprazolam (Xanax)

No matter which medication is selected or combined, each patient's comorbidities need to be assessed and evaluated before adding a new medication to the pain management medication regimen. The following sections of the chapter will discuss different classes of coanalgesics that can be used for additional pain relief.

ANTIDEPRESSANT MEDICATIONS

Antidepressant medications are classed into several different types:

■ Tricyclic antidepressants (TCAs)
■ Selective serotonin reuptake inhibitors (SSRIs)
■ Serotonin norepinephrine reuptake inhibitors (SNRIs)

Antidepressant medications have several different mechanisms of action. The TCAs (Table 8.1), such as amitriptyline (Elavil), inhibit presynaptic uptake of norepinephrine and serotonin, as do the SNRIs, such as duloxetine (Cymbalta). Other less-studied actions for TCAs include a mild opioid action at the mu binding sites, sodium and calcium channel blockade, NMDA site antagonism, and adenosine activity (Lynch & Watson, 2006). The SSRI medications, such as fluoxetine hydrochloride (Prozac), inhibit serotonin at the presynaptic junction site (Ghafoor & St. Marie, 2009). The effect of this inhibition decreases the ability of the pain stimulus to be transmitted higher up the central nervous system (D'Arcy, 2007). These medications are most commonly used as adjunct medications for neuropathic type pain, such as postherpetic neuralgia, painful diabetic neuropathies, and neuropathic syndromes (Lynch & Watson, 2006). They are also a good adjunct in patients with cancer and neuropathic pain when opioids have provided suboptimal pain relief (APS, 2008).

The TCAs were at one time considered to be the first line for treating neuropathic pain such as postherpetic neuralgia or postmastectomy pain syndromes. The starting doses are low, 10 to 25 mg titrated up to 150 mg per day (APS, 2008; Wallace & Staats, 2005). Escalating to higher doses to obtain an

Table 8.1 ■ *Tricyclic Antidepressants (TCAs)*

Common TCAs	Starting Dose	Effective Dose
amitriptyline (Elavil)	10–25 mg hs	50–150 mg hs
desipramine (Norpramin)	10–25 mg hs	50–150 mg hs
nortriptyline (Pamelor)	10–25 mg hs	50–150 mg hs

Abbreviations: hs, at bedtime. *Source:* American Pain Society (2008).

additive effect for pain relief should take place every 3 to 7 days (Chen et al., 2004). The pain management doses are lower than the antidepressant doses of 150 to 300 mg per day. Of note, the pain relief action of these medications is independent of any effect on mood (Lynch & Watson, 2006).

A meta-analysis of the TCA medications indicates that TCAs are effective for use in treating neuropathic pain (APS, 2008). Elavil is the best known and most studied of the TCAs. It is also a primary recommendation for the treatment of fibromyalgia pain (D'Arcy & McCarberg, 2005). Analgesic response is usually seen within 5 to 7 days (APS, 2008). Adverse effects of TCAs include the following:

- Sedation
- Dry mouth
- Constipation
- Urinary retention
- Orthostatic hypotension
- Anticholinergic side effects
- Caution in patients with heart disease, symptomatic prostatic hypertrophy, neurogenic bladder, dementia, and narrow angle glaucoma
- Increased suicide behavior in young adults (Institute for Clinical System Improvement [ICSI], 2007)

These side effects make the medications undesirable for use in the elderly, especially when they are used in combination with opioid analgesics.

Additionally, the TCAs can increase the risk of cardiac arrhythmias in patients with underlying conduction abnormalities. Caution with the use of desipramine hydrochloride (Norpramin) in children where anecdotal reports of sudden death have been reported (APS, 2008). Although these drugs are cheap and readily available, they do have some very significant adverse effects. At the opposite end of the spectrum, they also have the best profile for use in treating neuropathic pain conditions. However, each patient being considered for TCAs should have a thorough assessment for any risk factors, such as cardiac conduction abnormalities. When starting TCA therapy, the current recommendation is to screen all patients older than 40 years with an electrocardiogram (ECG) to evaluate the patients for conduction abnormalities (APS, 2008).

The TCA medications are not recommended for use in elderly patients because of the high incidence of undesirable side effects and the potential for increased fall risk related to early morning orthostatic hypotension (American Geriatrics Society [AGS], 2002; Lynch & Watson, 2006). The biggest benefits of using TCAs for pain relief are improved sleep (Wilson et al., 1997) and the relief of neuropathic pain—pain that is described by patients as burning, shooting, or painful numbness (D'Arcy, 2007).

When caring for a patient who is taking TCAs as adjuvant pain medication, health care providers should be aware of the potential for early morning orthostatic hypotension and caution patients to sit on the side of the bed for a few minutes before trying to stand. Some patients complain of sleepiness with these medications, and if this is problematic, the patient should be instructed to take the medication earlier in the evening rather than at bedtime, to decrease the early morning sedation that can be experienced. For elderly men, urinary retention can be problematic and urinary status should be carefully checked. For the dry mouth associated with TCA use, hard candies or gum can ease the dry feeling.

Patients should always be told the rationale for prescribing an antidepressant medication for pain so they are comfortable taking the medication. The onset of analgesic effect may take up to 2 weeks, and patients should be encouraged to extend a trial of these medications to this period to see if analgesia occurs.

Of all three groups of antidepressants, the SSRI group (Table 8.2) has the poorest profile for pain relief (American Pain Society [APS], 2006). When compared with placebo, these medications did not have any significant advantage for pain relief. Given the lack of efficacy for pain relief in these medications and the profile of side effects (e.g., sexual dysfunction, anxiety, sleep disorder, and headache), the SSRIs are not the medications that should be given unless there is a specific indication for use. The recommended use for this group of medications is for patients who have concurrent depression, anxiety, or insomnia (APS, 2008).

The pain relief mechanism of the SNRI group of antidepressants (Table 8.3) is the inhibition of serotonin and norepinephrine at therapeutic

Table 8.2 ▦ *Selective Serotonin Reuptake Inhibitors (SSRIs)*

	Starting Dose	*Effective Dose*
paroxetine (Paxil)	10–20 mg daily	20–40 mg daily
citalopram (Celexa)	10–20 mg daily	20–40 mg daily

Source: American Pain Society (2008).

Table 8.3 ▦ *Serotonin and Norepinephrine Reuptake Inhibitors (SNRIs)*

	Starting Dose	*Effective Dose*
venlafaxine (Effexor)	37.5 mg daily	150–225 mg daily
duloxetine (Cymbalta)	20 mg daily	60 mg daily

Source: American Pain Society (2008).

doses (APS, 2008). The SNRI medications do not have the same anticholinergic side effect profile as TCA medications. They are effective for various neuropathic pain conditions, such as diabetic neuropathy, postherpetic neuralgia, and atypical facial pain (Lynch & Watson, 2006). Venlafaxine (Effexor) has shown an effect on hyperalgesia and allodynia, both preventing the occurrence of and decreasing pain (APS, 2008; Wallace & Staats, 2005). Effective doses of venlafaxine for pain relief range from 150 to 225 mg, with a starting dose of 37.5 mg.

Duloxetine (Cymbalta) has received FDA approval for treating painful diabetic neuropathy (PDN). For duloxetine, the starting dose of 20 mg daily may decrease the incidence of side effects with pain relief being experienced at a dose range from 60 to 120 mg daily. Careful titration of the medications and slow dose increases will help decrease some of the side effects, such as somnolence, nausea, and sweating. There have been no identified increased cardiovascular risks associated with the use of duloxetine (APS, 2008).

There are some drawbacks with both venlafaxine and duloxetine. There is an increased risk of suicidal ideation and behavior in children and adolescents with major depressive disorders, and neither is approved for pediatric patients. Care should also be taken with patients who have liver disease or use alcohol consistently (Cymbalta package insert, prescribing information; Nurse Practitioner Prescribing reference, Winter 2006–2007, available at www.PrescribingReference.com). There is also the potential for the development of sick serotonin syndrome, which occurs when patients taking SNRI medications take other medications that affect serotonin production, such as SSRI medications.

Cardiac changes are also possible with atrioventricular (AV) block and increases in blood pressure (Lynch & Watson, 2006). Of venlafaxine-treated patients, 5% developed changes on ECG (APS, 2008). As a result, patients taking venlafaxine who also have diabetes mellitus, hypertension, or hypercholesterolemia, or are currently smoking should have ECG monitoring while on the antidepressant medication (APS, 2008). Patients who are taking these medications for adjunct pain relief should have regular blood pressure screenings and should be assessed regularly for any signs of cardiac changes. Careful dose tapering should take place when these medications are being discontinued to avoid discontinuation syndrome, insomnia, lethargy, diarrhea, nausea, dizziness, or paresthesia (APS, 2008).

ANTICONVULSANT MEDICATIONS

Anticonvulsants (Table 8.4) are commonly used to treat neuropathic pain of different types, such as postherpetic neuralgia, painful diabetic neuralgia (PDN), and trigeminal neuralgia (APS, 2006). The original premise for use

Table 8.4 ▧ *Anticonvulsant Medications*

Commonly Used Anticonvulsants	Starting Dose	Effective Dose
gabapentin (Neurontin)	100–300 mg hs	300–1200 mg tid
pregabalin (Lyrica)	150 mg daily	300–600 mg daily
carbamazepine (Tegretol)	100–200 mg daily	300–800 mg bid
topiramate (Topamax)	25 mg daily	100–200 mg bid
phenytoin (Dilantin)	300 mg hs	100–150 mg tid

Abbreviations: bid, two times a day; hs, at bedtime; tid, three times a day.

was that if these medications could control the erratic neuronal firing or seizures, it could be applied for controlling neuronal discharge from pain stimuli. Research has shown that this is essentially true, and one of the primary mechanisms of these medications is to reduce neuronal excitability and spontaneous firing of cortical neurons (APS, 2008). When applied to pain management, these drugs are thought to decrease the neuronal firing for neuropathic pain and to decrease neuronal sensitization (APS, 2008).

Anticonvulsant agents are commonly used for treating neuropathic pain. Gabapentin (Neurontin) is one of the medications used to treat a multitude of neuropathic pain syndromes; however, it is particularly effective with postherpetic neuralgia, diabetic neuropathy, phantom limb pain, Guillain-Barré syndrome, neuropathic cancer pain, and acute and chronic spinal cord injury (APS, 2008; ICSI, 2007). Syndromes that do not respond to gabapentin include HIV-related neuropathy and painful peripheral chemotherapy-induced neuropathies (APS, 2008).

Both gabapentin (Neurontin) and pregabalin (Lyrica) act by blocking neuronal calcium channels, the alpha 2-delta subunit specifically reducing the release of glutamate, norepinephrine, and substance P (APS, 2008). Because the drugs are renally excreted, dose reductions are advised for patients with renal impairment. The drawback to gabapentin is the length of time needed to reach effective dose strength; it is only 10% bioavailable. Because medication response is patient dependent, it may take several weeks or months to reach a dose of gabapentin that will provide pain relief. Pregabalin, as an alternate option, can provide a faster response for pain relief because therapeutic doses can be given earlier in the treatment and it has a 90% bioavailability.

For acute pain, gabapentin and pregabalin have demonstrated an opioid-sparing effect of up to 60% when the medications are given preoperatively at doses of 300 to 1200 mg. The drawback is the increased sedation that has also been reported.

The older anticonvulsants, such as phenytoin (Dilantin), have not been studied for pain relief as fully as the newer gabapentin medications and thus have only weak evidence for their use as coanalgesic medications for pain. There is a need for further research data. One early meta-analysis (McQuay et al., 1995, in APS, 2008) determined that four anticonvulsants, including phenytoin, carbamazepine (Tegretol), clonazepam (Klonopin), and valproate (Depacon), were effective for relieving the pain of trigeminal neuralgia, diabetic neuropathy, and migraine prophylaxis. Given the high profile for serious adverse side effects, the new gabapentin medications are indicated as first line for treating neuropathic pain (APS, 2008).

One of the major drawbacks to anticonvulsant medications is their high profile for adverse side effects. These include the following:

- Somnolence
- Dizziness
- Fatigue
- Nausea
- Edema
- Weight gain
- Stevens-Johnson syndrome
- Increased risk of suicidal behavior or ideation
- Aplastic anemia and agranulocytosis (ICSI, 2007)

The serious nature of the adverse side effects of this class of medications makes it imperative that when starting these medications, a full baseline history is taken from the patient. Careful monitoring is required, and the patients should be instructed to report the occurrence and severity of any adverse effect if it happens.

TOPICAL ANALGESICS

Lidocaine 5% Patch (Lidoderm)

When the patient has a specific tender point or has an area of pain that is limited, it is tempting to use a type of pain relief that will affect only the painful area. The lidocaine patch (5%) is a soft, flannel-backed patch with 5% lidocaine that can be applied over the painful area. It has an indication for use with postherpetic neuralgia and has been studied in painful diabetic neuropathy, complex regional pain syndrome, post-mastectomy pain, and HIV-related neuropathy (APS, 2008).

The patch is designed to be used for 12 hours on and 12 hours off, although patients have worn the patch for 24 hours with no ill effects (APS, 2008; D'Arcy, 2007). The maximum dose of Lidoderm is up to three patches at one time. The patches should be replaced daily and placed only on intact skin. Active serum levels of lidocaine with patch use are minimal (APS, 2008). Patients tolerate this type of therapy very well and, because it is noninvasive, if the patient does not like the feeling of the patch or effect, the patch can be easily removed. The only side effect from the Lidoderm patch that has been reported is rare instances of skin irritation at the site of patch application.

Capsaicin Cream (Zostrix)

Capsaicin is a topical cream that can reduce the secretion of substance P at peripheral nerve ending and is derived from hot peppers. It is sold over the counter in two different strengths as Zostrix cream. The neuropathic conditions for which this cream has been most helpful include postmastectomy pain, other peripheral neuropathic conditions, and neck and arthritis pain (APS, 2008).

When the cream is applied, it causes a burning sensation in the application area. Patients should be warned to expect the sensation. Gloves should be used to apply the cream to the painful area; other parts of the body, such as the eyes, should not be touched until all the cream is removed from the hands. This technique requires a dedicated patient who is willing to persevere and apply the cream 3 to 4 times per day for 2 weeks to see if there is any analgesic benefit.

A new 8% capsaicin patch called Qutenza is used for postherpetic neuralgia. It needs to be applied by a health care provider who has been trained in the technique. Local anesthetic is applied over the site of the pain, and the patch is applied for an hour and removed. This form of capsaicin can provide up to 12 weeks of pain relief.

Targeted Analgesic-Diclofenac Epolamine Patch (Flector)

The Flector patch is a nonselective NSAID patch that is applied directly over the site of the pain on intact skin. It is especially useful for strains and sprains. The recommended dose is one patch to the affected area twice a day (*Nursing*, 2013, 2012). Because this is a new use for NSAIDs, the research support is limited and data on systemic absorption are open to change when clinical usage increases. Currently, the medication has the same black box warning of all nonselective NSAIDs.

There are compounded gels and over-the-counter NSAID gel formulations as well. These can be very effective if used as directed in the prescribed surface area. However, with continued use and application over large areas, there is an increased potential for systemic absorption. Patients are advised to use the application card supplied with the medication and wear gloves when applying the gel (*Nursing 2013 Drug Handbook*, 2012).

MUSCLE RELAXANTS

Muscle relaxants are a good addition to a pain regimen for conditions, such as low back pain, in which muscle spasms occur regularly. They are also useful for conditions, such as fibromyalgia, for which cyclobenzaprine is considered a first-line option (APS, 2005; D'Arcy & McCarberg, 2005). The group of medications, generically called skeletal muscle relaxants, consists of several different groups of medications: benzodiazepines, sedatives, antihistamines, and other centrally acting medications (Tables 8.5 and 8.6) (APS, 2008).

Although there is no indication that these medications relax skeletal muscles, they are commonly used for spasm and muscle tightness (APS, 2008). After 1 to 2 weeks, the action of the medication shifts to a central activity rather than skeletal muscle activity (APS, 2008). The most common side effect of this group of medications is sedation. If they are being used concomitantly with opioid analgesic, the sedative effect is cumulative. There is the potential for abuse in patients who are predisposed to this problem, so intermittent or short-term use is advised.

Table 8.5 ■ *Skeletal Muscle Relaxants*

	Starting Dose	*Effective Dose*
cyclobenzaprine (Fexeril)	5 mg tid	10–20 mg tid
carisoprodol (Soma)	350 mg hs-tid	350 mg tid-qid
orphenadrine (Norflex)	100 mg bid	100 mg bid
tizanidine (Zanaflex)	2 mg hs	Variable
metaxalone (Skelaxin)	400 mg tid-qid	800 mg tid-qid
methocarbamol (Robaxin)	500 mg qid	500–750 mg qid

Abbreviations: bid, twice daily; hs, at bedtime; tid, three times a day; qid, four times a day. *Source:* American Pain Society (2008).

Table 8.6 ■ *Other Types of Relaxants*

	Starting Dose	*Effective Dose*
antispasmodic (Baclofen)	5 mg tid	10–20 mg tid
benzodiazepine (Diazepam)	1 mg bid	2–10 mg bid-qid

Abbreviations: bid, two times a day; qid, four times a day; tid, three times a day. *Source:* American Pain Society (2008).

OTHER TYPES OF COANALGESICS

There are various other medications that can be used as coanalgesics, ranging from cannabinoids, such as dronabinol, which are recommended for neuropathic pain from multiple sclerosis, to NMDA receptor blockers, such as ketamine, dextromethorphan (Benylin, Robitussin), and amantadine (Symmetrel), used for centrally mediated neuropathic pain and hyperalgesia. These agents are not recommended for first- or second-line use, but rather for patients who have failed all other attempts for pain relief. They have a high profile but little research support and rely more on anecdotal and single-study support.

These medications also have a high profile for significant adverse side effects. Dronabinol use can cause cognitive impairment, psychosis, and sedation (APS, 2008).

The NMDA receptor blockers have significant adverse side effects, such as ketamine-induced hallucinations, memory problems, and abuse potential; amantadine and dextromethorphan have less severe side effects, such as dizziness, insomnia, and nausea (*Nursing 2013 Drug Handbook*, 2012).

When considering the use of a coanalgesic, the health care provider needs to fully assess the patient and consider all the comorbidities and potential drug-drug interactions. The use of these medications is highly individualized, and doses may vary according to the patient's ability to tolerate the medications. Starting a lower dose and escalating slowly can help reduce the seriousness of the side effects. Because analgesic effect can take time to become apparent, patients should be encouraged to use these medications for at least 2 weeks before deciding if they are not effective for pain relief.

Case Study

Jonathan is a construction worker who had a construction truck rollover and crush his foot. He has been in excruciating pain since his accident. He has a history of needing heavy anesthesia doses when he has surgery and waking up during surgery. He has been reporting pain in the severe range for several days postoperatively. Nothing seems to control the pain. He is on Dilaudid PCA set at 0.3 mg every 6 minutes. He recently has been describing the pain in his foot as constant, feeling like a blow torch is burning his foot, and shooting sharp pain. He cannot sleep well and is not able to move out of bed well. How will you control his pain?

Questions to Consider

1. What types of pain does Jonathan have?
2. Will increasing his PCA doses control his pain?
3. What type of co-analgesics would be helpful for Jonathan's pain?
4. In the event that Jonathan does not get enough pain relief with one co-analgesic what type of co-analgesic combinations can you provide that would give better pain relief?
5. Would an interventional pain intervention work as a co-analgesic?

REFERENCES

American Geriatrics Society Panel on Persistent Pain in Older Persons. (2002, 2009). The management of persistent pain in older persons. *Journal of the American Geriatrics Society, 50,* S205–S224.

American Pain Society. (2006). *Pain control in the primary care setting.* Glenview, IL: Author.

American Pain Society. (2008). *Principles of analgesic use in the treatment of acute and cancer pain.* Glenview, IL: Author.

Chen, H., Lamer, T. J., Rho, R. H., Marshall, K. A., Sitzman, B. T., Ghazi, S. M., & Brewer, R. P. (2004). Contemporary management of neuropathic pain for the primary care physician. *Mayo Clinic Proceedings, 79*(12), 1533–1545.

Dalton, J. A., & Youngblood, R. (2000). Clinical application of the World Health Organization analgesic ladder. *Journal of Intravenous Nursing, 23*(2), 118–124.

D'Arcy, Y., & McCarberg, B. (2005). New fibromyalgia pain management recommendations. *The Journal for Nurse Practitioners, 1*(4), 218–225.

D'Arcy, Y. (2007). *Pain management: Evidence-based tools and techniques for nursing professionals.* Marblehead, MA: HCPro.

Ghafoor, V., & St. Marie, B. (2009). *Overview of pharmacology in core curriculum for pain management nursing.* Indianapolis, IN: Kendall Publications.

Institute for Clinical System Improvement. (2007). *Assessment and management of chronic pain.* Bloomington, MN: Author.

Lynch, M. E., & Watson, C. P. (2006). The pharmacotherapy of chronic pain: A review. *Pain Research & Management, 11*(1), 11–38.

Nursing 2013 Drug Handbook. (2012). Philadelphia, PA: Lippincott Williams & Wilkins.

Wallace, M. S., & Staats, P. S. (Eds.) (2005). *Pain medicine and management.* New York, NY: McGraw-Hill.

Wilson, P., Caplan, R., Connis, R., Gilbert, H., Grigsby, E., Haddox, D., . . ., Simon, D. (1997). Practice guidelines for chronic pain management: A report by the American Society of Anesthesiologists Task Force on Pain Management, Chronic Pain Section. *Anesthesiology, 86*(4), 995–1004.

9

Complementary and Integrative Therapies for Pain Management

USING COMPLEMENTARY TECHNIQUES

Patients like to have some control over the way their pain is treated, and many of them like and are interested in using techniques that are called integrative or complementary. This does not mean that patients forego standard medical care, but that they add these additional treatment options into their pain relief regimen. Patients will use hot or cold compresses, yoga, or just walking to help stay in shape and increase their ability to function. Some of the advantages of these integrative techniques include the following:

- Low or no cost
- Patients can control many of the options
- Readily available and many do not require a prescription

Many patients have a favorite, tried-and-true pain relief measure that they use before they consider seeking help for a pain problem. Other patients are focused on wellness and have techniques they use to relieve stress, such as yoga or relaxation, that can also be very beneficial for pain relief. Patients who have arthritis or a muscle strain or sprain will try a mild analgesic they may have in their medicine chest and a little light exercise, or heat or ice to relieve the pain. Topical creams, such as Ben Gay or Icy Hot, are very popular with older patients who have this type of pain complaint (Khatta, 2007).

Because these types of treatments are over the counter, seen on television, or promoted by word of mouth for effectiveness, there is little research to recommend one treatment option over the other. Looking for the research base in this area of medicine can be confusing to say the least, because the research may be very broad and patient outcomes may not be clearly identified. One of the best resources for information on complementary treatments is the Cochrane Study Group database (available at www.cochrane.org).

Because of the confusing research and outcomes information, the National Institutes of Health (NIH) is studying the use of alternative treatments and has a group called the National Center for Complementary and Alternative Medicine (NCCAM; www.nccam.nih.gov) with a goal to review all the literature support and develop recommendations about how effective and safe these treatments are. Because there is such a big interest in using organic substances such as teas, herbal remedies, and vitamin supplements for promoting health and alleviating some forms of pain such as arthritis, this group has started a review of the herbs and supplements being used to treat common conditions. Other areas of study include energy therapies and treatments such as chiropractic manipulation and acupuncture.

The general term that refers to these methods has been shortened to complementary and alternative medicine (CAM). CAM is defined as "a group of diverse medical and health care systems, practices, and products not presently considered to be a part of conventional medicine" (American Pain Society [APS], 2006). These techniques are meant to supplement, not to replace, standard medical therapies and medication.

Most patients are a bit shy about informing their health care practitioner about extra supplements and home remedies they are using. They feel the health care provider may make them feel uncomfortable about trying something that has not been prescribed for the condition. Many patients will openly tell the health care staff about their special supplements and herbal remedies if they are asked in a nonjudgmental way. Because some of these compounds can have a drug-drug interaction with the medication, it is important for the health care provider to ask questions about these types of remedies and supplements so that a full medication/supplement history is taken. Patients may not even consider this information important; however, for the health care provider, this can be an integral piece of the patient's history.

CAM techniques are attractive options for most patients. They do not require a prescription, the patient controls the use, and side effects are not common. Most medications for pain can have side effects such as constipation, sedation, or dizziness, to name a few. Cost can also be a factor—there is little to no cost for relaxation, biofeedback, or imagery.

Although it is hard to find a good set of CAM therapies for acute pain, there are some that are easy to use. Hot and cold compresses and massage can be used for both acute pain in the outpatient setting and for inpatients. Aromatherapy is popular with inpatients because most hospitals have an institutional/clinical odor that can be offset with essential oils. Ginger drops on a cotton ball inserted into the pillow can provide some relief from nausea and vomiting. Lavender oil used in the same way can help calm patients. Energy therapies, such as Reiki and relaxation tapes, can provide relief and decrease stress. Some patients come into the hospital looking for and expecting to have access to CAM therapies to help with relaxation and pain relief.

Where do the patients get information about CAM therapies? Many publications, such as women's magazines and the *American Association of Retired Persons* magazine, have articles on yoga, pool therapy, or relaxation for health and stress management. Patients are also very Internet savvy. They can search the Internet for information about any therapy or supplement of interest to them. Older patients are no exception. They can find information as easily as younger patients and may be willing to try something that seems to offer a quick and easy way to relieve pain (American Geriatrics Society [AGS], 2002). Health care providers should never underestimate the power of word of mouth. Something discussed at the bridge game last evening may show up in the examining room today.

Because many Americans are open to using CAM therapies to help relieve pain, practitioners of various therapies, such as yoga or acupuncture, have become commonplace. Patients should be encouraged to ask these practitioners about their training and expertise in the technique they are providing. There are schools for massage and certificates for practitioners of therapy such as Reiki that are given to those who have completed the classes required to practice the technique. For a patient to go to an acupuncturist who has little or no training or expertise, for example, may be more harmful than helpful.

In a 1997 survey, Americans reported that they made 629 million visits to CAM practitioners (Eisenberg et al., 1993). In Europe and Australia, about 20% to 70% of all patients use CAM therapies (O'Hara, 2003). Primary care practitioners responded that they do not ask patients about the use of CAM therapies. Only 40% of patients volunteer information on their use of CAM therapies (O'Hara, 2003). In a 2002 survey, the NCCAM determined that the most common conditions for which patients used CAM to help relieve pain were the following:

- Back pain
- Neck pain
- Joint pain
- Arthritis
- Headache (Pierce, 2009)

There can be no doubt that many patients, both old and young, find CAM modalities helpful for pain relief.

TYPES OF COMPLEMENTARY
AND ALTERNATIVE MEDICINE

Long-term pain is one of the primary reasons why patients try CAM therapies. There are some techniques, however, that can also be used in acute
care or a referral to a clinic practicing CAM can also be made. Many of the
techniques are minimally invasive, such as acupuncture, or noninvasive,
such as the energy therapies of Reiki or therapeutic touch (TT). Because
many patients are attracted to this type of therapy, incorporating it into
the plan of care can help track outcomes and determine benefit. Because
the use of these therapeutics is controversial and research is limited, it is
helpful to monitor the benefit of these therapies when they are added to a
plan of care. If the patient is referred for treatment to a CAM-type clinic,
it is important to communicate with the CAM practitioner to ensure that
the selected treatment is meeting the patient's goals of care.

Many terms are applied to CAM therapies. Terms have changed
through the years and some common terms are listed in the following.
Currently, "integrative" is the term most often used with this category of
therapeutic options.

Complementary: Techniques or additional therapies that are used in
conjunction with recognized mainstream medical practices; for example,
when acupuncture is used concurrently with medication for low back pain.

Alternative: This term means foregoing recognized medical therapy
and using other treatments for a condition; for example, when vitamin
supplements and imagery are used in place of radiation or chemotherapy
for cancer treatment.

Integrative: A term coined by CAM practitioners to indicate the
combined use of pharmacotherapy and nonpharmacologic methods
for medical treatment. This term was first used by Dr. Andrew Weil
and it is the most common term applied to CAM therapies at this time
(O'Hara, 2003).

There are many different types of CAM therapies that are available
for treating pain. Some are very simple to use, such as heat or cold therapy,
but others require patients to be educated about using the technique, such
as with biofeedback, and some require a trained practitioner to administer
them, such as with TT.

The four main areas or types of CAM as defined by the NCCAM are
the following:

1. **Body-based therapies**, such as heat and cold therapy, massage, and
   acupuncture
2. **Cognitive-behavioral approaches**, or mind-body work, such as relaxation, biofeedback, and imagery

3. **Energy medicine**, including Reiki and TT
4. **Nutritional approaches** that incorporate the use of herbs and vitamin supplements

Body-Based Therapies

Heat and Cold Therapy

Heat and cold applications are common home remedies and they are one of the most basic types of CAM therapy. Patients are comfortable with the idea of using a heating pad for back pain or applying a cold pack for a minor muscle injury. Every household has an assortment of heating pads, ice packs, and the newer versions of microwave heating pads and wraps. Most patients find more comfort in heat and prefer it over cold packs. As for research support, a Cochrane Report of patients with low back pain indicates that the therapies have limited support (D'Arcy, 2007; French, Cameron, Walker, Reggars, & Esterman, 2006). However, additional information demonstrates that using a heat wrap can increase functionality in this patient population (D'Arcy, 2007; French et al., 2006).

Using a heating pad or hot pack can increase circulation to the affected area, decrease stiffness, reduce pain, and relieve muscle spasms (American Society of Pain Management Nursing [ASPMN], 2010; D'Arcy, 2011). When using heat, patients should be cautioned as follows:

- Use it for short periods.
- Monitor use carefully over areas of decreased circulation to avoid burns.
- Avoid placing it over areas where mentholated creams such as Ben Gay or Icy Hot have been used, which can increase the potential for skin damage.
- Heat should never be placed over a patch delivering medications such as fentanyl, medications for hypertension, or smoking cessation patches. Heat over these patches will increase the delivery of the medication to the patients and put them at risk for overdose (D'Arcy, 2010).

Ice baths, cold packs, or ice massage is helpful for decreasing the pain of sprains and strains, low back pain, and muscle spasms. Many older patients do not like the cold sensation and defer using the therapy, although it would be an effective adjunct for pain relief. The cold applications work by the following:

- Decreasing nerve conduction
- Cutaneous counterirritation
- Vasoconstriction
- Muscle relaxation
- Reduction of local and systemic metabolic activity (ASPMN, 2010)

To improve the use of heat and cold and avoid tissue damage, they should be used only for a short period. Allowing the patient to use ice as a massage can be helpful and limit application time. Patients with desensitized skin, such as those with cardiovascular disease or diabetes, should take care to monitor the application sites for skin damage. Deeper application of heat can be performed using ultrasound or diathermy. Using these techniques for deep heat applications can be helpful for spasticity, muscle spasm, edema, sprains, or contusions. Again care should be taken with areas that have tissue that does not have a normal pattern of sensitivity (ASPMN, 2010).

A common approach used by health care providers for patients with a minor ache or sprain is RICE therapy.

- **R**est
- **I**ce
- **C**ompression
- **E**levation (Berry, Covington, Dahl, Katz, & Miaskowski, 2006)

For patients with chronic pain, this technique may be less useful; however, during exacerbation of musculoskeletal pain, it may provide some added relief.

Acupuncture

Acupuncture is one of the oldest CAM therapies. It originated in China, where it was used to balance the yin and yang or energy of life forces (O'Hara, 2003). The Chinese believe that life energy forces move through chakras located in various areas of the body. If the flow of energy is blocked, weak, or in a state of imbalance, an illness or pain will occur (Khatta, 2007). Acupuncture can restore balance by opening up the chakras that are blocked and allowing the life energy to flow naturally.

Acupuncture has several different variations in practice, depending on the part of the world where the practice originates. The classic approach is Chinese, and there are medical artifacts from history that indicate that acupuncture was used as a regular part of Chinese medicine for many centuries. Acupuncture relates to the use of thin needles and other needling techniques. For pain relief, acupuncture activates the A-delta fibers in skin and muscles, which are then conveyed to the spinal cord. It stimulates the beta endorphenergic system regulating sympathetic tone. Endorphins and other pain-blocking substances such as serotonin are released (Mamtani & Frishman, 2008).

Conditions in which acupuncture has been found to be helpful include low back pain, dental pain, and the relief of nausea associated with treatment such as chemotherapy (Mamtani & Frishman, 2008). Thin needles are inserted through the skin into acupuncture points (Dillard & Knapp, 2005; NCCAM, 2004). In some cases, once the needles are in place, they are manipulated by hand or electrically stimulated to release neurotransmitters that are helpful for pain relief (Dillard & Knapp, 2005).

Conditions for which acupuncture has been used include:
- Fibromyalgia
- Osteoarthritis
- Labor pain
- Dental pain (American Pain Society [APS], 2005; Dillard & Knapp, 2005).

In a study with 570 patients with osteoarthritis receiving acupuncture, the patients in the study had improvements in function and decreased pain levels (Khatta, 2007). In a review of the therapy used for relief of low back pain, acupuncture and dry needling were found to be better than sham acupuncture or no treatment for pain relief and improved function (Furlan, Brosseau, Imamura, & Irvin, 2002). For low back pain, acupuncture was found to be more effective than sham acupuncture (Chou & Huffman, 2007). In acute care, finding the right location and time frame to perform acupuncture may be the most challenging aspect.

Massage

The NIH/NCCAM defines massage as pressing, rubbing, and otherwise manipulating muscles and soft tissue in the body (NCCAM, 2004). Massage has existed in many different cultures and was perceived to be healing in nature. Massage can take several different forms, from deep tissue massage to a lighter technique. Aromatherapy can be combined with massage to make the experience more relaxing. Massage is thought to relax and lengthen muscles, allowing oxygen and increased blood flow into the affected area (NCCAM, 2004). When massage is compared with other noninvasive interventions, it produces similar effects for pain relief (Chou & Huffman, 2007). Conditions that can benefit from massage include stress, pain management, improving mobility and movement, edema, postoperative care, and preoperative settings (Calenda & Weinstein, 2008). In the United States, not all insurance plans cover massage and over 90% of respondents to a survey on massage report paying for the treatment out of pocket (Calenda & Weinstein, 2008). For the purpose of pain management in a study with 500 patients, the respondents self-reported reduced pain, reduced analgesic consumption, and improved physical functioning. Since massage is basically a noninvasive technique, a trial of efficacy is warranted in the acute care setting even if the area of the body is limited to hand or foot massage.

Chiropractic

For outpatients, chiropractic treatment or adjustments, which consist of spinal manipulation and other techniques, align the body to reduce pain. The findings on using chiropractic for pain relief are mixed. For low back pain, however, there is good evidence that chiropractic therapy is effective for chronic or subacute low back pain (Chou & Huffman, 2007). When using this type of therapy it is always wise to have the patient go to an accredited therapist so that the best outcome can be expected.

Transcutaneous Electrical Nerve Stimulation (TENS)

For some acute care patients, using a TENS unit can decrease pain to more tolerable levels. To use this technique, a small battery pack is attached to leads with electrodes at the end. The electrodes are placed around the painful area, sometimes adjacent to a surgical incision, and a mild current is passed over the painful area. This activates large afferent fibers that stimulate dorsal horn neurons, releasing endorphins (Sharma, 2005). Since the technique is noninvasive, if the patient feels there is no benefit to the therapy, the leads can just be removed.

Other Types of Body-Based Therapies

Other forms of body-based therapies are not well supported by research. These therapies include magnets and copper bracelets. However, those that do have support can be useful to help relieve pain.

Physical therapy for reconditioning and improving balance can help maintain the mobility and functionality of older patients (AGS, 2002; Bruckenthal & D'Arcy, 2007). A regular physical therapy program has been found to reduce pain and improve mood (Bruckenthal & D'Arcy, 2007). For low back pain, exercise has good evidence to support it for pain relief (Chou & Huffman, 2007). Yoga, a form of gently stretching exercise, has also been found effective for pain relief. Viniyoga has been found superior to regular exercise for improving functional status and the use of pain medications (Chou & Huffman, 2007). Using pool therapy, in which the patients perform the physical therapy exercises in a swimming pool, can lessen the strain on sore muscles and help support the patient's body during exercise.

| *Clinical Pearl* | The use of cognitive behavioral therapy, progressive relaxation, exercise, interdisciplinary rehabilitation, functional restoration, and spinal manipulation have produced differences of 10 to 20 points on a 100-point visual analog pain scale (Chou & Huffman, 2007). |

Cognitive-Behavioral Therapy

Many patients are interested in using the complementary methods of relaxation, biofeedback, self-hypnosis, and imagery to provide additional pain relief (AGS, 2002; D'Arcy, 2007). Not all patients are open to trying these techniques. For those patients who are willing to invest the time and energy in learning how to use these methods, a good outcome can be expected.

Music

For acute care patients, one simple and easy technique to use is music. It can provide a distraction and provide relaxation for patients of all ages. Music therapy is defined as the use of specific music techniques to meet physical, emotional, social, and psychologic goals and objectives (Codding & Hanser, 2008). For pain management, music has a greater effect when pain is present, but as pain intensities increase the positive effect of music tends to diminish. It is thought that patients who listen to music to relieve pain are providing a competing stimulus to distract themselves from the pain they are experiencing. When using music in acute care, matching the patient's preference for music type provides the best outcome. Older patients may enjoy Benny Goodman or big band tunes while younger patients may prefer more modern songs.

Relaxation

Various types of relaxation techniques can be used to help relieve pain.
- Regulating breathing for decreased respiratory efforts
- Relaxation tapes for progressive relaxation
- Relaxation exercises (D'Arcy, 2007, 2010)

Relaxation techniques have been effective for decreasing pain (Cole & Brunk, 1999). These techniques result in the reduction of physical tension, muscle relaxation, and the promotion of emotional well-being (NCCAM, 2004). Relaxation is beneficial for patients who had chronic pain or cancer pain, and for surgical patients (Dillard & Knapp, 2005). For acute care patients, relaxation can be done as a one-on-one intervention by a provider trained in relaxation techniques or relaxation tapes can be provided for patients to listen to as they feel the need. Relaxation can provide an improved sense of well-being and higher scores on quality-of-life scales (Dillard & Knapp, 2005).

When patients use relaxation, they are asked to either progressively relax their muscles, starting from the top of the body and progressing to the lower extremities, or they can focus on one process, such as controlling breathing. There are prerecorded tapes with relaxation exercises on them that patients can purchase to use at certain times of the day, such as when they feel stress building or as a help for relaxing to fall asleep. The patient can keep track of progress with a pain diary or journal.

Imagery

Imagery is a form of relaxation using a mental image. When a patient uses imagery, he or she is encouraged to create a peaceful or soothing image. The patient can enjoy the feeling of comfort that the scenario provides. Images can be created by the patient or provided by tapes if the patient has difficulty developing the mental images. For example, a patient could be asked to relax and picture a beautiful beach. They are asked to smell the sea air, feel the sun on their body, and hear the sound of the surf. This image is peaceful and pleasant. The patient should choose an image that can be easily called up from memory so the technique can be used very easily when it is needed for pain relief or stress reduction.

Using imagery for pain relief can also include the use of an image that locates the area of pain, such as a headache. The patients can picture the headache as a red or dark color when pain is present. Working with the image, the patients can use relaxation and cognitive restructuring to see the headache lifting from the head, getting smaller in size, or seeing the color turning to a more peaceful and restful blue tone. This type of imagery is a little more complex, but patients can learn to use it effectively to help decrease pain.

The Arthritis Self-Management Program (ASMP) uses some mind-body techniques (AGS, 2002). These include the following:

- Education
- Cognitive restructuring
- Physical activity to reduce pain
- Problem solving
- Relaxation
- Development of communication skills to help interact with health care professionals (D'Arcy, 2010)

This program has demonstrated reduced pain that lasted more than 4 years and a cost savings of 4 to 5 times the cost of the program (Khatta, 2007)

Biofeedback, hypnosis, and meditation are other forms of relaxation techniques. Meditation or mindfulness has been found to reduce pain and help patients with chronic pain learn to cope more effectively with the condition (Khatta, 2007). If the patient can learn to quiet or center him- or herself to go through a series of images or relaxation techniques, or to focus on an object, meditation can be a useful adjunct for pain control. All of the mind-body techniques discussed earlier have research support for their use and which technique works for a specific patient depends on the type of approach the patient prefers (O'Hara, 2003).

Another type of therapy that may fit into this category of treatment options is animal-assisted therapy. In some cases these are just informal visits by animals such as dogs that are suited and cleared to visit patients in hospitals. In other cases the animals receive training in goal-directed therapy with a specific outcome as the end result. There are guidelines for this type of intervention developed by the Delta Society. Overall, pet therapy (no matter what type of pet) is designed to provide an outside focus, increase feelings of safety, and create a source of comfort. Given the large number of pets in the United States, most patients would welcome a visit from a pet while they are in pain or ill.

Energy Therapy

Asian cultures have used energy healing for many centuries. The idea of channeling energy from the universe through the patient to open blocked chakras is derived from the concept of Qigong, an external and internal energy life force. To use these therapies with patients today, several newer energy therapies were developed, including Reiki, TT, and healing touch (Pierce, 2009).

There are some differences in the practices, but the overall concepts have a similar intent.

- The human body has an energy field that is generated from within the body to the outer world.
- There is a universal energy that flows through all living things, and it is available to them.
- Self-healing is promoted through the free-flowing energy field.
- Disease and illness may be felt in the energy field and can be felt and changed by the healing intent of the practitioner (D'Arcy, 2010; Pierce, 2009).

These energy therapies are effective for pain relief and relaxation. Two of the most commonly practiced are Reiki and TT.

Reiki

The Reiki practitioner who is performing a therapeutic session on a patient uses the natural energy of the universe and channels through the patient's body to unblock chakras or energy points. The techniques used by Reiki practitioners were developed and taught by the Buddhist monk Mikao Usui from Japan beginning in 1914 (Pierce, 2009). In basic Reiki, the Reiki practitioner places his or her hands in specific configurations on the patient's body to channel the universal energy through the chakras, opening up blocked points. In more advanced levels of practice, a Reiki practitioner transmits energy a long distance to benefit a specific person (NCCAM, 2004).

Reiki has been used in Eastern cultures to ease both the mind and body. There are three levels of Reiki practice. Each level includes some additional form of energy transfer. Even with the basic level, the patient feels relaxed and experiences emotional and physical healing. The Reiki practitioner who channels the energy for the patient also receives benefit. He or she feels more relaxed and in tune with his or her own body energy after the session is completed (D'Arcy, 2010).

Studies trying to show positive benefit from Reiki have focused on patients with cancer. In a study of 24 cancer patients using Reiki or rest periods, the Reiki patients had a significant decrease in pain (Pierce, 2009).

Therapeutic Touch

Therapeutic touch (TT) was developed by two nurses who hoped it would become a part of mainstream nursing care. It is similar to Reiki but the TT practitioner does not place the hands onto the patient but holds the—over the patient to do an assessment for blocked energy.

Smoothing the aura by the energy transfer from the practitioner to the patient can help provide healing energy. TT should not be mistaken for the more religious practice of the laying on of hands as a healing practice. The premise of TT is that the practitioner's healing force transfers or channels energy, thereby positively affecting the recovery of the patient (NCCAM, 2004). As the TT practitioner allows his or her hands to move over the patient, blocked energy is identified and, through the practitioner's hands, healing forces are directed to the area to promote healing and pain relief.

There are some studies that indicate greater pain relief with the use of TT in patients with chronic pain and fibromyalgia, when compared with patient groups not receiving the energy treatment option (Pierce, 2009). It is difficult to conduct a study with TT because the recipient knows that they are not receiving the actual treatment, but only a sham. Because randomized placebo-controlled studies are not possible with TT, it is difficult to measure the true effect of the practice.

Nutritional Approaches

Folk medicine and natural healing have long been a part of most cultures. Many patients feel uncomfortable sharing information on their use of supplements and herbal remedies with their health care provider. It is important to ask about these supplements and allow for an open discussion of the pros and cons of this type of therapy. Herbal remedies are some of the most common forms of complementary therapeutics (Khatta, 2007). The advantage of these therapies is that they are simple and easy to use, viewed as noninvasive, and are benign with few side effects, but on the negative side, they have little or no quality control mechanism. From 1990 to 1997, herbal remedy use increased by 380% (Khatta, 2007). Cost-wise, the annual expenditure on herbal remedies in the United States exceeded $1.5 billion (Khatta, 2007).

Many of the tonics and elixirs peddled in early American towns and settlements had cocaine or high alcohol content with flavorings to make them palatable. Laudanum was a popular elixir used for pain relief, from childbirth to war injuries. Today, all dietary supplements are categorized under the Dietary Supplement Health and Education Act of 1994, which requires quality, safety, and efficacy standards. However, there are still discrepancies in contents of some of the supplements and herbal remedies sold over the counter, so, as always, buyers should be wary of what they are purchasing. This is especially true for pregnant and compromised patients. Common herbal remedies include the following:

- **Cayenne (Capsicum).** Cayenne can be made into plasters and placed over the painful areas. Capsaicin is the active ingredient of cayenne peppers (Khatta, 2007). Capsaicin is sold as an over-the-counter cream as a generic product or with the brand name Zostrix. The cream produces a strong sensation of heat, and it can also burn and sting. It comes in two strengths and should be carefully applied while the patient is wearing gloves to protect the areas that are not painful. Patients who are using capsaicin should apply the cream 3 to 4 times daily over at least 2 weeks to see any improvement. When applying capsaicin cream, wearing gloves is advised and care with touching other parts of the body, especially the eyes, is recommended. A new 8% topical capsaicin patch has been developed (Quetensa) for topical application in herpes zoster patients who develop postherpetic neuralgia (PHN), a very painful condition. This patch needs to have a local anesthetic applied over the application area prior to patch placement. The patch must be placed by a medical professional and removed in exactly one hour. The benefit is a good level of pain relief that can last for up to 12 weeks.
- **Devil's claw (Harpagophytum procumbens).** Use of this herb in patients with osteoarthritis resulted in a reduction in pain levels and an increase in mobility (Khatta, 2007).
- **Willow bark (Salix alba).** The results for this herb are inconsistent, and only short-term improvement has been demonstrated (Khatta, 2007).
- **Corydalis.** A frequently used herb, *Corydalis* is an alkaloid with potent analgesic properties (Dillard & Knapp, 2005). It traditionally has been used for menstrual pain.

Nutritional supplements include the following:

■ One of the most popular and disputed supplements for arthritis pain is glucosamine and chondroitin. Studies have shown a slowing of disease progression over time and that combination medications can affect pain in osteoarthritis patients (Khatta, 2007).

■ Omega-3 fatty acids affect prostaglandin metabolism, thereby affecting the inflammatory process. Fish oil has been found to have anti-inflammatory effects in patients with rheumatoid arthritis, whereas flaxseed oil has no similar effect (Khatta, 2007).

Patients who are taking nutritional supplements and herbal remedies should tell their primary care provider that they are using the substances. Because there is the potential for interactions with mainstream medications, every patient should be asked if they are taking a supplement or herbal remedy. Only those supplements and herbs that have shown efficacy in clinical trials and are recommended by the NCCAM should be used for complementary pain relief.

SUMMARY

Acute care can be a difficult place to use complementary therapies. Outpatient settings offer much more opportunity for a trial of these therapies. Trying the techniques one at a time and choosing one that the patient feels may be effective is a way to introduce the patient to the idea of using a different approach to pain control. Once the patient is comfortable with a new idea about pain control, the patient may be more open to trying a variety of techniques that will in the end provide a better outcome than medication alone.

Case Study

Your neighbor Susanne tells you she has hurt her back recently in a motor vehicle accident. She says the pain is about a 6/10 and it stays there all the time. Her doctor told her there was nothing wrong with her back and it would be better in time. She can barely bring herself to get out of bed in the morning. She is stiff and her muscles just seem to be tight in her lower back. She tries to stay up on her feet, but the pain has gotten to be such a problem for her, and it does not seem to get any better. She has been taking acetaminophen for the pain, and she wonders if there is some kind of home remedy or nonpharmacologic technique that would help her. She hates pain medicine and gets sick every time she takes it. What would you suggest for her pain?

> ### Questions to Consider
>
> 1. Because Susanne has been seen by her doctor who has not found any cause for her pain, what types of CAM therapies could be used?
> 2. Would Susanne be a candidate for acupuncture, TENS, or chiropractic manipulation?
> 3. After Susanne finds a way to decrease her pain, what types of mind-body or cognitive-behavioral techniques could she use?
> 4. Would any of the topical agents or supplements help Susanne's pain?
> 5. After Susanne's pain improves, would a regular yoga class help maintain her muscle strength and flexibility?

REFERENCES

American Geriatrics Society. (2002). The management of persistent pain in older persons. *Journal of the American Geriatrics Society, 50*(Suppl. 6), S205–S224.

American Pain Society. (2005). *Guideline for the management of fibromyalgia syndrome pain in adults and children.* Glenview, IL: Author.

American Pain Society. (2006). *Pain control in the primary care setting.* Glenview, IL: Author.

American Society of Pain Management Nursing. (2010). *Core curriculum for pain management nursing.* Dubuque, IA: Kendall Hunt Publishing.

Berry, P., Covington, E., Dahl, J., Katz, J., & Miaskowski, C. (2006). *Pain: Current understanding of assessment, management, and treatments.* Reston, VA: National Pharmaceutical Council.

Bruckenthal, P., & D'Arcy, Y. (2007). A complementary approach to pain management. *Topics in Advanced Practice Nursing eJournal, 7*(1). Retrieved from http://www.medscape.com/viewarticle/556408

Calenda, E., & Weinstein, S. (2008). *Therapeutic massage in complementary and integrative medicine in pain management.* New York, NY: Springer.

Chou, R., & Huffman, L. (2007). Nonpharmacologic therapies for acute and chronic low back pain: A review of the evidence for an American Pain Society/American College of Physicians clinical practice guideline. *Annals of Internal Medicine, 147*(7), 492–504.

Codding, P., & Hanser, S. (2008). *Music therapy in complementary and integrative medicine in pain management.* New York, NY: Springer.

Cole, B. H., & Brunk, Q. (1999). Holistic interventions for acute pain episodes: An integrative review. *Journal of Holistic Nursing, 17*(4), 384–396.

D'Arcy, Y. (2007). *Pain management: Evidence-based tools and techniques for nursing professionals.* Marblehead, MA: HCPro.

D'Arcy, Y. (2010). *How to treat pain in the elderly.* Indianapolis, IN: Sigma Theta Tau.

D'Arcy, Y. (2011). *Compact clinical guide to chronic pain management: An evidence-based approach for nurses.* New York, NY: Springer.

Dillard, J. N., & Knapp, S. (2005). Complementary and alternative pain therapy in the emergency department. *Emergency Medical Clinics of North America, 23*(2), 529–549.

Eisenberg, D. M., Kessler, R. C., Foster, C., Norlock, F. E., Calkins, D. R., & Delbanco, T. L. (1993). Unconventional medicine in the United States: Prevalence, costs, and patterns of use. *New England Journal of Medicine, 328*(4), 246–252.

French, S. D., Cameron, M., Walker, B. F., Reggars, J. W., & Esterman, A. J. (2006). Superficial heat or cold for low back pain. *Cochrane Database of Systemic Reviews* (1), Art. CD004750.

Furlan, A. D., Brosseau, L., Imamura, M., & Irvin, E. (2006). Massage for low back pain. *Cochrane Database of Systematic Reviews* (2).

Khatta, M. (2007). A complementary approach to pain management. *Topics in Advanced Practice Nursing eJournal, 7*(1). Retrieved from http://www.medscape.com/viewarticle/556408

Mamtani, R., & Frishman, W. (2008). *Acupuncture in complementary and integrative medicine in pain management.* New York, NY: Springer.

National Center for Complementary and Alternative Medicine. (2004). *Expanding horizons of health care strategic plan 2005–2009.* Bethesda, MD: U.S. Department of Health and Human Services, National Institutes of Health. Retrieved from www.nccam.nih.gov

O'Hara, D. A. (2003). Pain management. In P. Iyer (Ed.), *Medical–legal aspects of suffering.* Tucson, AZ: Lawyers and Judges Publishing.

Pierce, B. (2009). A nonpharmacologic adjunct for pain management. *The Nurse Practitioner, 34*(2), 10–13.

Sharma, M. (2005). Complementary and alternative medicine. In M. Wallace & M. Staats (Eds.), *Pain medicine and management: Just the facts* (pp. 227–282). New York, NY: McGraw-Hill.

10

The Effect of Opioid Polymorphisms and Patient Response to Medications

Today's critical care patient most often presents to the health care provider as an unknown. They do not arrive at the emergency department, critical care unit, or cardiac unit with a list of current medications, information on how medications work for them, or a history of adverse reactions. What they do bring to the process is their own genetic uniqueness and gender-related differences. This chapter examines the current literature concerning the role of gender and genetics on the patient's response to pain medications.

PATIENT DIFFERENCES IN PAIN MANAGEMENT

One of the newest pieces of pain management research is focused on the effect of the patient's gender and genetic makeup on pain medication binding and utilization. For many years there has been speculation by clinicians as to why some patients responded well to small doses of opioids and got excellent pain relief while other patients required large doses to get just minimal relief.

In early research using mouse models, there was much research related to the nociceptive sensitivity of some strains or genetic mutations of mice (Mogil, 1999). In a variety of studies with various mouse strains, the differences in nociception ranged from 1.2- to 54-fold (Lotsch, Geisslinger, & Tegender, 2009). Not surprisingly, the response of the different mouse stains to morphine varied as well.

In human trials the results were similar. In a placebo-controlled study with controlled-release oxycodone with postherpetic neuralgia patients, 42% of the participants did not respond to the treatment, with responders reporting a variety of response rates (Watson & Babul, 1998). In a study of extended release oxymorphone for low back pain, 93% of the study participants had a clinically significant response while 72% of the placebo group also had a clinically meaningful response (Katz et al., 2007). This wide variation in response to medication and placebo indicates that each patient is unique and that medication efficacy may be based on genetic predisposition over which the patient has no control.

For many years a patient was considered to be drug seeking if large doses of medication were required to control pain. Patients were considered to be exemplary if they could manage pain relief with small amounts of medication. Little concern was given to the individual differences that all patients bring to the pain management setting. Because little was known about how genetics, gender, and pain were related, the patient often felt that he/she was being blamed for any lack of success with pain management regimens.

Today we know that pain relief is not a simple process of putting the right medication into the right patient, but rather, a process dependent on patient genetics and pathophysiology. Not all patients can utilize certain pain medications such as codeine because they lack the liver enzyme needed to convert the codeine to morphine, the active form. As research progresses findings indicate that there are many genetic factors that play an important role in how pain medications work for the individual patient.

Patients with chronic pain also have a changed response to subsequent pain stimulus because the repeated pain stimuli cause the nervous system to modify its function to react more comprehensively. This is called **neuronal plasticity** (Rowbotham, Kidd, & Porreca, 2006). Neuronal plasticity can result in the phenomenon called peripheral sensitization where nociception in peripheral neurons is heightened and pain stimuli are felt to be more severe than is indicated by the stimulus. As the pain input continues, pain facilitating substances such as cytokines and substance P are recruited to the area leading to increased pain sensation, inflammation, and the development of hyperalgesia and allodynia.

Wind-up is another physiological change that occurs when the central nervous system pain response is activated as a result of continued peripheral pain input. As the pain continues, the wind-up phenomenon allows the patient to experience pain that is more intense, prolonged, and much more difficult to treat. With wind-up the *NMDA* receptors are activated and help accelerate and increase the intensity of the pain stimuli. Examples of diseases where wind-up becomes very problematic are osteoarthritis and rheumatoid arthritis (Rowbotham et al., 2006).

	• Hyperalgesia is a heightened response to a normally painful sensation, e.g., IV needle insertion.
Clinical Pearl	• Allodynia is a painful response to a sensation not normally perceived as painful, e.g., painful hugs.

Over the years, as more has become known about the effect of pain, how pain is processed, and how pain response is formulated, there is a rich area of research that has now begun to look at the role of genetics, gender, and race in how pain is perceived and processed. Although the area is still very new, the information in this chapter provides some early insight into what is known about the differences we cannot control that affect pain modulation and medication effectiveness.

GENDER AND PAIN

Since the days of Adam and Eve, who were doomed to experience physical suffering because of their errors in judgment, pain has been a topic of great discussion. How pain is produced, why it occurs, and what treatment options are effective have been discussed by both academics and the average citizen. One topic that continues to be debated is the question of differences in pain sensation between men and women: Does it exist? And if so what is causing these suspected differences? Recent research into the differences between men's and women's pain has provided some interesting information and created a need for much more research on the topic.

Do men and women experience pain differently? Yes, they do; it is a result of their hormonal variation and differences in pain pathway activation when a pain stimulus is presented for interpretation. Are there differences in the way that men and women respond to pain medications? Again the answer is yes, for a variety of reasons. Some of these differences include:

- Specific, different pain pathways for men and women
- Differences in the way pain is processed
- Effect of sex hormones
- Differences in response to opioid medications
- Lower threshold and tolerance for some pain stimulus in women (Wilson, 2006)

For many years, women were eliminated from research because it was thought that there was an estrogenic effect on pain that would skew research results. An additional consideration was the fact that estrogen levels in women fluctuated during menstrual cycles causing data to be skewed depending on the time of the month. Because of these suspicions most of the early research in breast cancer was done with male subjects. Animal studies on pain were performed with desexed animals hoping to avoid any hormonal effect on the study results. Now research focuses on these differences and uses them to advantage, such as research into the causes and treatment options for menstrual migraines.

There are some pain conditions that are more specific to women than men. Examples of these syndromes include:

- Fibromyalgia
- Temporomandibular joint (TMJ) pain
- Phantom breast pain
- Postmastectomy pain syndrome
- Menstrually related migraine
- Irritable bowel syndrome
- Interstitial cystitis
- Vulvodynia

In a study to compare the analgesic effect of morphine in both men and women, three important conclusions were derived:

- Morphine is more potent in women than men
- The onset and offset of morphine is slower in women than men
- Plasma concentrations of both the active drug and two metabolites were identical for both sexes (Dahan et al., 2008)

These findings are particularly important for acute pain and postoperative pain management. Since morphine is considered the gold standard for pain management medication and commonly used in postoperative pain relief, these differences in potency and onset are important considerations when pain relief is assessed. As an interesting addendum, the sex effect with morphine disappears with older patients, leading to the speculation that hormones have an effect on morphine's ability to pass through the blood-brain barrier (Dahan et al., 2008)

In addition to the differences in morphine with men and women, the side effects from opioid medications tend to have some sex-related relationships. The most common side effects with opioid medications are nausea/vomiting, sedation, cardiovascular effects, and respiratory depression. These differences include:

- More nausea/vomiting with women using opioids for postoperative pain control
- Increased risk for opioid induced respiratory depression in women
- Morphine associated with lower heart rate in women but the development of hypertension in men
- With opioid use, women reported more feelings of euphoria (a high feeling) and reported more instances of dry mouth (Dahan et al., 2008)

Other differences with pain medications were related to differences seen with kappa agonist medications such as nalbuphine, butorphanol, and pentazocine.

The melanocortin-1 receptor gene *Mc1r* has a specific role in modulating a pain pathway that exists only in women. This gene is commonly associated with people who have red hair, fair skin, freckles, and a high predisposition to melanoma (Dahan et al., 2008)

- Tested by giving pentazocine to both men and women
- No pain relief in men but pain relief in redheaded, fair skinned women
- The hypothesis is that men and women have separate pain pathways that are created by different genes and neurochemicals (Mogil, 1999)

The study of differences in pain response and to pain medications in men and women is a very new area of research. Much more research is needed to confirm these early findings. The early research is promising and points the way to finding the true differences between men and women in both pain response and medication efficacy.

GENETIC RESPONSE VARIABILITY AND OPIOID POLYMORPHISMS

We already know that genetics plays a big role in the production of physical characteristics—eye color, for example. Some people have blue, green, gray, or brown eyes based on the dominant gene expression in their individual physiology. What we are just learning is that people can also respond to opioids differently based on their genetic make-up.

One of the most promising targets for study is the A118G single nucleotide polymorphism in the mu opioid receptor *MOR* gene (Janicki et al., 2006; Landau, 2006). Differences in this section of genetic code are hypothesized to create differences in opioid needs and pain relief.

In a research study with patients (n = 74) who were undergoing total knee replacement, patients were genetically profiled by opioid binding site types. One group was AA homozygous patients that had a genetically efficient morphine metabolism pattern; another group had an AG heterozygous genetic variant, and group three, GG, was a homozygous nonsensitive genetic variant with reduced or impaired morphine sensitivity. The findings of morphine use via PCA and analgesia in the first 48 hours postoperatively were significantly different for both morphine consumption and pain relief among these groups.

- AA used 25 mg of morphine and had good pain relief
- AG used 25 mg of morphine and had good pain relief

■ GG used 40 mg of morphine and had many more attempts on their PCAs trying to achieve better pain control (Chou et al., 2006)

What does this mean for the clinician? It does explain some of what we see in the clinical setting with variation in patient response to opioids. Some patients may be genetically programmed to have a good, efficient response to morphine, while other patients might benefit from another medication that they are more suited to by their genetic make-up. In fact, the individual response to opioids may vary by as much as 40-fold (Argoff, 2010).

In a prospective, observational study with both acute care patients (n = 101) and patients with chronic noncancer pain (n = 121) the results were somewhat different. The patients were either typed as having *A118MOR* (major) or as variant *G118MOR* (minor) alleles. The results of the acute pain, postoperative group showed no statistical difference in pain scores or in morphine consumption in either group (Janicki et al., 2006). The patients with chronic pain did have some differences between the two groups of patients. In that group, the carriers of the major allele required significantly higher doses of opioids when compared to the opioid use of the patients with the minor allele (Janicki et al., 2006).

Clinical Pearl	*Opioid polymorphism* is differences in opioid response and effect based on genetic and gender differences.

The variation in study results could be expected. The area of research is so new that not many replications have been performed and study protocols are widely variant. As more research is done there should be some consistent findings to illustrate the differences between patient groups, medications, and pain medication delivery systems, e.g., PCA versus oral.

What does this mean for clinicians? The results of the studies do seem to indicate that genetic differences can cause a patient to need more morphine to control pain. They seem to indicate that the patients with the major gene expression (*A118MOR*) had a higher need for pain medication when compared to the minor allele group (*G118MOR*) if the pain was chronic. However, does genetics account for all the differences? In reality morphine use on a PCA can be a somewhat unreliable way to measure a patient's desire for using morphine for pain relief, need for medication, fear of addiction, or occurrence of side effects. If a patient is nauseated, the patient may defer using the PCA because the pain is less burdensome than the nausea. Research indicates that not only is the opioid response controlled by genetics but the incidence of adverse effects is affected by genetics and gender, affecting both health care costs and patient outcomes (Argoff, 2010).

The biggest indication from these very basic and early studies is that there is a need for more research to better define and confirm the findings of the first studies. There is an element of excitement here that the findings could really lead to a breakthrough about why patients have such variation in response to opioids and possibly lead to the creation of a way to predetermine what type of medication or dose would be best for each individual patient. Only more research can prove or disprove these early studies and determine if we will ever be able to know which pain medication will give each patient the best pain relief.

OPIOID ROTATION AND EQUIANALGESIA

Many endogenous and exogenous substances, including opioids, bind to specific sites in patients' bodies. Early research identified the site for opioid binding as the mu receptor and then followed groups of studies to determine just how the binding was accomplished. As research progressed, various differences in the opioids receptors were discovered and current research indicates that there are as many as 45 different subtypes at the mu receptor sites (Pasternak, 2005).

Because of these variations, it is not uncommon to try one medication, have it fail, trial another medication and have it work well to relieve the patient's pain. The ability of the medication to relieve pain is truly a function of the patient's genetics and the binding ability of the medication. If the patient's best binding potential is set up for morphine, giving the patient fentanyl for pain will result in poorer outcomes and diminished pain relief.

As the binding sites become accustomed to certain pain medications the pain relief response can be decreased. These are patients who report less effective pain relief with one medication after dose escalations and interval adjustment. As the doses go up, the side effect profile becomes more burdensome, so little is gained in the way of pain relief while side effects increase. In these cases a technique called opioid rotation can help increase pain relief and decrease side effects, all at lower doses of a new medication.

Opioid rotation is defined as the clinical practice of substituting one strong opioid for another strong opioid in an attempt to achieve a better balance between pain relief and side effects (Quigley, 2006). Another way to describe the rotation effect is switching opioids from one to another when treatment-limiting toxicity establishes poor responsiveness

(Indelicato & Portnoy, 2002). Simplistically the opioid receptor gets a little tired and overly accustomed to seeing one drug all the time and will "perk up" and accept (bind) to a new drug more efficiently providing a higher level of pain relief with fewer side effects.

Which patients are candidates for opioid rotation? Chronic cancer patients who are heavily opioid dependent are excellent candidates for opioid rotation and may have a group of medications that they rotate through regularly. Chronic pain patients who have taken opioids for an extended period of time are also very good candidates for opioid rotation. This may include trauma patients with multiple injuries that create chronic pain conditions. This phenomenon was first seen in chronic pain patients when their opioid use had continued over the course of several years (Indelicato & Portnoy, 2002)

What do these patients look like clinically? These are the patients who complain of poor pain relief; even though you escalate the dose, they continue to complain of pain at the same level with no improvement. In addition, as the doses continue to increase there is a potential for side effects such as nausea, pruritis, or other unwanted side effect. The risk/benefit ratio of medication use is reached and further dose escalation would not be useful.

In a study with patients who had cancer (n = 164) changes in opioid medication were tracked. In this patient group, 56% of the patients required opioid rotation related to side effects and ineffective pain relief. The medications being manipulated in this study were morphine, hydromorphone, methadone, fentanyl, and oxycodone (Walsh et al., 2004).

The end result of opioid rotation is improved pain relief with a lower dose of medication. In order to perform an opioid rotation there are several steps to follow. Using the equianalgesic table (Table 10.1), convert the old medication dose to an equianalgesic dose of the new medication. Equianalgesic just means equal in analgesic strength. The one warning with using these tables is to remember that the doses were set in single dose studies with opioid naïve patients in acute care settings (Sternak, 2005). They do not fully capture medication differences over the long term and cannot account for patient variability.

To perform the opioid rotation, calculate the correct conversion of the medication using the table and then decrease the new dose by 25% to 50% and offer adequate breakthrough medication (Indelicato & Portnoy, 2002). The reduction in dose is needed because of the anticipated incomplete cross tolerance (caused by the differences in mu receptor and binding) that leads to greater effect and increased side effects if the dose were converted at full strength (D'Arcy, 2009).

Additionally, the individual patient needs to be considered along with comorbidities and patient age (Indelicato & Portnoy, 2002).

> ### *Clinical Pearl*
>
> **OPIOID ROTATION CONVERSION**
>
> **ORIGINAL MEDICATION: MS CONTIN**
>
> MS contin 120 mg twice per day with MSIR 30 mg every 4 hr as needed for pain.
>
> **NEW MEDICATION: OXYCONTIN**
>
> MS Contin 120 mg twice per day (240 mg/day) is equal to oxycontin 80 mg twice per day (160 mg/day).
> MSIR 30 mg is equal to oxycodone 20 mg every 4 hr.
>
> **DECREASE THE NEW DOSE BY 25% TO 50%**
>
> 25% = oxycontin 60 mg twice per day with 15 mg oxycodone every 4 hr for breakthrough.
> 50% = oxycontin 40 mg twice per day with 10 mg of oxycodone every 4 hr for breakthrough.
> (From D'Arcy, 2009)

There is no hard and fast rule about using morphine for breakthrough pain with morphine ER or oxycodone with oxycontin, but the illustration helps to show an additional conversion by also including the breakthrough option. As a prescriber you can choose to mix and match morphine with other drugs and vice versa. The key here is to choose medications the patient has not seen in a while and to monitor the effect closely so that you can see if the change has made any difference. If you choose to go with the conservative option (50%), you can always increase the new medication up to the 25% reduction to improve pain relief if the patient starts to have increased pain. If the patient is someone who could tolerate a bigger dose, considering previous medication history, age, and comorbidities, the 25% option may work best. Always offer adequate breakthrough medication so the patient can more easily convert to the new medication regimen and retain pain control.

OTHER FACTORS

There are other factors that contribute to the use of and response to opioids in the body that can also affect pain management outcomes. The liver has a group of enzymes that affect how medications are metabolized and inactivated, or provide a diminished or exaggerated response. The CYP 450 system in the liver transforms some opioids to usable metabolites. If this system is

Table 10.1 ■ *Equianalgesic Conversion Table*

Generic	Brand Name	Dose	Dose	Dose	Dose	Dose	Schedule	Route
Immediate-Release Analgesics								
morphine	Roxanol, MSIR	5 mg	10 mg	15 mg	25 mg	30 mg	Q 4 hrs	PO
oxycodone	Roxicodone, Oxy IR	3 mg	7 mg	10 mg	17mg	20 mg	Q 4 hrs	PO
hydromorphone	Dilaudid	1 mg	3 mg	4 mg	6 mg	8 mg	Q 4 hrs	PO
meperidine *	Demerol	60 mg	100 mg	150 mg	250 mg	300 mg	Q 4 hrs	PO
methadone	Dolophine	2 mg	4 mg	6 mg	10 mg	12 mg	Q 4 hrs	PO
Extended-Release Analgesics								
morphine	MS Contin, Oramorph	5 mg	30 mg	45 mg	75 mg	90 mg	Q 12 hrs	PO
morphine	Kadian	30 mg	60 mg	90 mg	150 mg	180 mg	Q 24 hrs	PO
fentanyl transdermal	Duragesic **	25 mcg	50 mcg	75 mcg	100 mcg		Q 3 days	Topical
Breakthrough IR morphine		*3 mg*	*6 mg*	*9 mg*	*15 mg*	*18 mg*	*Q 1-2 hrs prn*	*PO*

(continued)

Table 10.1 ■ *Equianalgesic Conversion Table (continued)*

Generic	Brand Name	Dose	Dose	Dose	Dose	Dose	Schedule	Route
oxycodone	Oxycontin	10 mg	20 mg	30 mg	50 mg	60 mg	Q 12 hrs	PO
Breakthrough Oxy IR		*2 mg*	*4 mg*	*6 mg*	*10 mg*	*12 mg*	*Q 1-2 hrs prn*	*PO*
Parenteral Analgesics								
Morphine	Astromorph, Duramorp	0.4 mg	0.8 mg	1.3 mg	2.1 mg	2.5 mg	Q 1 hr	SQ/IV
Hydromorphone	Dilaudid	0.1 mg	0.1 mg	0.2 mg	0.3 mg	0.4 mg	Q 1 hr	SQ/IV
Meperidine*	Demerol	3 mg	6 mg	9mg	16 mg	19 mg	Q 1 hr	SQ/IV
Fentanyl	Sublimaze	4 mcg	8 mcg	13 mcg	21 mcg	25 mcg	Q 1 hr	SQ/IV

* This drug is not recommended for use but is included for comparison only.

** Dosage from Levy MH, NEJM 1996; 335(15) 1124–1132.

Basic IV Conversion: Morphine 1 mg = Dilaudid 0.2 mg = Fentanyl 10 mcg.

impaired or inactivated by another medication, the opioid effect will be directly affected. Additionally genes responsible for encoding proteins that activate opioid transport affect opioid responsiveness. P-glycoprotein is affiliated with encoding controlled by the ATP-binding B1 of the multidrug resistance gene (*MDRI*). This process affects the bioavailability of opioid medications such as fentanyl, morphine, and methadone, causing a variation in individual patient medication efficacy (Argoff, 2010).

Some patients have different metabolism profiles for medication utilization. If the patient has a rapid or ultra rapid medication metabolism, medication will be used quickly. These are the patients who tell you that a standard does of opioid medication just does not last long enough. In the medication section of this book, the warning for codeine was highlighted for rapid metabolizers since several incidents of morphine overdose were detected in nursing infants whose mothers had taken codeine and rapidly metabolized the codeine to morphine.

Conversely, at the other end of the spectrum, patients who metabolize medication slowly are at risk for increased effects of opioids with repeated doses. These are the patients who may tell you a small dose of opioid medication lasts a long period of time or they request low dose opioids since they report being "sensitive" to opioids. These patients may also have a higher profile for oversedation, nausea/vomiting, and so on, because the medication stays in their systems for longer periods of time.

No matter what aspect of genetic variability you encounter in clinical practice, there are options to counteract the effect. Switching medications, trying different types of medications, adding in co-analgesics or complementary methods may increase the potential for optimal pain relief. This is one area where pain management is truly an art and science, and in this case the science is helping to facilitate the chances of finding the right medication for the individual patient.

Case Study

Sally Jane is a 49-year-old patient who was admitted to the ICU step down after a motor vehicle accident in which she sustained a pelvic fracture, fractures of her femur, and a shoulder separation. She complains about the medication being used for her pain. She becomes quite agitated when physical therapy tries to move her. She says "I don't know what you are using for my pain but it not working. What little pain relief I do get does not last long enough. I refuse to do any kind of therapy until you find a medication that works for me. Demerol used to work great. Why can't I have that?"

Questions to Consider

1. As the nurse you are looking for better outcomes for Sally. Right now Sally is using morphine PCA to control her pain. What can you try to increase Sally's pain relief? Change medications? Change doses?
2. What does being a fair skinned red-headed woman have to do with Sally's pain management?
3. Does Sally's gender have a role in her lack of pain relief with opioids?
4. In order to get a good idea of what types of medications have not worked for Sally, she gives you a list of medications she has tried with only fair results: morphine caused nausea/vomiting; Percocet caused lightheadedness; Vicodin; and Tylenol #3. Would you consider trying Ultram/Ultracet, Dilaudid, or Oxymorphone? Would you consider going back to one of her old medications and trying a lower dose? Would you rotate opioids?
5. What kinds of non-opioids would you suggest? NSAIDs, APAP, anticonvulsants, antidepressants, etc.?
6. What role does Sally's statement about the pain medication not lasting long enough play in the plan of care? Could you consider her opioid metabolism? She may be a rapid opioid metabolizer. Should you consider scheduling some opioid medication for her or adding a continuous infusion?
7. Would adding a complementary method to her pain management regimen be helpful? What would you suggest for a low back pain patient with poor pain relief and sleep dysfunction?

REFERENCES

Argoff, C. (2010). Clinical implications of opioid pharmacogenetics. *The Clinical Journal of Pain, 26*, S16–S20.

Chou, W. Y., et al. (2006). Association of mu opioid receptor gene polymorphism (*A118G*) with variation in morphine consumption for analgesia after total knee arthroplasty. *Acta Anaesthesiologica Scandinavica, 50*(7), 787–792.

Dahan, A., Kest, B., Waxman, A., Sarton, E., Durieux, M., & Gin, T. (2008). Sex-specific response to opiates: Animal and human studies. *Anesthesia & Analgesia, 107*(1), 83–95.

D'Arcy, Y. (2007). *Pain management: Evidence-based tools and techniques for nursing professionals.* Marblehead MA: HcPro.

D'Arcy, Y. (2007). One pain medication does not fit all: Using opioid rotation in your practice. *The Nurse Practitioner, 32*(11), 7–8.

D'Arcy, Y. (2009). Opioid therapy: Focus on patient safety. *American Nurse Today, 4*(5), 18–22.

Janicki, P., Schuler, G., David, F., Bohr, A., Gordin, V., Jarzembowski, . . . Mets, B. (2006). A genetic association study of the functional A118G polymorphism of the human mu-opioid receptor gene in patients with acute and chronic pain. *Anesthesia & Analgesia, 103*(4), 1011–1017.

Indelicato, R. A., & Portnoy, R. (2002). Opioid rotation in the management of refractory cancer pain. *Journal of Clinical Oncology, 20*(1), 348–352.

Katz, N., Rauck, R., Abdieh, H., et al. (2007). A 12-week, randomized placebo-controlled trial assessing the safety and efficacy of xylophone extended release for opioid naïve patients with chronic low back pain. *Current Medical Research & Opinion, 23*, 117–128.

Landau, R. (2006). One size does not fit all: Genetic variability of mu opioid receptor and postoperative morphine consumption. *Anesthesiology, 105*(2), 235–237.

Lotsch, J., Geisslinger, G., & Tegender, I. (2009). Genetic modulation of the pharmacological treatment of pain. *Pharmacology & Genetics,* 124:168–184.

Mercadante, S., & Bruerae, E. (2006). Opioid switching: A systemic and critical review. *Cancer Treatment Reviews, 32*, 304–315.

Mogil, J. S. (1999). The genetic mediation of individual differences in sensitivity to pain and its inhibition. *Proceedings of the National Academy of Sciences of the United States of America, 96*, 7744–7751.

Pasternak, G. W. (2005). Molecular biology of opioid analgesia. *Journal of Pain and Symptom Management, 29*(5S), S2–S9.

Quigley, C. (2006). Opioid switching to improve pain relief and drug tolerability. *The Cochrane Database of Systemic Reviews,* (4).

Rowbotham, M., Kidd, B., & Porecca, F. (2006). Role of central sensitization in chronic pain: Osteoarthritis and rheumatoid arthritis compared to neurop. In H. Flor, E. Kalso, & J. Dostrovsky (Eds.), *Proceedings of the 11th World Congress on Pain. August 21 – 26th 2005, Sydney, Australia.* Seattle WA: IASP Press.

Walsh, D., Davis, M. P., Estfan, B., Legrand, S. B., Lagman, R. L., & Shaheen, P. (2004). Opioid rotation prospective longitudinal study: 8258. *Journal of Clinical Oncology, 22*(Sup14), 793s.

Watson, C. P., & Babul, N. (1998). Efficacy of oxycodone in neuropathic pain: A randomized trial in post herpetic neuralgia. *Neurology, 50,* 1837–1841.

11

Surgical and Procedural Pain Management in Critical Care

When a patient is admitted to the critical care area the primary concern is the preservation of life. As such, the focus of intensive care providers is to save and maintain life while trying at the same time to provide adequate pain relief. Sources of pain in the intensive care unit (ICU) include:

- Therapies and interventions designed to preserve life such as intubation
- Invasive procedures such as chest tubes and line insertion
- Pain from surgery
- Pain related to trauma
- Inflammation
- Immobility (Mularski, Sessler, & Schmidt, 2010)

The patient who is in critical care can often have pain management needs overlooked given the severity of the medical condition. The surgical patient who is being admitted to a critical care area has had a significant surgery that requires close monitoring or continued intubation. Most patients, when asked about their experience with pain management in the ICU, respond that their pain was inadequately assessed and that pain management was not sufficient to relieve their pain (Topolovec-Vranic et al., 2010).

Intravenous opioids have long been used in these patients but medical conditions such as renal disease or liver dysfunction can limit their use. Further hampering adequate pain relief for the critical care patients is the difficulty of adequate pain assessment in patients who are intubated, on end of life care, or are delirious or demented. Using a team approach to developing a comprehensive treatment plan that includes pain management is essential to ensure that the patient's pain management needs do not get overlooked by the severity of the health care needs.

It is important to remember that patients come into the critical care setting bringing all their current pain management issues. All critically ill patients have the right to adequate analgesia and management of their pain (Jacobi et al., 2002). Some of the patients will have low back pain, rheumatoid arthritis or other chronic painful conditions that are not helped by immobility plus the pain of surgery or trauma. The procedures and care being provided can also be painful, as illustrated in the Thunder II Project (Puntillo et al., 2001) where procedures such as line insertion or chest tube insertion and a simple turn in bed had pain scores that were higher than expected.

In order to detect pain and delirium in patients who are unable to respond, using tools such as the Adult Nonverbal Pain Scale (ANVPS) and the Confusion Assessment Method-ICU (CAM-ICU) can be helpful. In a study where the ANVPS was trialed, patients reported increased assessments and decreased time to medication administration, while staff reported increased confidence in assessing pain in nonverbal patients, and found the tool simple and easy to use (Topolovec-Vranic et al., 2010).

In order to get an accurate assessment of pain, critical care patients should also be assessed for delirium. Delirium is an acute onset confusion condition that can be caused by infections, medications, surgery, or changes in location. In surgical patient, often delirium is unrecognized and undiagnosed, especially given the multiple tasks, monitorings, and assessments that need to be performed by nurses in the ICU. Once a patient has been determined to have delirium, pain medications are often discontinued or reduced in an effort to diagnose the cause of the delirium. To assess a patient for delirium a tool such as the CAM-ICU can give an accurate assessment. In a study with 156 surgical patients in the ICU comparing the CAM-ICU to other delirium tools, the CAM-ICU scored the highest validity of all scales in determining delirium in ICU patients (Luetz et al., 2010). Screening and assessment for delirium are important for ventilated ICU patients since there is a correlation between delirium and higher mortality, increased ventilator days, and longer hospital stays in the ICU with critical care patients (Ely et al., 2004; Robinson et al., 2008).

Using tools that can provide an accurate assessment for pain and can diagnose the presence of delirium for critical care patients can move the critical care team toward developing a plan of care that will both relieve pain and identify delirium. No matter if the patient is a trauma, surgical, or older patient with chronic pain; providing accurate pain assessment, realizing that the critical care patient needs pain management, and assessing for an unrecognized effect such as delirium can help the patient receive adequate pain relief.

SEDATION AND ANALGESIA IN THE INTENSIVE CARE UNIT

A large number of patients in the critical care setting will be ventilated, which has been identified as painful by patients. The surgical patient who is admitted to critical care after surgery may need extended ventilation, which requires sedation. To maintain the ventilation, patients are sedated with a sedative agent such as propofol, midazalam, or dexmedetomidine combined with an opioid such as morphine or fentanyl. Because the patient in ICU is under physiological stress, normal organ function is impaired at some level. The oral route for medication administration is often not an option. Using medications on a continuous basis can also impact the way the drug is being processed. For example, fentanyl is noted to have a quick onset and quick offset when given as a bolus dose but the half-life of the medication when used as a continuous infusion for sedation can stretch to 13 hours (Erstad et al., 2009).

When pain is unrelieved in the critical care unit, there can be consequences that reach beyond the pain itself. Some systemic and physiologic effects include:

- *Immune system*: decreased immune response and ability to fight infection
- *Cardiovascular:* increased oxygen demand on heart muscle creating stress and ischemia
- *Renal:* water and sodium retention
- *Endocrine:* hyperglycemia and hypotension
- *Respiratory*: hypoxia, ventilator dysfunction, increased pneumonia risk, and telecasts
- *Psychological*: depression, fatigue, and anxiety
- *Hematological*: gastrointestinal bleeding and thromboembolic disease (Mularski et al., 2010).

Given the serious nature of the consequences, providing adequate analgesia for critically ill patients is highly important. However, the critical care patient can present a challenge when opioids are being used; for example, patients with hepatic or renal dysfunction can experience oversedation. Even patients with normal physiology can have protracted periods of sedation with the extended use of opioids.

No analgesic or sedative agent has been shown to be superior over the others (Mularski et al., 2010). The choice is based on provider preference and suitability for the individual patient. Commonly used opioids and sedative agents include:

Opioids	Dose
Fentanyl	25–100 mcg IV push until pain is controlled or as a continuous infusion to accompany sedation
Morphine	2–5 mg IV push until pain is controlled or

continuous infusion to accompany sedation. Extreme caution in patients with hepatic or renal dysfunction

Sedation	Dose
Midazolam	2–5 mg IV push every 10–20 min until goal achieved; then as-needed doses or as a continuous infusion for sedation with an opioid
Propofol	Start at 5 mcg/kg/min; titrate every 5 min until at goal; use as a continuous infusion with an opioid (Mularski et al., 2010)
Dexmedetomidine	Start as a 1 mcg/kg loading dose with a continuous infusion of 0.2–0.7 mcg/kg/hr. May be used for more than 24 hour at rates of up to 1.5 mcg/kg/hr (Gerlach, Murphy, & Dasta, 2009)

The alpha 2-adrenergic receptors clonidine and dexmedetomidine (Precedex) have been used in critical care for adjuvant pain relief, with Precedex being used as a sedative agent as well. This bi-modal effect has prompted the use of Precedex for both pain and sedation. To date, the literature is not fully explored as to the benefit of using the medication for both uses. It may be restricted to patients who have failed other types of sedation (Anger, Szumita, Baroletti, Labreche, & Fanikos, 2010). In part, this is due to the incidence of hypotension, hypertension, and bradycardia that are side effects frequently seen with Precedex (Gerlach et al., 2009). A study comparing 56 cardiac surgery patients sedated with Precedex or Propofol found there was no difference for all patients in ICU length of stay or duration of ventilation, but hypotension was seen more frequently in the Precedex group (Anger et al., 2010).

Just because a critically ill patient is sedated does not mean pain is controlled. As well, sedation does not mean that patients will have no memory of events when under sedation. In a study of critical care patients who were sedated and ventilated, 55% of the patients had recall of the events and pain while they were perceived as too sedated to be aware of their surroundings or happenings (Puntillo, 1994).

Patients are often set up on a daily wakening protocol where sedation is decreased to determine suitability for weaning the patient from the ventilator. In a study with 104 mechanically ventilated patients where one-half of the patients were awakened daily and participated in range of motion and physical therapy, findings indicated that in the intervention group, those that were awakened daily and participated in exercises, 35% had a return to a higher physical functioning on discharge and a higher return to participation in transfers and activities of daily living (Frontera, 2011).

Clinical Pearl   A point to remember: Sedation is not analgesia. The use of sedative agents without an analgesic will leave the patient unable to communicate pain but experiencing pain. Combining a sedative agent such as propofol with an analgesic agent is a better combination to provide some element of pain relief. Additional analgesic may be needed after assessment with a BPS indicates the presence of pain in a ventilated sedated patient.

If the critically ill patient is restless and agitated, it may mean that they are having pain. As always it is prudent to provide an analgesic trial if the patient has a condition that is painful to others who have it. Monitoring the effect of the analgesic in reducing the restlessness or agitation can help determine if the patient was experiencing unrelieved pain.

Monitoring the critically ill patient for the presence of pain is an important part of the care being provided. By assessing and providing pain medication for these patients who are too ill to self-report pain, these patients will have less stress and continue to discharge with a better physical and mental condition.

THE SURGICAL PATIENT IN CRITICAL CARE

Any patient who has cardiac surgery, neurological surgery, or a significant abdominal or orthopedic surgery may find they are sent to the ICU to recover. Patients in need of opioids with significant comorbidities such as obesity may also find they spend some of their recovery time in the ICU to receive more intense monitoring for respiratory depression with opioid use in the postoperative time period. Trauma patients with significant orthopedic repairs may need some time in ICU after surgery to stabilize.

For most of these patients, the oral route for pain medications is not an option and mechanical ventilation may be used. Since these patients have had a serious surgery and pain management is needed, a variety of techniques can be used to provide adequate pain relief after surgery.

For all surgical patients, a history of prior pain medication use, doses taken daily, and use of alcohol and illicit substances is needed. If the patient has chronic pain and is opioid dependent, higher doses of medication for pain will be needed. It is not enough to rely on regular analgesic doses for accompanying sedation to control pain. The patient who is opioid dependent or is using illicit substances such as heroin will need additional doses of medication to ensure adequate pain relief in the acute postoperative period because of the tolerance to opioids. For the opioid-dependent patient, it may be necessary to contact the prescriber of these medications since the patient may not have been able to provide this information.

Intravenous Opioids

For some surgical patients the use of intermittent IV opioids will provide adequate pain relief. However, when the doses need to be given frequently or the pain relief is not sufficient, another form of medication administration such as patient-controlled analgesia (PCA) is needed. Common IV opioid medications used in the critical care setting for postoperative pain relief include fentanyl, morphine, and hydromorphone. Doses are set by considering the patient's opioid use status, the condition of the patient, and physiologic considerations such as hepatic and renal function.

Patient-Controlled Analgesia (PCA)

PCA is good option for pain relief for patients who are able to activate the control button to deliver pain medication. If the patient is opioid tolerant, a continuous infusion may be needed if the patient is not able to take oral pain medications. Even if the PCA is set for only bolus dosing, there is an option to have additional bolus doses; that is, clinician-administered boluses that can provide increased pain relief when needed. Once the patient is off ventilation, a PCA that the patient can use to control pain is a good option. For patients in critical care, it is important to assess their ability to activate the machine correctly to get the pain medication they need to control pain. More information on PCA use will be provided in Chapter 12.

Epidural Analgesia

Epidural analgesia is an ideal option for critically ill surgical patients since it provides the highest level of pain relief using the smallest amount of opioid medication. This has the effect of decreasing unwanted side effects

(Mularski et al., 2010). Most postoperative epidurals such as those used for thoracotomy patients have solutions of both an opioid such as fentanyl, hydomorphone, or morphine combined with a local anesthetic such as bupivacaine or ropivacaine. The epidural is placed into the dermatomal area where the innervation of the surgical area is located. Once the patient has bolus doses to achieve pain relief, a low dose continuous infusion can keep the patient comfortable. Another option is to use a continuous infusion with a demand dose patient-controlled epidural analgesia (PCEA).

Thoracotomy patients have good outcomes when epidural analgesia is used. The pain of thoracotomy can be quite severe and optimizing pulmonary function postoperatively is critical. Using epidural analgesia can help control pain, increase pulmonary function, and shorten the return to physical functioning. Using a thoracic epidural with a combined local anesthetic and opioid epidural solution is the recommended method for treating postoperative pain in thorocotomy patients as compared to other regional techniques, per a systematic review of randomized trials by Joshi et al. (2008). Also recommended was a paravertebral block with a similar profile for efficacy as the thoracic epidural.

Other patient types that benefit from the use of an epidural analgesia for postoperative pain control are:

- Abdominal aortic aneurysm repair
- Large abdominal surgeries such as colon resection
- Large orthopedic surgeries

In a recent study of 200 patients undergoing off-pump coronary artery bypass surgery, thoracic epidural analgesia used for 72 hours after surgery with general anesthesia reduced hospital stay, improved pain control and quality of recovery, and reduced the incidence of dysrhythmias (Caputo et al., 2011)

The use of epidural analgesia is common and there are side effects that should be considered when the technique is being used. Patients who are anticoagulated are not good candidates for epidurals. There is a significant risk of epidural hematoma when anticoagulation is being used with an epidural. The use of epidural with Lovenox is not recommended and the placement of an epidural with an INR greater than 1.5 is also not recommended. Other side effects that can be anticipated include:

- Loss of sensation or paresthesia over the dermatomal area, treated in most cases by reducing the infusion rate of the epidural
- Motor blockade, treated by stopping the epidural for a short period of time and reducing the rate of the epidural
- Urinary retention
- Other opioid-related side effects such as pruritis, nausea, and vomiting

More information on regional analgesia techniques such as epidural will be provided in Chapter 13.

Procedural Pain Management

There are a large number of procedures performed in the many areas addressed in critical care. Procedural pain has been an area that has been overlooked since most procedures are felt to be quick and relatively painless by those that are performing them. From the patient's perspective, however, procedural pain is something to be dreaded and time seems to lag while they are being treated.

In a study of pain related to procedures being performed in an emergency department, researchers questioned approximately 1,200 patients about the pain they experienced with their procedure. The patients ranked the most painful procedures as:

▪ Nasogastric intubation
▪ Abscess incision and drainage
▪ Fracture reduction
▪ Urinary catheter insertion (Singer, Richman, Kowalska, & Thode, 1999)

The practitioners who performed the procedures ranked them in a similar fashion. When the two groups, patients and practitioners, were asked which procedures were less painful the responses were ranked as:

▪ IV insertion
▪ Drawing blood gases
▪ Local anesthesia
▪ Lumbar puncture
▪ Blood drawing
▪ Suturing (Singer et al., 1999)

Of the group of 1,200 patients only 12.8% had been offered analgesics prior to the procedure. The information from patients compared to providers was highly variable when estimating pain. These findings indicate that is it critical to ask patients about pain when performing a procedure of any type and to offer analgesia (Singer et al., 1999).

In the critical care setting, a large multi-center study with 6,200 patients (Puntillo et al., 2001) including both adults and children studied the intensity of pain during several different types of procedures. The researchers had the patients rate the pain using a 0 to 100 pain intensity for children and the 0 to 10 NRS for adults.

▪ For children, turning in bed was rated as 28 to 60 on the 100-point scale and tracheal suctioning was rated as 52 to 56.
▪ Adolescents reported pain ratings of wound drain removal at 5 to 7 on the NRS.

■ Adults reported that turning in bed was most painful at an NRS rating of 4.93.

It is clearly seen in this group that procedures caused significant pain. The distress ratings for procedures was also quite high with adolescents, rating their distress at 4.83 to 6.0, and with adults, at 1.89 to 3.47. The pain these patients experienced was described as sharp, stinging, stabbing, shooting, and awful (Puntillo et al., 2001) Of note is that less than 20% of all patients received opiates before any of the procedures (Puntillo et al., 2001).

In other research, a descriptive study of 31 surgical patients reported that pain was the most common sensation during drain removal and they rated the pain at 4 on the NRS (Mimnaugh, Winegar, Mabrey, & Davis, 1999). In another descriptive study 45 adult patients reported their pain at 7 on the NRS with endotracheal suctioning (Puntillo, 1994).

Based on patient reports, most of the procedures that are performed on patients are painful. However, most of the patients receive very little in the way of analgesics or local anesthetics. Recommendations for pain relief during procedures include:

■ Regular pain assessment and reassessment
■ Use a behavioral pain scale if the patient is nonverbal and note any recognized pain behaviors such as grimacing, moaning, or increases in body tension
■ Use a topical anesthetic cream or a local intradermal anesthetic to decrease the pain associated with the insertion of an IV cannula
■ Use a lidocaine spray or combine it with a lidocaine jelly when inserting a nasogastric tube
■ Medicate the patient for pain or ensure that the patient receives an anesthetic agent before a procedure such as a bone marrow aspiration
■ Make sure the patient receives an analgesic before a procedure such as a chest tube removal

In some cases procedural sedation is needed to perform the procedure. This is a new area of practice and hospitals have set up procedures and policies surrounding the practice that define who may provide this service and what types of medication can be used. Minimal and moderate sedation can be used. Moderate sedation is defined as patent airway and responsive to verbal commends or light tactile stimulation. Monitoring parameters are required, with oxygen saturation, cardiac monitoring, and blood pressure measurements done throughout the sedation period (Todd & Miner, 2010). Patients who undergo mild, moderate, or even deep sedation may be amnesic about the events during the procedures. Common medications used for sedation are propofol, ketamine, etomidate, and a combination of fentanyl and midazolam (Todd & Miner, 2010).

For most patients who are undergoing a procedure, providing pain medication or some type of local anesthetic/numbing medication will make the experience less painful and distressing. For other procedures, sedation at some level will be required. Using complementary methods with analgesics can help the patient relax when the procedure is being performed. Providing pain relief during procedures is an important aspect of clinical care in critical care or emergency department settings.

Case Study

Peter Smith is a 56-year-old patient who is having a thoracotomy. He knows the surgery is serious and he is anxious about the outcome. He tells you about his concerns and then says "In spite of everything, I am really concerned about pain control. I had a friend who had the same surgery and he said the pain was terrible. Is there anything you can give me to make the pain less severe?" You provide Peter with some information about the surgery and then tell him about the types of analgesic options he has for pain control after surgery. You indicate that the decision about the type of postoperative analgesia is a decision that he can make with his surgeon and the anesthesiologist. What do you tell Peter about pain relief after his surgery?

Questions to Consider

1. What type of analgesia would provide the best pain relief for Peter?
2. If Peter has a heart condition for which he is taking coumadin, would he be a good candidate for an epidural?
3. What are the benefits of using an epidural for a thoracotomy patient?
4. What impact can the lack of adequate pain management have on the outcome of Peter's hospitalization?

REFERENCES

Anger, K. E., Szumita, P. M., Baroletti, S. A., Labreche, M. J., & Fanikos, J. (2010). Evaluation of dexmedetomidine versus proprofol-based sedation therapy in mechanically ventilated cardiac surgery patients at a tertiary academic medical center. *Critical Pathways in Cardiology, 9*(4), 221–226.

Caputo, M., Alwair, H., Rogers, C. A., Pike, K., Cohen, A., Monk, C., . . ., Angelini, G. D. (2011). Thoracic epidural anesthesia improves early outcomes in patients undergoing off-pump coronary artery bypass surgery: A prospective, randomized, controlled trial. *Anesthesiology, 114*(2), 380–390.

Ely, E. W., Shintani, A., Truman, B., Speroff, T., Gordon, S. M., Harrell, F. E. Jr., . . ., Dittus, R. S. (2004). Delirium as a predictor of mortality in mechanically ventilated patients in the intensive care unit. *JAMA, 291*(14), 1753–1762.

Erstad, B. L., Puntillo, K., Gilbert, H. C., Grap, M. J., Li, D., Medina, J., . . ., Sessler, C. N. (2009). Pain management principles in the critically ill. *Chest, 135*(4), 1075–1086.

Frontera, J. A. (2011). Delirium and sedation in the ICU. *Neuro Critical Care, 14,* 463–474.

Gerlach, A. T., Murphy, C. V., & Dasta, J. F. (2009). An updated focused review of dexmedetomidine in adults. *Annals of Pharmacotherapy, 43,* 2064–2074.

Jacobi, J., Fraser, G., Coursin, D., Riker, R., Fontaine, D., Wittbrodt, E., . . ., Lumb, P. (2002). Clinical practice guidelines for the sustained use of sedatives and analgesics in the critically ill adult. *Critical Care Medecine, 30*(1), 1–42.

Joshi, G. P., Bonnet, F., Shah, R., Wilkinson, R. C., Camu, F., Fischer, B., . . ., Kehlet, H. (2008). A systematic review of randomized trials evaluating regional techniques for postthoracotomy analgesia. *Anesthesia and Analgesia, 107*(3), 1026–1040.

Luetz, A., Heymann, A., Radtke, F. M., Chenitir, C., Neuhaus, U., Nachtigall, I., . . ., Spies, C. D. (2010). Different assessment tools for intensive care unit delirium: Which score to use? *Critical Care Medicine, 38*(2), 409–418.

Mimnaugh, L., Winegar, M., Mabrey, Y., & Davis, J. E. (1999). Sensations during removal of tubes in acute postoperative patients. *Applied Nursing Research, 12*(2), 78–85.

Mularski, R., Sessler, C., & Schmidt, G. (2010). Pain management in the intensive care unit. In *Bonica's management of pain* (4th ed.). Philadelphia, PA: Lippincott Williams & Wilkins.

Puntillo, K. A. (1994). Dimensions of procedural pain and its analgesic management in critically ill surgical patients. *American Journal of Critical Care, 3*(2), 116–122.

Puntillo, K. A., White, C., Morris, A. B., Perdue, S. T., Stanik-Hutt, J., Thompson, C., Wild, L. (2001). Patients' perceptions and responses to procedural pain: Results form the Thunder Project II. *American Journal of Critical Care, 10*(4), 238–251.

Robinson, B. R., Mueller, E. W., Henson, K., Branson, R. D., Barsoum, S., & Tsuei, B. J. (2008). An analgesia-delirium-sedation protocol for critically ill trauma patients reduces ventilator days and hospital length of stay. *Journal of Trauma, 65*(3), 517–526.

Singer, A. J., Richman, P. B., Kowalska, A., Thode, H. C. Jr. (1999). Comparison of patients and practitioner assessments of pain from commonly performed emergency department procedures. *Annals of Emergency Medicine, 33*(6), 652–658.

Todd, K. H., & Miner, J. (2010). Pain management in the emergency department. In *Bonica's pain management.* Philadelphia, PA: Lippincott Williams & Wilkins.

Topolovec-Vranic, J., Canzian, S., Innis, J., Pollmann-Mudryj, M. A., McFarlan, A. W., Baker, A. J. (2010). Patient satisfaction and documentation of pain assessments and management after implementing the adult nonverbal pain scale. *American Journal of Critical Care, 19*(4), 345–355.

12

Using Patient Controlled Analgesia (PCA) in Critical Care

Patient controlled analgesia (PCA) is more than the machine used to deliver the medication; it is a process. This process consists of the patient, the delivery system, and the medications with dosing parameters. If any one of these elements is eliminated, the process should no longer be considered PCA.

Because the use of PCA requires an alert patient who is able to activate the medication delivery system, the use of the classic PCA where bolus doses are used to control pain may be limited. For the surgical or trauma patient or in opioid tolerant patients, after a comprehensive assessment the use of continuous infusion as an adjunct to sedation may be indicated. For patients who are alert enough and able to push the PCA button, PCA can provide an excellent method for achieving pain relief.

The PCA system consists of a computerized pump that delivers opioid medication through IV tubing into the patient's IV access. When pain increases, the patient is able to activate the machine using a push button device. Once the button is pushed, the pump delivers a preset dose of medication to the patient. The pump is programmed by the nursing staff according to PCA orders written by a licensed prescriber. The pump can be set to deliver several different types of pre-filled opioid syringes or bags and can be programmed to deliver a continuous or basal dose along with a patient-activated bolus dose.

Most patients prefer PCA to other forms of postoperative analgesia because they have some control over the system. They can use the medication when they feel pain and not have to wait for the nurse to answer a call light, get the medication from a medication machine (PYXIS), and then return to the patient's room to deliver the medication. The ease of PCA and quick response time for medication delivery are very attractive for patients. A Cochrane Review of 55 studies with 2,023 patients reported that PCA provided better pain relief and increased patient satisfaction compared to as-needed medication dosing, but the patients also had a higher medication use and increased pruritis compared to patients using standard means of postoperative pain management (Hudcova, McNicol, Quah, Lau, & Carr, 2006).

The first PCAs were developed in the 1970s in an effort to improve upon the current forms of postoperative pain control; i.e., IM injections and intermittent injections of opioids provided by a nurse. The older forms of medication administration allowed for a period of oversedation, then a period of pain relief, followed by a period of pain as the medication dissipated. Because of the potential for irregular medication absorption, IM injections are no longer recommended for pain management (APS, 2008). Blood levels of medication fluctuated and exceeded the patient's needs and then as blood levels decreased the patient began to experience pain. Very often, as pain returned, the patients would be told that "it is not time for your medication" and would be forced to wait in pain until the stipulated time was reached. Studies conducted on PCA in the early 1970s indicated that small doses of medication given at regular intervals provided superior pain relief to the standard IM injections and eliminated the variation in pain relief with intermittent injections (Grass, 2005).

Each patient has an individual level of medication that will provide pain relief. With PCA, the patient can be medicated with loading doses until a satisfactory level of pain is reached. Once this level is reached, the patient can then use the PCA boluses to remain comfortable. With most PCA machines, no matter how often a patient pushes the button they will receive only the dose that is programmed into the pump in the preset lockout time.

PCA MEDICATIONS AND ORDERS

There are several medications and medication combinations that can be used in PCA pumps (Table 12.1). The most common opioids are morphine, hydromorphone (Dilaudid), and fentanyl (Sublimaze). Other medications, such as methadone (Dolophine) and buprenorphine (Buprenex), can also be used but have more specific actions such as extended half-life for methadone and mixed agonist-antagonist activity for buprenorphine. Each medication has a benefit that can be used to maximize pain relief for a patient and each patient has a genetic uniqueness that makes some types of medication work most effectively. Pairing the right medication with the patient's genetic predisposition and metabolism characteristics can provide the best pain relief possible.

Clinical Pearl	The binding ability and activity of a medication being used for PCA is in part related to its chemical structure. For example, morphine is hydrophilic (water loving) and tends to spread throughout the body in the aqueous regions. Since the spread is so wide, morphine tends to remain active for longer periods of time. Fentanyl, on the other hand, is lipophylic (fat loving), crosses the blood brain barrier easily, and tends to move in and out of the body more quickly, making it necessary for repeated doses in short periods of time to maintain pain relief.

Table 12.1 ■ *Medication Doses for Use in PCAs*

Medications	Bolus dose	Lockout
morphine	1–2 mg	6–10 min
hydromorphone	0.2–0.4 mg	6–10 min
Fentanyl	10–20 mcg	5–10 min
Buprenorphine	0.03–0.1 mg	8–20 min
Methadone	0.5 mg	8–20 min
Meperidine*	—	—

Basal infusions not recommended for opioid naïve patients.

*Not recommended for use.
Sources: From Hurley, Cohen, & Wu, 2010; Grass, 2005.

As stated, medication choice and dosing for PCA is extremely important and individual. In critical care areas the use of opioids combined with other sedating agents makes careful monitoring for respiratory depression a necessity. The patient must receive enough loading medication either through intermittent injection of doses through the PCA or through the IV so that the patient reaches a comfort level that can be maintained by bolus doses. Medications that can be used in PCA pumps include:

Morphine: Considered the gold standard for IV PCA and equianalgesic conversions. Excreted by glucuronidation, it has a metabolite called morphine-6-glucuronide that is renally excreted, creating the potential for accumulation and delayed excretion. This increases the potential for increasing and delaying sedation in patients with renal impairment. Hydrophilic activity with maximum serum levels is reached within 6 minutes and steady state within 16 to 20 hours (Thomas & von-Gunten, 2006).

Hydromorphone: Considered to be six times more potent than morphine (Grass, 2005). It is metabolized in the liver and excreted as an inactive glucuronide metabolite, which is a benefit for patients with renal impairment. Small doses can provide a high level of pain relief, thus decreasing the potential for adverse effects such as nausea or pruritis. Hydrophilic action is similar to morphine. Hydromorphone is more midrange than morphine and it reaches peak effect in 30 minutes to an hour (Fine & Portneoy, 2007).

Fentanyl: Considered to be 80 to 100 times more potent than morphine with single doses, and with repeated dosing 33 to 40 times the potency of morphine (Grass, 2005). It is metabolized in the liver and not renally excreted, making it a suitable medication for patients with renal failure. Its lipophilicity provide high bioavailability and it can easily penetrate the blood-brain barrier but also has a rapid offset (Thomas & vonGunten, 2006). Peak effect is reached in less than 10 minutes (Fine & Portnoy, 2007).

Methadone: Has lipophilic action with mu receptor agonism, coupled with NMDA receptor antagonist activity (Hurley, Cohen, & Wu, 2010). Prescribing should be reserved for pain specialists or those familiar with methadone prescribing. The half-life of methadone is 8 to 72 hours with 1 to 15 days required to a steady state (Thomas & vonGunten, 2006). This time delay creates a significant potential for delayed respiratory depression (American Pain Society [APS], 2008). Because of the extended half life it may be considered a good choice for highly opioid tolerant oncology patients. Peak effect with methadone is variable but is generally considered to be within 1 to 2 hours (Fine & Portnoy, 2007). Extreme caution should be used in opioid naïve patients. There is also potential for cardiac arrhythmias with long-term use. High-dose oral medication patients will need an electrocardiogram (ECG) as a baseline at medication initiation with a monitoring ECG every 6 months to monitor for any Q-T interval changes (APS, 2008).

Buprenorphine: Mixed agonist-antagonist activity, mu opioid receptor partial agonist coupled with a kappa opioid receptor antagonist (Hurley et al., 2010). Not a first-line option for pain relief, but it has been used successfully for gynecological surgeries. May provoke an acute withdrawal syndrome when a pure opioid agonist has been used for pain control before the mixed agonist-antagonist. High potential for psychotomimetic side effects such as hallucinations (Grass, 2005).

Ketamine: A NMDA receptor antagonist, it blocks activation of NMDA receptor sites that are activated with continued pain stimulus. Combined with opioids in PCA, low-dose ketamine has been shown to reduce opioid consumption (Subramaniam, Subramaniam, & Steinbrook, 2004), but other studies have shown little to no effect on reducing pain, opioid consumption, or side effects (Svetici, Farzanegan, Zmoos, et al., 2008). Additionally, ketamine has a high profile for side effects such as hallucinations, memory problems, abuse, and addiction (APS, 2008). Given the mixed results of the current studies, more research with more consistent positive results would be necessary to make a positive clinical recommendation.

One medication that has fallen out of favor for use in general pain management as well as PCAs is meperidine (Demerol). For many years it was a mainstay for pain relief in postoperative patients. Now, pain management societies have moved the medication from a first-line pain medication to a second-line option and discourage its use altogether. Meperidine has the potential for seizures associated with a toxic metabolite called normeperidine that can accumulate in the CNS fluid. For these reasons it is not recommended for use with patients who have a renal impairment or CNS disease. It should not be used long term and if used at all, the cumulative daily dose should be no higher than 600 mg/24 hr and it should be used for the shortest period of time possible. The best choice is to eliminate the use of this medication and select one of the other medications such as morphine or hydromorphone for PCA use.

The Joint Commission recommends that all hospitals have standard or pre-printed orders that can be used by any practitioners licensed to prescribe opioids. Listed on the order set should be the drug, concentration, loading dose, bolus or demand dose, PCA lockout, and 1 or 4 hour totals. The Joint Commission also recommends the use of standardized concentrations so that fewer medication errors are made when unusual or nonstandard concentrations are ordered. Included on the order set should be a monitoring protocol for frequency of vital signs, oxygen saturation, and respiratory status. Some order sets include an order for naloxone (Narcan), an opioid reversal agent that is used to reverse oversedation in patients. An additional section listing treatments for adverse effects such as nausea, vomiting, pruritis, and urinary retention should be included.

Setting up a PCA requires knowledge of the patient's opioid use prior to the surgery, any prior difficulties with particular opioids, and knowledge of what medications are commonly used for PCA. The use of a basal rate on PCA where medication is delivered continuously is not recommended for opioid naïve patients (Acute Pain Management Scientific Evidence, 2005; APS, 2008; Grass, 2005; Hurley et al., 2010; Institute for Safe Medication Practices [ISMP], 2009). It has been found to have little additive effect for pain relief, but it is considered to be a high risk factor for increasing sedation (APS, 2008; ISMP, 2009). The use of basal infusions on PCAs is more appropriate—in fact, a necessity—when opioid tolerant patients are not taking oral medications and need to have their usual daily oral medication dose changed to PCA delivery postoperatively.

To order a PCA for a patient, first select the opioid with a standard concentration, select the doses and lockout, and add any additional order for anti-emetics, laxatives, etc., and doses.

For example, a PCA prescription might read:

Drug	Morphine 1 mg/mL
Mode	PCA only; no basal rate selected
Loading dose	2 mg
Dose	1 mg
Lockout	6 min
1 hour total	10 mg
Clinician bolus	2 mg every 4 hr as needed for increased pain or activity
Monitoring parameters	Respiratory rate, oxygenation, vital signs Laxatives, antiemetics

An example of a standardized order sheet is provided in Exhibit 12.1. Other important elements of PCA ordering to consider are:

- The loading doses for morphine should be patient dependent and range between 2 to 4 mg (Grass, 2005). An equianalgesic conversion can be used to order loading doses with other medications, e.g., hydromorphone (0.4 mg to 0.8 mg).
- The 1 or 4 hour total is controversial at this time. There are differing opinions as to the necessity of the parameter or whether a 1 or 4 hour total is more effective. The advantage one of using a 1 hour total, which should equal the total number of doses available to the patient in the hour, is that you can quickly determine if there is a need for adjusting PCA doses. By waiting 4 hours the patients may be underdosed or overdosed for a longer period of time.
- Using clinician or supplemental boluses allows the nurse to give an extra dose of medication when the patient needs it. For example, if a patient falls asleep and does not push the button and wakes in pain, the nurse can administer the extra dose after assessing that the patient is stable enough to tolerate the additional medication. These doses are also helpful for providing the patients with additional medication for activity such as physical therapy or walking around the unit.

Patient Controlled Analgesia (PCA)
PHYSICIAN'S ORDERS

| ALLERGIES ➤ | ☐ NKDA |
| | ☐ Other |

I HEREBY AUTHORIZE THE PHARMACY TO DISPENSE A GENERIC EQUIVALENT
UNLESS THE PARTICULAR DRUG IS CIRCLED.

PATIENT PLATE

Physicians: Please draw a line through any orders not desired.

Patient Controlled Analgesia (PCA) Standard Physician Orders

Discontinue all opioids or sedatives unless ordered for use WITH PCA by MD writing PCA orders.

☐ IV Fluid _____ (solution) at _____ ml/hr.

☐ Analgesic: ☐ Morphine   ☐ Dilaudid   ☐ Fentanyl
         1 mg/ml   1 mg/ml   12.5 **micrograms**/ml.

☐ Method of administration:
   ☐ IV PCA only   ☐ IV CONTINUOUS only   ☐ IV PCA and CONTINUOUS

☐ Medication to be administered via PCA pump: (indicate **milligrams** or **micrograms**)
   LOADING DOSE (optional): _____ ☐ mg ☐ **micrograms** (by pump)
   (Suggested adult morphine 2 mg, Dilaudid 0.5 mg., Fentanyl 25 **micrograms**)

   CONTINUOUS INFUSION (optional): _____ ☐ mg or ☐ **micrograms** per hour
   (suggested adult Morphine 1 mg/h., Dilaudid 0.2 mg/h., Fentanyl 12.5 **micrograms**/h)
   *Caution for elderly > 65 y of age, or opioid naïve patients

   ON DEMAND DOSE (PCA dose): _____ ☐ mg or ☐ **micrograms**
   (suggested starting adult dose Morphine 1 mg., Dilaudid 0.2 mg., Fentanyl 12.5 **micrograms**)

   LOCKOUT INTERVAL: _____ minutes   (suggested 6 or 8 minutes)

   1 HOUR LIMIT (Maximum amount of drug in 1 hour. Should equal total amount of hourly doses.)
   _____ ☐ mg or ☐ **micrograms**
   (suggested adult Morphine 10 mg., Dilaudid 3 mg., Fentanyl 200 **micrograms**)

☐ **Clinician bolus:** For increased pain or pain related to increased activity, nurse may bolus patient
   with selected medication above ____ ☐ mg or ☐ **micrograms** every _____ hours. No more
   than 4 doses in a 24 hour period.

☐ In case of IV failure and inability to restart IV give _____ ☐ SQ ☐ IM
   ☐ PO every _____ hour prn and call physician.

☐ Assessment: Documented on the Pain Documentation Sheet.
   *Vital signs, O2 saturation and sedation level every 15 minutes x 4 at start and then every ____
   hrs and each time analgesic dose is increased.
   *For **respirations** less than 8 per minute, stop PCA pump.
   • Narcan Administration:
      1. Dilute one amp of Narcan (0.4 mg.) in 10 ml of normal saline.
      2. Once Narcan is diluted as above:
         For **unarousable** patients give 2.5 ml (0.1mg.) slow IV push. If no response in 90 seconds repeat dose.
         For **apneic patients or resp. rate < 4 per minute** give 5 ml (0.2 mg.) of diluted Narcan
         solution slow IV push. If no response after 90 seconds repeat dose. Continue to repeat dose
         until resp. rate > 14 or O2 saturation 94% or greater.
   *Get STAT ABGs oxygen saturation and apply O2 at 2 liters nasal cannula for saturation less than 94%.
   *Notify Pain Specialist for all occurrences of sedation requiring Narcan administration - send
   computer consult.

☐ Antiemetic: _____ ____ mg ☐ IV ☐ IM ☐ PO ☐ Rectal every ____ hrs prn nausea/vomiting

☐ Laxative: _____ ____ (dose) every ____ hr ☐ PO ☐ Rectal PRN constipation.

| SIGNATURE | TITLE | DATE | TIME | PRINTED | SIGNATURE | TITLE | DATE | TIME | PRINTED |

PATIENT SAFETY ALERT

	USE	Do not use
	DAILY	QD
	EVERY OTHER DAY	QOD
	UNITS	U
0.5 MG.		Lack of leading zero (e.g. .5 mg)
10 MG.		Trailing zero (e.g. 10.0 mg)
MORPHINE SULFATE		MS or MSO4
MAGNESIUM SULFATE		MgSO4
MICRO-GRAM OR MCG.		µg or µ for microgram
INTER-NATIONAL UNITS		IU
LEFT EAR; RIGHT EAR; BOTH EARS		A.S.; A.D.; A.U.
LEFT EYE; RIGHT EYE; BOTH EYES;		O.S.; O.D.; O.U.

Exhibit 12.1 ■ Example of standardized PCA order sheet.

■ Monitoring parameters help to ensure that the patient is being carefully watched while using PCA. If supplemental oxygen is being used,
electronic monitoring with pulse oximetry may be skewed with blood
oxygen levels in the 70s while oximetry readings may be much higher
(Vila, 2005). Having the nurse assess the patient regularly (every 2 to
4 hr) provides a trained eye on the patient's real status. Additionally,

capnography, which monitors end tidal carbon dioxide levels (etCO$_2$), has been found to provide a more accurate reading on blood oxygen levels in postoperative patients and is being used more frequently in the postoperative setting. Some national guidelines recommend the use of both capnography and pulse oximetry (Institute for Safe Medication Practices [ISMP], 2003).

MONITORING AND TREATING ADVERSE EFFECTS WITH PCA

Sedation/Oversedation

Respiratory depression, sedation, and oversedation can occur with any patient. Although these events are though to occur frequently, the actual level of occurrence is thought to be less than 5% (Hurley et al., 2010), 0.19% to 5.2 % (Hagle, Lehr, Brubakken, & Shippee, 2004), 0.25% (Grass, 2005), respectively. Compared to the incidence of respiratory depression of 0.9% for intermittent IM injections, PCA compares favorably (Grass, 2005). Monitoring parameters are set by order on the PCA form. Using a simple numeric sedation scale, the Ramsey on general nursing units or the RASS in critical settings, may find early stages of sedation and avoid progression to over sedation. Conditions that contribute to respiratory depression with PCA use include concomitant administration of other sedating agents such as sleeping medications, obesity, the use of a basal rate, advanced age, and pulmonary conditions such as sleep apnea (Hurley et al., 2010). Additionally, Hagle et al. (2004) report that risk factors for sedation with PCA include: age greater than 70, basal infusion with IV PCA; renal, hepatic, pulmonary, or cardiac impairment; sleep apnea; concurrent central nervous system depressants; obesity; upper abdominal or thoracic surgery; and an IV PCA bolus dose greater than 1 mg.

If the patient becomes oversedated, the use of naloxone is recommended to reverse the effects of the opioid and to restore normal respiratory status. For patients with sleep apnea, the ASA and the Joint Commission both recommend more aggressive monitoring when opioids are used in the postoperative setting.

Postoperative Nausea/Vomiting (PONV)

All opioid medications have the potential to create nausea and vomiting. A Consensus Guideline by the American Society of Anesthesiologists (2004) indicates that some patients are at a higher risk of developing PONV, including female sex, history of motion sickness or PONV, nonsmokers, and use of postoperative opioids. The use of antiemetics is needed for these patients to control PONV. For many patients the use of antiemetics start in the operating room in an effort to control PONV.

Constipation

As with PONV, constipation is the natural outcome of regular opioid use. For all patients using opioids for postoperative pain, control laxatives and stool softeners are recommended to maintain adequate bowel function. Constipation is the only adverse effect for which patients cannot develop tolerance. The use of stool softeners such as Colace and laxative such as Senokot, Miralax, or milk of magnesia can restore normal bowel function despite opioid use.

Pruritis

All opioids can cause pruritis and some patients are more prone to pruritis with opioids. The occurrence of pruritis does not mean that the patient has an allergy to the medications. The generalized itching felt by that patient with opioid use is the result of histamine release. It follows, therefore, that the use of an antihistamine, such as diphenhydramine (Benedryl), is recommended. Unfortunately, if diphenylamine is used, it can add to the cumulative sedation potential for the patient and lower doses are considered appropriate, especially if used for the elderly.

Delirium, Confusion

With older patients taken out of familiar surroundings and receiving medications for pain and surgery, confusion and delirium can occur. Some practitioners confuse the demented patient's progressive decline in cognitive function with delirium, a sudden onset of an acute confused state. Although most often considered to be a condition that affects the older patient, delirium can happen to any patient who receives opioids or surgical medications, or who undergoes a form of sedation. The incidence of delirium in the general hospital population is felt to range from 10% to 60% of all patients (Vaurio, Sands, Wang, Mullen, & Leung, 2006). Patients who are taking oral pain medications have less delirium while older patients and those who receive IV pain medications have a higher rate of delirium (Vaurio et al., 2006). It is also important to note that unrelieved pain can contribute to delirium.

If a patient on PCA becomes confused, changing medication to the oral route may possibly help, but adding other nonopioid interventions such as NSAIDs, blocks, and neural blockade may be helpful while eliminating other contributing medications such as benzodiazepines and other medications with CNS effects.

RECOMMENDATIONS FOR SAFE PCA USE

The Joint Commission and the ISMP have tracked PCA use for many years. They have found that there are significant safety issues with PCA and have issued some recommendations to make the practice safer for all, prescribers and patients.

One of the issues that has emerged from safety monitoring systems include cases of overdose and death, with the PCA found to play a role in each case (ISMP, 2003; Joint Commission on Accreditation of Healthcare Organizations [JACHO], 2005). Current estimates of risk with PCA indicate that death from user programming errors was estimated to be 1 in 33,000 to 1 in 338,800, resulting in an estimate of 65 to 667 deaths in the history of use of the device (Vicente, Kada-Bekhaled, Hillel, Cassano, & Orser, 2003). Other concerns are linked to operator error and misprogramming. In one quality improvement study, 71% of the errors found were related to misprogramming causing either overmedication or undermedication; 15% were related to human factors, resulting in the administration of the wrong medication; and 9% were related to equipment problems (Weir, 2005).

Breaking down the programming errors, the most common errors were found to be:
■ Confusion over milliliter and milligram
■ Confusing the PCA bolus dose with the basal dose
■ Entering the loading dose instead of the bolus dose
■ Wrong lockout setting selected
■ Wrong medication concentration selected (ISMP, 2003)

Because of the errors that were found in the monitoring systems, the Joint Commission and the ISMP have made recommendations about PCA that can help to ensure the safest possible PCA practice. The current recommendations include two independent nurse checks of medication, concentration, and dose settings; clear identification of the IV line where the PCA is infusing; use of pre-filled syringes or bags; and use of standardized order sets.

The Joint Commission has also addressed some pertinent practice issues and has made recommendations for practice in these areas.

Proper Patient Selection

Choosing the correct patient type and limiting PCA use to those patients who are good candidates can ensure that PCA is properly used. PCA is a fairly simple concept to understand and children as young as five years of age have demonstrated that they can safely activate a PCA pump. The Joint

Commission and the ISMP have listed several patient groups that they feel are not good candidates for PCA use, Including:
- Infants and young children
- Confused older adults
- Patients who are obese or have sleep apnea or asthma
- Patients taking other medications with sedating effects, such as muscle relaxants antiemetics, and sleeping medications (Cohen & Smetzer, 2005)

PCA by Proxy

The term PCA by proxy is usually defined as the activation of the PCA pump by someone other than the patient, usually a friend or family member who perceives the patient to be in pain but unable to activate the pump independently. Most hospitals have a policy that prevents anyone but the patient from activating the PCA. This prohibition includes nurses or other staff members. Once the patient him- or herself is removed from the PCA process, the possibility of potentially fatal over sedation is very real. Of the 460 PCA errors reported to the PCA errors database of the United States Pharmacopeia, 12 were related to PCA by proxy with one fatal event.

PCA Pump Safety

Since the PCA pump is an integral piece of the PCA process, safe pump design can help minimize the occurrence of adverse events, medication errors, and misprogramming. PCA pump buttons should not resemble call lights, so that the patient can discriminate which button brings the nurse and which one delivers pain medication. Intuitive programming features can make it easier for nurses to enter prescriptions and monitor medication usage. Free flow protection should be a part of every pump that is designed for use as a PCA.

Human Error

Human error is always possible when interacting with machines but designing pumps that are simple and easy to use while protecting the patient can help to decrease error. Nurses are also responsible for learning to correctly enter PCA orders and for maintaining competency in PCA practice. Using root cause analysis after PCA-related incidents can help pinpoint areas in the PCA process that need correction so that future errors can be avoided.

PATIENTS NEEDING SPECIAL CONSIDERATION WITH PCA USE

Although the Joint Commission has set recommendations for patient selection with PCA use, there are other patient populations that require special consideration. Cognitively intact older patients, patients with a history of substance abuse, and patients who use opioids for relief of chronic pain require special consideration when PCA is being considered as a means of pain control. Other factors such as weight play no role in PCA dosing, although men have been found to require more morphine than women (Burns et al., 1989).

Older Patients

Patients who are older than 65 years of age require special considerations when PCAs are being used for pain management. Despite their older age they can be excellent candidates for PCA use, especially during major orthopedic procedures such as total joint replacements. The majority of these patients are opioid naïve and have some level of organ dysfunction related to age. For these patients, opioids can be prescribed but the doses should be reduced by 25% to 50% and monitoring should be more frequent. In a study comparing morphine consumption in younger versus older patients, for patients 20 to 30 years of age, morphine consumption was 75 mg, while for those patients aged 60 to 70, morphine consumption was 30 mg (Macintyre & Jarvis, 1996).

Patients With Chronic Pain

Patients who have chronic pain or are taking regular opioids for pain relief present another difficult-to-treat patient group. These patients have advanced pain processing pathophysiology that may make their pain more intense, may increase sensitivity to pain, and may reduce the effectiveness of opioids. For these patients, their normal daily doses of opioids should be restarted as soon as possible and continued through their hospitalization. They will also need additional medication for the new acute pain. If the usual oral medications cannot be restarted in a timely fashion, the conversion to IV or PCA will need to be made but the efficacy of these doses may also be reduced. For these patients, a continuous infusion using an equianalgesic conversion and allowing for the PCA demand dose medication will have to be performed. Many pharmacists are skilled at these conversions and are willing to help the prescriber with conversion doses.

Patients With a Substance Abuse History

For patients with a history of substance abuse or active drug use, treating pain either from acute injury or surgery is a challenge. Since there is no equianalgesic conversion for street drugs, a best-guess estimate will be needed and a full history of how much drug is being used daily is essential. The actively addicted patient will need a continuous infusion with generous bolus doses to account for any underdosing.

Patients with a history of substance abuse have used drugs in the past, but even though they are not using them now, they still have pathophysiologic changes that make treating the pain more difficult. Such patients also have increased sensitivity to pain stimulus and decreased efficacy of opioid medications. For these patients, a continuous rate may be needed and the doses will need to be higher than the surgery or acute pain might indicate. Although these patients are highly opioid tolerant, it is still possible to have them become oversedated if the doses are large enough so it is important to maintain the frequent monitoring parameters.

For all of these patients PCA is a good option although there are adjustments that will need to be made. It is important to set up reasonable expectations about medication use and pain relief. Postoperative patients cannot expect to be pain free and although some patients have chronic pain, the focus in the postoperative setting is on the surgical pain.

> *Clinical Pearl*
>
> In order to use the 0 to 10 nonverbal pain scale (NPS) for difficult-to-treat patients, ask the patient with chronic pain what his or her average daily pain score is and set a realistic pain goal of 2 or 3 points lower for the new acute pain. For older patients, set an achievable pain goal and ask the patient what pain rating would be reasonable that would allow the patient to participate in activities and physical therapy. For addicted patients or patients with a history of substance abuse, set parameters around medication use and set a reasonable goal for pain relief. Explain that no pain or 0/10 pain is not reasonable for the type of surgery/injury the patient has sustained. Also indicate that purposeful sedation is not the goal of PCA therapy; pain relief is the focus and goal.

Charles Sands is admitted to the critical care unit after a motorcycle accident on the interstate highway. He was going at high speed and hit the guardrail full on. He has sustained a concussion and multiple orthopedic injuries that include a fractured pelvis and fractures of both the right arm and leg. He is sent to surgery to repair his arm and leg fractures. He is alert and oriented after waking from his anesthesia and complains of severe level pain in his leg and pelvis, cannot stand to be repositioned because of pain, and tells you he has a headache. His morphine PCA is set at 1 mg every 8 minutes and he says it feels like he is getting no medication when he pushes the button. You ask Charles about his opioid use preadmission and he tells you he has been taking 6 Percocet a day for chronic low back pain prescribed to him by his primary care practitioner. When you ask him about other substances and alcohol he denies ever using them. You review his admission urine drug screen and find he has shown a positive response for marijuana and benzodiazipines for which he has no prescription, as well as opioids. What can you do to improve the pain relief for Charles so you can reposition him without severe pain?

1. What would be the first option for improving Charles's pain? Change the setting and increase the dose? Add a basal rate since he is opioid tolerant? Provide clinician boluses for activities such as repositioning?
2. Would changing the medication to another opioid be beneficial?
3. NSAIDs may be contraindicated due to the increased risk of bleeding but what other adjuvant medications could be used to help control the severe pain?
4. Does the fact that Charles has a concussion affect his use of opioids?
5. What do you do about the fact that Charles is taking benzodiazepines for which he has no prescription and had been smoking marijuana? Do you confront him or have an open conversation about the need to know about his substance use? Do you question his Percocet use since he has failed to tell you about his substance use and may be underestimating his Percocet use?

REFERENCES

Acute Pain Management: SE Working Group of the Australian and New Zealand College of Anesthetists and faculty of Pain Medicine. (2005). *Acute pain management: Scientific evidence* (2nd ed.). Melbourne, Australia: Author.

American Pain Society. (2008). *Principles of analgesic use in the treatment of acute pain and cancer pain* (6th ed.). Glenview, IL: Author.

American Society of Anesthesiologists. (2004). *Practice guidelines for acute pain management in the perioperative setting.* Park Ridge, IL: Author.

Burns, J. W., Hodsman, N. B., McLintock, T. T., Gillies, G. W., Kenny, G. N., McArdle, C. S. (1989). The influence of patient characteristics on the requirements for postoperative analgesia. A reassessment using patient-controlled analgesia. *Anaesthesia, 44,* 2–6.

Cohen, M. R., & Smetzer, J. (2005). Patient-controlled analgesia safety issues. *Journal of Pain and Palliative Care Pharmacotherapy, 19*(1), 45–50.

Grass, J. A. (2005). Patient controlled analgesia. *Anesthesia and Analgesia, 101,* S44–S61.

Hagle, M. E., Lehr, V. T., Brubakken, K., & Shippee, A. (2004). Respiratory depression in adults patients with intravenous patient-controlled analgesia. *Orthopedic Nursing, 23*(1), 18–27.

Hudcova, J., McNicol, E., Quah, C., Lau, J., & Carr, D. B. (2006). Patients controlled analgesia versus conventional opioid analgesia for postoperative pain. *Cochrane Database of systematic reviews,* (4), CD003348.

Hurley, R. W., Cohen, S. P., & Wu, C. L. (2010). Acute pain in adults. In S. M. Fishman, J. C. Ballantyne, & J. P. Rathmell (Eds.), *Bonica's Management of Pain* (4th ed., pp. 699–706). Philadelphia, PA: Wolters Kluwer Health-Lippincott Williams & Wilkins.

Institute for Safe Medication Practices. (2003). *Patient controlled analgesia: Making it safer for patients.* Retrieved from http://www.ismp.org/profdevelopment/PCAMonograph.pdf

Institute for Safe Medication Practices Medication Safety Alert. (2009). Beware of basal opioid infusions with PCA therapy. *Nurse Advis-ERR, 7*(10). Retrieved October, from http://www.ismp.org/Newsletters/nursing/issues

Joint Commission on Accreditation of Healthcare Organizations. (2005). Focus on five: Preventing patient controlled analgesia overdose. *Joint Commission Perspective on Patient Safety, 5,* 11.

Macintyre, P. E., & Jarvis, D. A. (1996). Age is the best predictor of post-operative morphine requirements. *Pain, 64,* 357–364.

Subramaniam, K., Subramaniam, B., & Steinbrook, R. A. (2004). Ketamine as an adjuvant to opioids: A quantitative and qualitative systematic review. *Anesthesia and Analgesia, 99,* 482–495.

Thomas, J., & vonGunten, C. F. (2006). Pharmacologic therapies for pain. In J. H. Von Roenn, J. A. Paice, & M. E. Preodor (Eds.), *Current diagnosis & treatment of pain* (pp. 21–37). New York, NY: Lange Medical Books/McGraw-Hill.

Vicente, K. J., Kada-Bekhaled, K., Hillel, G., Cassano, A., & Orser, B. A. (2003). Programming errors contribute to death from patient-controlled analgesia: case report and estimate of probability. *Canadian Journal of Anaesthesia, 50,* 328–332.

Vaurio, L. E., Sands, L. P., Wang, Y., Mullen, E. A., & Leung, J. M. (2006). Postoperative delirium: The importance of pain and pain management. *Anesthesia and Analgesia, 102*(4), 1267–1273.

Weir, V. L. (2005). Best practice protocols: Preventing adverse drug events. *Nursing Management, 36*(9), 24–30.

13

Regional Techniques and Epidural Analgesia for Pain Relief in Critical Care

EPIDURAL BASICS

Epidural pain management can provide the largest amount of pain relief with the least amount of medication. This is because equianalgesically the doses of opioids delivered to the epidural and intrathecal spaces are several times more potent than the same medications given intravenously. Adding a local anesthetic such as bupivacaine or ropivacaine to the epidural solution creates a synergistic effect that enhances the overall analgesic effect of the epidural.

For patient in critical care areas, the use of epidurals can provide excellent pain relief with less opioid than usually required. It can allow the patient with a thoracotomy or flail chest to cough and deep breathe more effectively and, for other patients, increase mobility. Trauma patients can benefit greatly from the use of an epidural or other regional technique in order to control pain that can last for several weeks at high intensity levels.

In most cases the epidural is placed perioperatively and either used during surgery as an alternate to general anesthesia but also as postoperative analgesia. The opioid medications used for epidural pain management bind to opioid receptors in the dorsal horn of the spinal cord and can produce effective analgesia at greatly reduced doses. The addition of local anesthetic allows the nerve roots closest to the placement site to be bathed in the epidural solution, causing localized pain relief. In most cases epidurals used for postoperative pain relief have solutions that contain both low dose opioids and local anesthetic.

Some patients are resistant to epidural catheters fearing that they will have a needle in their backs during the entire time of infusion. Patients should be reassured that the needle is only used for placing the catheter and the tubing that remains is very small and soft.

Patients who are good candidates for epidural analgesia are patients with major surgeries or procedures such as:

- Thoracotomy
- Large abdominal surgeries
- Aortic aneurysm repair
- Orthopedic patients (total joint replacements)
- Labor and delivery patients (used for delivery)
- Trauma patients with multiple rib fractures or flail chest (Level 1; Evidence from Guidelines for Blunt Force Trauma, 2004)

In a study of 226 thoracotomy patients randomized to thoracic epidural and general anesthesia or general anesthesia only, length of stay was significantly reduced in the combined group and median intubation time and the incidence of arrhythmias were both significantly lower (Caputo et al., 2011). Additional findings indicated that although there was an increased use of vasoconstrictors intraoperatively in the combined anesthesia/analgesia group, impairment from pain was lower and morphine consumption was also lower in the combined group (Caputo et al., 2011).

To place an epidural catheter, the patient is placed into a sitting or side lying position with the back flexed in an outward curve. The anesthesiologist or certified nurse anesthetist inserts a beveled hollow needle through the skin of the back into the epidural space, which is really a potential space between the ligament flavum and the dura mater. Once fluid enters the epidural space it expands, much like blowing air into a flat paper bag expands the bag. Once the needle is placed at the correct dermatome, the epidural catheter is threaded through the needle and placement is confirmed by a technique called loss of resistance. This means that the resistance felt by the tissue at the tip of the catheter is relieved once an open space such as the epidural space is reached. For epidural placement, the needle itself does not extend into the cerebral spinal fluid (CSF) or the spinal cord.

Once the anesthesiologist or certified nurse anesthetist feels a loss of resistance it is fairly certain that the catheter has entered the epidural space. After the catheter is determined to be placed properly, the practitioner can then bolus the catheter to determine the effect. The epidural space contains a variety of structures that include spinal nerve roots, fat, areolar tissue, lymph tissue, and blood vessels including a rich venous plexus (Rockford & Deruyter, 2009). Since the analgesic effect is so localized, the catheter is placed at the level of the expected surgical incision with catheter placement being done commonly in the thoracic and lumbar spinal levels. The medication "spread" is determined by the site of injection. "Spread" is defined as the spread of the medication either rosteral or caudal from the expected dermatomal level. Additional factors that may influence the spread of the medication are the patient's age and the volume of drug being infused (Rockford & De Ruyter, 2009).

It is important to note that once the epidural catheter reaches the epidural space, it can migrate upward (rostral) or downward (caudal). This migration can affect the way the patient feels the analgesic effect. In some cases the epidural catheter provides analgesia to a nonoperative lower extremity when the intent is to provide analgesic to the operative extremity. This effect is caused by the curling of the catheter in the epidural space leading to a reduced effect in the desired location.

Spinal or Intrathecal Differences

It is more precise to use the terms epidural and intrathecal analgesia although the term spinal, when used, is closely associated with intrathecal placement. For some patients a single dose of preservative-free morphine is used as an adjunct to postoperative analgesia. These doses are commonly referred to as "single shots." They are given one time only and an extended-release morphine such as Astromorph, Duramorph, or DepoDur is used to extend the action of the medication for 24 hours. Since morphine is a hydrophilic medication, it can spread throughout the CSF and extend the action of the medication. A single shot Duramorph injection is done using 0.1 to 0.3 mg with the dose being dependent on the patient's history and prior opioid use (APS, 2008; ASPAN, 2003).

When an intrathecal catheter is placed for continuous infusion, the catheter extends directly into the thecal space and the medication flows into the CSF. Either opioids or local anesthetics can be used intrathecally, but continuous infusion of local anesthetics is associated in some cases with the development of cauda equina syndrome (Scientific Evidence, 2005).

Since medications inserted into the epidural space need to cross the dura, onset of action of epidural analgesia is slower when compared to intrathecal administration. A hydrophilic medication such as a morphine is more useful as medications infused into the intrathecal space spread through the CSF. Uptake can take place locally at the site of the insertion through spinal blood vessels, fatty tissue, and CSF, and doses lower than those used epidurally may produce effective analgesia.

EPIDURAL MEDICATIONS

All medications used for epidural analgesia should be preservative free since many preservatives such as alcohol can damage neural tissue. The opioid medications used for epidural analgesia are basically the same as those used with PCA, but there are also different local anesthetic agents that are used in combined solutions. When epidural is compared to intrathecal medication administration, the epidural route has fewer side effects and a lessened potential for respiratory depression (Rockford & DeRuyter, 2009).

Opioids

Morphine, hydromorphone, and fentanyl are the three most common medications used for epidural analgesia. The two drugs recommended for use in epidurals are morphine and fentanyl with hydromophone having less evidence for use (American Society of Anesthesiologists [ASA], 2004).The choice of which medication to use for infusion is provider dependent and patient specific. If the patient has allergies to morphine, another medication is selected and adequate pain relief is the measure of effectiveness.

When comparing the use of morphine versus fentanyl, the pharmacokinetics shows a differentiation of action. Morphine is a hydrophilic medication. When morphine is used in epidural solutions there is a rapid rise in morphine serum concentration, and the action is similar to IV PCA (Rockford & DeRuyter, 2009). Conversely, when fentanyl, a lipophilic medication, is used in epidural solutions, the serum concentration of the medication rises more slowly due to medication uptake by epidural fat and other epidural tissues. To approximate the action of IV medication administration, it takes about 25 hours for the lipid uptake of fentanyl to allow the drug to freely enter the circulatory system (Rockford & DeRuyter, 2009). Morphine has a naturally occurring longer action, while fentanyl has a shorter period of activity making it more suitable for use as an epidural PCA that is called patient controlled epidural analgesia (PCEA). Hydromorphone is a midrange medication whose action falls somewhere between morphine and fentanyl.

Clinical Pearl	To compare equivalent doses of morphine, consider that morphine 30 mg orally is equivalent to 10 mg intravenously, 1 mg epidural, and 100 mg intrathecal (APS, 2008).

Local Anesthetics (LAs)

The two most commonly used local anesthetics (LAs) for epidurals are preservative-free bupivacaine and ropivacaine. These medications are used because of all the possible LAs, they have the longest action, which makes them more suitable for continuous infusion. When used in an epidural solution, the role of the LA is to bathe the nerve roots, dorsal root ganglia, spinal nerves in the paravertebral space, and nerve rootlets creating paresthesia and analgesia. Combining a LA with an opioid produces a synergistic effect and superior pain relief (APS, 2008; Hurley, Cohen, & Wu, 2010; Scientific Evidence, 2005). Ropivacaine is thought to have a lessened effect on muscles and is commonly used in epidurals for patients who will be actively engaged in physical therapy or early ambulation postoperatively such as total joint replacement patients.

Additional Medications

Clonidine is an alpha 2-agonist used to treat pain. For neuropathic pain, a continuous infusion of clonidine at 30 mcg per hour demonstrated a positive effect (Eisenach, DuPen, Dubois, Miguel, & Allin, 1995). Other studies demonstrated an analgesic effect when clonidine is used alone and a synergistic effect to prolong epidural blockade (Forster & Rosenberg, 2004). Side effects of clonidine include hypotension, sedation, and bradycardia (Hurley, Cohen, & Wu, 2010). In order to stop a clonidine infusion, careful titration downward over several days is recommended to avoid rebound hypertension (Rockford & DeRuyter, 2009).

Medications Used for Epidural Infusions

Medication	Loading Dose	Continuous Infusion	Bolus Dose-PCEA	Lockout	Onset	Duration of Single Dose
Morphine	1–6 mg (age dependent)	0.1–1.0 mg/hr	50–200 mcg NR	30–45 min	30 min	6–24 hr
Fentanyl	50–100 mcg	50–100 mcg/hr	15–20 mcg	10 min	5 min	4–8 hr
Hydromorphone	0.4–1.0 mg	30–120 mcg/hr	20–40 mcg	15 min	5–8 min	4–6 hr
Clonidine	NR	0.30	NR	NR	NR	NR
Local Anesthetic						
Bupivacaine 0.1%		3–10 mL/hr				
Ropivacaine 0.2%		3–10 mL/hr				NR
Clonidine	Used an adjuvant					

NR, not recommned due to delay of action.
Source: Hurley, Cohen, & Wu, 2010; Grass, 2005; APS, 2008; Rockford & DeRuyter, 2009.

MONITORING PATIENTS ON EPIDURAL ANALGESIA

Careful and consistent monitoring of patients on epidural analgesia is needed to not only ensure adequate analgesic, but the safety of patients using this method for postoperative pain relief. Vital signs, respiratory rates, and pain assessments will need to be done very frequently in the postoperative recovery unit and then hourly for the first few hours. Assessments can move to 2 hours after the initial postoperative time period and as the patient stabilizes.

Indicators that should be monitored are as follows.

Site Care

Inspect the site for swelling, drainage, infiltration, and any signs of redness. The dressing over the epidural site should remain dry and intact. Tubing connections should be secured and remain tight (ASPMN, 2009).

Pain Relief

The patient's level of analgesia should be assessed regularly and dose adjustments made as needed with the order of the anesthesiologist. Patients may need bolus doses after physical activity or as postoperative medication wears off.

Other elements that should be assessed regularly include:
- *Respiratory depression*: Reduce or stop the opioid infusion. For significant sedation and decreased respiratory rate below 8 or 10 breaths per minute, naloxone administration may be needed with an alternate method of pain management.
- *Motor block*: Stop or reduce the infusion.
- *Confusion related to opioid use*: Reduce or stop the infusion and ask for a trial of a LA infusion only to reduce the effect of the opioid.

TREATING SIDE EFFECTS AND SPECIAL CONSIDERATIONS

Sedation/Oversedation

As with all forms of opioids, oversedation with ensuing respiratory depression is a possibility. The overall rates of respiratory depression with epidural analgesia are 0.1% to 0.9% (Deleon-Cassola, Parker, & Lema, 1994). Hyrodrophilic medications such as morphine are thought to have the potential for delayed respiratory depression while lipophilic medications such as a fentanyl are believed to have more potential for early respiratory depression (Hurley, Cohen, & Wu, 2010). The use of supplemental oxygen can skew the mechanical reading of oxygenation provided by oxygen monitoring. For a more accurate reading of blood oxygen levels, the use of capnography or end tidal CO_2 monitoring is recommended. Patients with epidural analgesia will need consistent and frequent monitoring for the onset of respiratory depression.

Nausea/Vomiting

Nausea and vomiting are common side effects of opioid use. The occurrence is estimated to be between 45% and 80% of all patients (White, Berhausen, & Dumont, 1992). Using anitemetics such as ondansetron, dexamethsasone, and scopolamine patches can help reduce the effects of the nausea and vomiting but can also increase sedation.

Pruritis

Pruritis or generalized itching is one of the most common side effects of epidural analgesia occurring in about 60% of the patients (Hurley, Cohen, & Wu, 2010). The mechanism of pruritis with epidural opioids is not well understood. It was once thought to be caused by a histamine release but the source is now thought to be centered in the higher cerebral centers (Hurley, Cohen, & Wu, 2010). The one fact that can be confirmed is that pruritis is not a result of a true allergic reaction. It can be treated with a variety of medications that include hydroxyzine (Atarax), naloxone (Narcan), and nalbuphine (Nubaine) at reduced doses.

Hypotension

The hypotension found with epidural analgesia is the direct result of the LA combined with postoperative hypovolemia. With the LA, the blood vessels dilate and decrease the fluid pressure within the vessel. If the patient is hypovolemic, the effect will be more pronounced. Fluid bolus and epidural rate reduction, if possible, are the recommended actions for hypotension with epidural analgesia.

Motor Block

In some cases, epidural analgesia has a greater effect on motor function and a blockade may be produced as a result of the LA. The incidence of motor block is higher with lumbar epidural placement (Gwirtz et al., 1999), but the overall incidence is low at 2% to 3% of all patients (Hurley, Cohen, &

Wu, 2010). Patients may first experience numbness along the lateral thigh and if infusion rates are not decreased, the blockade can proceed across the thigh muscles causing a loss of quadriceps strength. Patients who are receiving epidural analgesia with LA and PCEA especially should always be tested for quadriceps strength before trying to stand.

Urinary Retention

Urinary retention for patients with epidural catheters receiving infusions with opioids and LA is the result of detrusor muscle weakness from the LA effect on the spinal cord opioid receptors. The average estimated rate of urinary retention is felt to be about 10% to 30% (Hurley, Cohen, & Wu, 2010). Urinary catheters may be needed for the first days of epidural analgesia therapy to avoid urinary retention.

Anticoagulants and Epidurals

Most patients who are on epidural analgesia may require anticoagulation either as prophylaxis for thrombus formation, or as a treatment as is the case with thoracotomy patients. Since many patients in critical care areas are anticoagulated, it is an important consideration when epidural catheter use is being considered. In either case, the use of anticoagulants must be carefully monitored in the postoperative period. Recommendations for catheter placement and removal to avoid the formation of an epidural hematoma are given in the following section.

Safety Issues With Epidural Infusions

One of the most dangerous and significant side effects with epidural analgesia is epidural hematoma. An epidural hematoma is created by bleeding into the epidural space by tissue damage, usually when the catheter is placed or removed. If the patient is anticoagulated, the potential for epidural hematoma formation is increased. Although infrequent, the seriousness of the hematoma formation cannot be minimized. Since the bleeding is taking place in a limited and confined area inside the spinal column, the expansion of the blood creates a clot that presses on the spinal cord leading to spinal cord compression. The cord compression can lead to a spinal cord injury and permanent paralysis if not detected in the early stages.

Patients with epidural hematoma complain of extremely severe back pain that progresses to loss of lower extremity function and loss of bowel and bladder control. Any patient with an epidural catheter who complains of extreme pain and is on anticoagulants should immediately be screened by CT or MRI for epidural hematoma formation.

Because of the significant consequences of an epidural hematoma, the American Society of Regional Anesthesiologists (ASRA, 2002) has drafted a position paper with criteria for use of anticoagulants with epidural patients.

These recommendations include:

Subcutaneous heparin:

No contraindication for placement or catheter removal

Warfarin:

INR required to be less than 1.5 for catheter removal, no placement with elevated INR

Low molecular weight heparins:

Thrombophylaxis: Placement 10 to 12 hours after last dose; removal either directly before daily dose or 10 to 12 hours after last dose. Medication can be resumed 2 hours after catheter removal

Treatment doses: Placement: 24 hours after last dose; removal of catheter prior to treatment

Antiplatelet medications:

Ticlopidine: Catheter placemen; discontinuation of medication in 14 days

Clopidogrel: Catheter placement; discontinuation of medication in 7 days

Fondaparinux: Avoid using indwelling catheters (ASRA, 2002)

Epidural Catheter Migration

Epidural catheter migration from the epidural space through the dura into the spinal canal is relatively rare. The clinical sign that this should be considered is continued sedation of the patient despite dose reductions. In order to confirm that the catheter has migrated, the catheter fluid can be aspirated and checked for the presence of glucose, which would indicate that the catheter has migrated into the CSF.

Epidural Abscess

The occurrence of epidural abscess is rare, cited as 1 in 1,930 in one study (Wang, Hauerberg, & Schmiodt, 1999) and infection rates listed as 1.1 in 100,00 in other reviews (Aromaa, Lahdensuu, & Coznaitits, 1997). The most recent recommendation by ASRA relate to careful use of aseptic technique when catheters are being placed to avoid any contamination that could allow for abscess formation (Horlocker, Wedel, & Benzon, 2003). Patients who are experiencing an epidural abscess present with much the same complaints as those with epidural hematoma—severe back pain, neurological changes, and, with abscess, fever. MRI can clearly identify the site of the abscess formation. A delay in diagnosis can lead to a greater risk of permanent motor impairment (Davies, Wald, & Patel, 2004).

Outcomes

The outcomes related to epidural analgesia are very good when compared to other techniques. In a Cochrane DARE review, epidural analgesia was superior for pain relief when compared to all other routes of postoperative pain control (Block, Liu, Rowlingson, Cowan, Cowan, & Wu, 2005). In a review article by Viscusi (2005), epidural analgesia was reported to improve analgesia, increase patient satisfaction, and improve clinical outcomes. Intrathecal analgesia for postoperative pain relief was studied in a large study with 5,969 adult patients by Gwirtz et al. (1999) and the finding indicated that over a 7-year period, with the large number of participants, patient satisfaction with the technique was very high and the occurrence of side effects and complications was very low.

As always, multimodal therapies are the best recommendation for postoperative pain management but using epidural analgesia as the base can provide high benefits with few negatives. As practice evolves and more becomes known about the way that the body perceives postoperative pain and analgesic actions, better outcomes can be expected with these techniques.

RATIONALE FOR USE OF REGIONAL ANALGESIA

Since 30% to 80% of surgical patients report moderate to severe pain after surgery (Apfelbaum, Chen, Mehta, & Gan, 2003; Mcgrath et al., 2004), it is important to provide the highest level of postoperative analgesia possible. This means the use of multiple techniques to control pain. The use of peripheral catheters with local anesthetic is particularly helpful for critical care patients who may have large incisions that are extremely painful. The use of regional anesthesia has been recommended by the American Society of Anesthesiologists (ASA, 2004) as a means of extending the superior pain management of the operating room. There are two main techniques or types that are used: intraoperative neural blockade, a one time procedure, and continuous peripheral nerve or wound catheters.

By using a blockade or continuous infusion, the use of opioids can be minimized in the postoperative setting resulting in fewer adverse effects such as nausea and vomiting. The level of pain relief with a regional analgesia technique is superior to opioids alone and reduces opioid-related side effects such as nausea, vomiting, sedation, and pruritis (Liu & Salinsa,

2003; Le-Wendling & Enneking, 2008; Richman et al., 2005). Pain relief and functionality are improved with the use of a peripheral catheter (PC) (Rosenquist & Rosenberg, 2003). There is also some indication that the use of regional anesthesia, epidurals, and regional analgesia has a positive impact on mortality and morbidity with high risk patients (Hanna, Murphy, Kumar, & Wu, 2009).

In a systematic review of regional techniques for postthoracotomy pain, there was equal support for the use of thoracic epidurals and continuous paravertebral block with local anesthetic (Joshi et al., 2008). The second recommendation with less support was for the use of intrathecal opioid or intercostal block, which was found to last less time than needed to fully control the pain (Joshi et al., 2008).

The current day anesthesia provider has many more options for increasing the effectiveness of postoperative analgesia, including extending the controlled anesthetic and analgesic techniques of the operating room into the postoperative time period. Using single injections for regional blockade and inserting peripheral nerve catheters (PCs) that can provide extended adjunct pain relief can help the surgical patient or the trauma patient recover faster with fewer side effects.

INTRAOPERATIVE BLOCKADE

Intraoperative blockade can be used to reduce pain in the immediate postoperative time period. There are a variety of blocks that can be used, such as plexus, illioinguinal, penile, axillary, or femoral to name a few. The use of a blockade can extend the analgesia of the operating room into the first hours of the recovery time period. The disadvantage of using a single block is the limited effect. Postoperative one-time blocks can last for up to 24 hours but tend to wear off in a relatively short period of time (Hurley, Cohen, & Wu, 2010). The use of epinephrine in the block solution can help extend the action of the block.

Solutions that are used for blocks are local anesthetics: 2% lidocaine and 1.5% mepivicaine have a rapid onset combined with a short duration of action (Wallace & Staats, 2005); 0.5% bupivacaine, 0.75% ropivacaine, and 0.5% levobupivacaine have extended action but a slower onset time (Wallace & Staats, 2005).

These single-dose intraoperative blocks can be placed in a wide variety of surgical locations. The blocks are designed to provide lack of sensation to the surgical area and use a local anesthesia such as bupivacaine that can have an extended action if epinephrine is included in the block solution.

Areas that commonly are used for blockade include:

Axillary: This block is used for upper extremity surgery such as shoulder surgery. It is used for procedures of the forearm, wrist, hand, chronic pain syndromes, and vascular diseases. It blocks the terminal branches of the brachial plexus.

Interscalene: This block is commonly used for open shoulder surgery, rotator cuff repair, acromioplasty, shoulder arthroplasty, and proximal upper limb surgery (May & DeRuyter, 2009). The block performed is a brachial plexus block. When performed as a surgical adjunct, this block may not produce analgesia for the ulnar nerve; the loading bolus may produce phrenic nerve block and the patient can develop hoarseness from laryngeal blockade as well as Horner's syndrome as a result of sympathetic blockade.

Femoral: The femoral block is commonly used for surgeries of the knee and femur. Anesthesia of the anterior thigh, femur, and most of the knee joint is produced with blockade. It can be combined with a sciatic block that effectively blocks both the anterior and posterior aspects of the knee. These blocks have been most effective when a continuous local anesthetic infusion is used leading to improved patient outcomes and side effects in the postoperative time period. Careful assessment is needed to determine if there is muscle weakness in the lower extremity, primarily quadriceps muscle weakness, with the block before getting the patient out of bed to avoid buckling of the extremity. Some of the more important patient outcomes when this block is used are increased ability to move the surgical joint, opioid sparing, decreased side effects such as postoperative nausea and vomiting (PONV), and increased patient satisfaction.

Sciatic: Sciatic blocks provide anesthesia to the skin of the posterior thigh, hamstring, biceps muscle, and part of the hip and knee joints, and the entire leg below the knee with the exception of the skin of the lower leg. It can be combined with a femoral block for knee surgery or lumbar plexus block for hip and femur surgery.

Thoracic Paravertebral: The thoracic paravertebral block is commonly used for breast, chest wall, and abdominal surgeries. Other uses for this type of block include anesthesia and/or analgesia for herniorraphy, iliac crest bone grafts, and soft tissue mass excisions, and as an analgesic adjunct for laparoscopic surgery, cholecystectomy, nephrectomy, appendectomy, thorocotomy, obstetric analgesia, minimally invective cardiac surgery, and hip surgery. Positive patient outcomes with this type of block include reduction in pain scores, opioid sparing effect, decreased PONV, and decreased length of stay (May & DeRuyter, 2009; Melton & Liu, 2010; Wallace & Staats, 2005).

PERIPHERAL CATHETERS (PC)
FOR POSTOPERATIVE ANALGESIA

In certain patient populations such as orthopedic total joint replacement patients where high levels of pain are expected, using pain medications in conjunction with a peripheral (perineural) catheter (PC) infusion has become the accepted practice. The prior practice pattern for these orthopedic patients was to use epidural catheters for postoperative analgesia. The change in practice was partially stimulated by the focus on prophylactic anticoagulation in these patients and the recognition of increased potential for adverse effects such as epidural hematoma. The ASRA (ASRA, 2002) developed a consensus statement related to anesthesiologist practice with epidural catheters and anticoagulation that outlines recommendations for practice when epidural catheters are used for postoperative pain relief in patients receiving anticoagulants. As a result of this paper and the recognition of the increased risk of epidural hematoma with the use of epidurals and anticoagulants, the use of epidural catheters decreased dramatically over a period of a year or two.

This decrease in epidural use made way for the development of alternate methods of pain control for total joint replacement patients using a combined medication and regional analgesia technique with PC. Since multimodal analgesia is always recommended as the best approach to postoperative pain management (ASA, 2004), this new technique is a good addition to the options that surgeons and anesthesia providers are able to offer patients.

The PC is a catheter that is similar to an epidural catheter that can be placed as a soaker hose configuration along the edge of a large incision to provide localized pain relief, or it can be placed along a nerve such as the femoral nerve, sciatic nerve, or both for total knee replacement patients, or along the interscalene brachial plexus to provide continuous pain relief. With either type of placement, the patient can expect to have the catheter remain in place while infusions of local anesthetic such as bupivacaine or ropivacaine infuse through the catheter.

Most PCs use some type of infusion device to provide continuous flow. One example is the On-Q pump, an elastomeric device that can be configured to deliver a preset rate of continuous flow but also has a device by which the patient can self-administer a bolus dose. During surgery the catheter is inserted into the area where blockade is desired. A ball-shaped reservoir is filled with a local anesthetic solution and a rate is set by adjusting a knob at the top of the ball by the surgeon or anesthesia provider. The On-Q infusion is complete in several days depending on the rate and

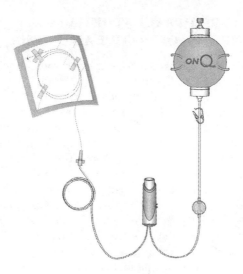

Figure 13.1 ▓ On-Q pump

when the ball containing the medication collapses and is no longer firm to touch. There are a variety of infusion devices available that work in basically the same fashion and each has its own advantages and disadvantages. The additional option of a patient-controlled device can allow the patient to provide a bolus dose of local anesthetic when needed.

PLACEMENT OF PCs

In order to place a peripheral nerve catheter, the anesthesia provider uses a hollow Touhy-type needle connected to a nerve stimulator or an ultrasound. Once placement has been confirmed, the provider threads the catheter down the hollow center of the needle to the area that needs analgesia. To test placement, the provider confirms location via one of two techniques:

▓ *Nerve stimulator (NS):* To locate the correct site for placement using a nerve stimulator, the anesthesia provider use a short, beveled, Teflon-coated needle inserted into the area for blockade attached to a nerve stimulator with a pulse duration of 0.15 msec. The correct nerves are located by the twitches elicited by the stimulation. The stimulation intensity is reduced after the block is injected, the catheter is inserted, and the needle is removed.

■ *Ultrasound guided peripheral nerve block:* To locate the correct site for placement with ultrasound, a short, beveled, Teflon-coated needle is inserted into the area for blockade so that the entire shaft of the needle is in the ultrasound beam and both the shaft and the tip of the needle are visualized. Once the site is located, the injection is completed and the catheter is threaded through the needle. Spread of local anesthetic is confirmed with continuous sonography.

The onset of blockade with ultrasound has been reported as faster compared with the older nerve stimulation technique. There is Level 1b evidence to make a grade A recommendation that the use of ultrasound improved onset and success of sensory blockade, decreased local anesthetic needs, and decreased time to perform lower extremity blockade (Salinas, 2010). Indications not entirely favorable to the use of ultrasound include the same effects noted for tissue damage to neighboring structures and inadequate analgesia in a small number of patients (Le-Wendling & Enneking, 2008). Nerves that can be blocked using continuous local anesthetic infusion for continued analgesia after surgery include those that were described earlier in the chapter for block locations.

The risks of using a PC are very low. Nerve injury with blocks is estimated to be 0% to 10% with upper extremity single shot blocks, and 0.5% with lower extremity blocks (Melton & Liu, 2010). Systemic local anesthetic toxicity is reported as rare (Bleckner et al., 2010). Pneumothorax rates are reported as low with both interscalene and paravertebral blocks. Infections with blocks and catheters are rare and ASRA has recommended the use of aseptic technique for catheter placements with monitoring of infections.

The use of local anesthetic catheters has moved into new areas and found acceptance in the popular press. In 2006, *The New York Times* reported an anesthesiologist who recognized the positive benefits of using local anesthetic infusions to help relieve battle wounds in the leg and arm. He used a small compact infusion pump with local anesthetic as adjunct pain relief for soldiers in military hospitals. This technique allowed for immediate decreases in pain and helped to continue pain relief as the soldiers were transported to other military facilities for surgery or rehabilitation.

A PC should always have a secondary method of pain relief such as PCA or intermittent IV analgesic in case of PC failure or dislodgment. The value of using a PC is related to the use of two different types of analgesia—multimodal analgesia using local anesthetic in the pump and intravenous opioids, providing an opioid sparing effect, and a reduction in side effects such as nausea. Increases in patient satisfaction, though difficult to determine, have been reported with the use of PCs as is decreased length of stay. Meta-analyses have shown a reduction of 1 day of hospitalization (Liu, Richman, & Thirlby, 2006). Technical failure is rare (1%), and local anesthetic toxicity (0%) with wound infection rates were below control group rates at 0.7% (Liu et al., 2006). Given that the cost of the pump is low ranging from $200–$280 dollars per patient (Ilfeld, Morey, & Enneking, 2004), and the outcomes are very good, this economical local anesthetic infusion option provides added benefit for patients, health care providers, and hospitals, and has dramatically improved postoperative pain management.

Case Study

Robert Smith is a 65-year-old patient who has had a thoracotomy. His surgeon felt that an epidural was indicated but did not use a peripheral catheter believing that the epidural should be sufficient to control pain. When you first visit Robert he is still in bed and will not move to the chair. He says it really hurts when he is asked to cough and deep breathe or move. He rates his pain as 6/10 and feels he really could use more analgesia. His epidural is fentanyl and bupivacaine and is running at 4 mL per hour with a PCEA of 2 mL every 15 minutes. You note that he has been activating the bolus dose 20 times per hour.

Questions to Consider

1. How can you improve Robert's pain relief?
2. Should you just increase the continuous infusion for Robert or would providing a clinician bolus first be indicated? What does his frequent use of the bolus dose indicate?
3. Robert says he has some nausea. Should this limit his doses of epidural medications?
4. Would combining a peripheral catheter or block have increased pain relief for Robert? If so what type of regional analgesia would have been useful?
5. What criteria would be helpful in determining the best outcomes for Robert's surgery? Respiratory status, pain intensity, and/or ability to move from bed to chair?

REFERENCES

Apfelbaum, J. L., Chen, C., Mehta, S. S., & Gan, T. (2003). Postoperative pain experience: results form a national survey suggest postoperative pain continues to be under managed. *Anesthesia and Analgesia, 97,* 534–540.

American Pain Society. (2008). *Principles of analgesic use in the treatment of acute pain and cancer pain.* Glenview, IL: The Society.

American Society of Anesthesiologists. (2004). Practice guidelines for acute pain management in the perioperative setting. *Anesthesiology, 100*(6), 1573–1581.

American Society of Regional Anesthesia and Pain Management. (2002). *Consensus Statement: Regional anesthesia in the anticoagulated patient: Defining the risks.* Retrieved from www.asra.com/consensus-statement/2.html

Aromaa, U., Lahdensuu, M., & Cozanitis, D. A. (1997). Severe complications associated with epidural and spinal anesthesia in Finland. *Acta Anaethesiology Scand, 41,* 445–452.

Bleckner, L., Bina, S., Kwon, K., McKnight, G., Dragovich, A., & Buckenmaier C. (2010). Serum ropivacaine concentrations and systemic local anesthetic toxicity in trauma patients receiving long-term continuous peripheral nerve block catheters. *Regional Anesthesia, 110*(2), 630–634.

Caputo, M., Alwair, H., Rogers, C., Pike, K., Cohen, A., Monk, C., . . . Angelini, G. (2011). Thoracic epidural anesthesia improves early outcomes in patient undergoing off-pump coronary artery bypass surgery. *Anesthesiology, 114*(2), 380–390.

Davies, D. P., Wald, R. M., & Patel, R. J. (2004). The clinical presentation and impact of diagnostic delays on emergency department patients with spinal epidural abscess. *Journal of Emergency Medicine, 26,* 285–291.

Deleon-Cassola, O. A., Parker, B. M., & Lema, M. J. (1994). Epidural analgesia versus intravenous patients controlled analgesia. Difference sin the postoperative course of cancer patients. *Regional Anesthesia, 19,* 307–315.

Eisenach, J. C., DuPen, S., Dubois, M., Miguel, R., & Allin, D. (1995). Epidural clonidine analgesia for intractable cancer pain. The epidural clonidine study group. *Pain, 61,* 391–339.

Hanna, M., Murphy, J., Kumar, K., & Wu, C. (2009). Regional techniques and outcome: What is the evidence? *Current Opinion in Anesthesiology, 22,* 672–677.

Joshi, G., Bonnet, F., Shah, R., Wiljkinson, R., Camu, F., Fishcher, B., . . . Kehlet, H. (2008). A systematic review of randomized trials evaluating regional techniques for postthoracotomy analgesia. *Anesthesia and Analgesia, 107*(3), 1026–1040.

Le-Wendling, L., & Enneking, F. K. (2008). Continuous peripheral nerve blockade for postoperative analgesia. *Current Opinion in Anesthesiology, 21,* 602–609.

Liu, S., & Salinsa, F. (2003). Continuous plexus and peripheral nerve blocks for postoperative analgesia. *Anesthesia and Analgesia, 96*(1), 263–272.

Liu, S., Richman, J., Thirlby, R., & Wu, C. (2006). Efficacy of continuous wound catheters delivering local anesthetic for postoperative analgesia: A Quantitative and qualitative systematic review of randomized controlled trial. *Journal of the American College of Surgeons, 203*(6), 914–932.

McGough, R. (2006, June 13). Pain pump tested in battle. *Wall Street Journal.*

Mcgrath, B., Elgendy, H., & Chung, F. (2004). Thirty percent of patients have moderate to severe pain 24 hours after ambulatory surgery: A survey of 5,703 patients. *Canadian Journal of Anesthesia, 51,* 886–891.

Melton, S., & Liu, S. (2010). Chapter 52. In S. Fishman, J. Ballantyne, & J. Rathmell (Eds.), *Bonica's management of pain* (5th ed.). Philadelphia, PA: Lippincott.

Rosenquist, R., & Rosenberg, J. (2003). Postoperative pain guidelines. *Regional Anesthesia and Pain Medicine, 28*(4), 279–288.

Salinas, F. (2010). Ultrasound and review of evidence for lower extremity peripheral nerve blocks. *Regional Anesthesia and Pain Medicine, 35*(2, Suppl. 1), S16–S24.

14

Managing Pain in Cardiothoracic Critical Care Patients

CHEST PAIN

There are approximately 8 million visits to emergency departments (EDs) for chest pain or other symptoms consistent with myocardial ischemia annually in the United States, which makes this the second most frequent cause of ED encounters in adults, although only a small percentage of these patients have a life-threatening condition (Amsterdam et al., 2010). Heart Disease and Stroke Statistics reported that in 2007 hospitalizations in the United States due to acute coronary syndromes were 1.57 million admissions per year; ST segment elevation myocardial infarction (STEMI), 0.33 million admissions per year; and unstable angina/non ST-elevation myocardial infarction (UA/NSTEMI), 1.24 million admissions per year. The incidence of NSTEMI/UA has continued to increase over the years. Heart disease is the leading cause of death in the United States.

Although not all chest pain is cardiac pain, it is important for the clinician to determine if the patient is presenting with cardiac etiology. Once coronary disease is excluded, then other noncardiac life-threatening disorders must be considered. Major causes of acute chest pain include cardiac, gastrointestinal, musculoskeletal, and pulmonary conditions.

Clinical Pearl	Three major causes of severe chest pain are acute myocardial infarction (MI), aortic dissection, and pulmonary embolus.

The myocardium requires adequate blood flow to the heart in order for the heart to pump effectively. If there is any restricted blood flow to the myocardium, such as a blockage in one of the vessels to the heart, the myocardium is deprived of oxygen resulting in ischemia to that area of the heart. Ischemia usually occurs as a result of thrombus formation at an atherosclerotic plaque rupture in the vessel wall.

ETIOLOGY

Chest pain is the presenting symptom in most patients with UA/NSTEMI and acute-STEMI. Chest pain generally produces retrosternal or midsternal pain that is diffuse, radiating to the arm, neck, or jaw. The pain can be described as chest heaviness, pressure, tightness, squeezing, or burning and can be triggered by various factors including exertion, emotional stress, or temperature extremes. The severity of the pain is variable. Other symptoms may include shortness of breath, diaphoresis, pain, and nausea (Leeper, 2010).

Diagnosis is based upon a focused clinical history, physical examination, 12-lead ECG, and initial cardiac biomarkers. The major factors increasing the likelihood of coronary artery disease (CAD) are often found in obtaining the initial history and physical exam:

- Chest pain assessment (nature, intensity, character, location, onset, and duration of chest pain)
- Prior MI or documented CAD
- Number of risk factors (diabetes, smoking, hypercholesterolemia, hypertension, postmenopausal)
- Age

When patients first present with chest pain to the ED, they should be triaged immediately. A rapid, targeted history must be taken and if suggestive of acute coronary syndrome, a 12-lead ECG must be done within 10 minutes of arrival to the ED. Based on the history and ECG findings, they should be triaged into the appropriate category:

- Acute STEMI
- UA / NSTEMI
- Low risk/noncardiac chest pain

Treatment

Aspirin should be administered to patients with acute coronary syndrome (ACS) as soon as possible unless contraindicated. Other antiplatelet medications and combinations of antiplatelet medications may be appropriate depending upon the overall treatment plan. Nonsteroidal antiinflammatory drugs (NSAIDs) should be discontinued on admission to the hospital in a patient with ACS (Kushner et al., 2009). Beta-blockers are instituted within the first 24 hours in absence of contraindications. Proceeding to coronary angiography is preferable in patients with ongoing symptoms or unstable vital signs.

Patients who are free of ACS symptoms and are otherwise stable can be managed with medications alone. If significant blockages are discovered at the time of angiography, the choice to proceed to angioplasty, stent implantation, or bypass surgery is determined based upon the individual's overall findings.

Various interventions are used to treat chest pain although some of the most common standards of practice have been questioned.

1. *Oxygen:* Routine oxygen is not warranted in all patients except those with respiratory distress or other high-risk features for hypoxemia. The theory behind using supplemental oxygen is that it may improve the oxygenation to the ischemic area of the heart and this could potentially reduce pain, size of the infarct, and ultimately reduce morbidity and mortality. In a recent Cochrane Review, the conclusion of the review was that there is no evidence to support the use of oxygen in every patient who experiences an acute myocardial infarction (Cabello, Burls, Emparanza, Bayliss, & Quinn, 2010). The exception would be if oxygen is clinically indicated based upon the patient experiencing respiratory distress or other conditions that warrant its use.

2. *Nitrates:* Patients with chest pain should receive sublingual nitroglycerin (NTG) 0.4 mg every 5 min for a total of 3 doses. For patients with continued unrelieved ischemic chest pain, a determination should be made if IV NTG should be used for the first 48 hours.

   NTG is considered the first line pain medication for patients with NSTEMI. Nitrates dilate the coronary arteries, which increases blood flow to the heart, relieving chest pain or angina. Nitrates also dilate veins throughout the body, which increases venous blood volume, reducing the amount of blood returning to the heart and reducing the heart's workload.

3. *Morphine:* Based upon the current recommendations, IV morphine sulfate should only be administered in unstable angina or NSTEMI patients for uncontrolled ischemic chest pain that is refractory to the use of nitroglycerin. It is also recommended that other therapies be utilized to manage any underlying ischemia. These recommendations were based on 2005 data gathered from the CRUSADE registry. In an analysis of the data, 57,039 patients who were high risk for NSTEMI and received morphine found a higher in-hospital mortality compared to those who did not receive morphine or those who received IV NTG (Meine et al., 2005). The researchers found that patients who received morphine were no more likely to exhibit symptoms of heart failure, even after they excluded patients from the analysis who died within 24 hours of admission. These results did not differ significantly from the overall findings. Meine et al. noted that morphine blunts angina severity without improving the underlying pathology. At the same time, morphine's side effects, which include hypotension, bradycardia, and respiratory depression, might result in harmful outcomes in ACS patients.

4. *NSAIDs:* No NSAID, nonselective or COX-2 selective (except ASA), should be given during hospitalization for patients with high risk of mortality, reinfarction, stroke, hypertension, heart failure, or myocardial rupture (Roumie et al., 2008; McGettigan & Henry, 2006; Anderson & Adams, 2011). These classes of medications contain black box warnings of the risks associated with use.

In a network meta-analysis, researchers reviewed 31 large-scale, randomized controlled trials comparing any NSAID with other NSAIDs or placebo. The overall data revealed that no conclusive evidence could be made that any of the drugs investigated were safe from a cardiovascular perspective. Compared with placebo, rofecoxib was associated with the highest risk of myocardial infarction (rate ratio 2.12, 95% credibility interval 1.26 to 3.56) and naproxen (rate ratio 0.82, 95% credibility interval 0.37 to 1.67) was the least harmful (Trelle, Reichenbach, Wandel, et al., 2011).

AORTIC DISSECTION

An aortic dissection is the most common disorder of the aorta that brings a patient to the ED because the pain associated is severe. Acute aortic dissection is the most common devastation of the aorta and is associated with high morbidity and mortality. According to the Vascular Disease Foundation, aortic dissection affects 2 out of every 10,000 people in the United States. African Americans are at higher risk for aortic dissection than Caucasians. Approximately 33% of patients with untreated aortic dissection die in the first 24 hours; 50% die within 48 hours (Chaikof et al., 2009) An aortic dissection lesion begins with a tear that is typically oblique that does not involve the entire circumference of the vessel. The tear in the aortic intima and media allows for the blood to flow into the aortic wall. The pressure can force the tear to open and allow blood to pass through, eventually splitting or dissecting the middle layer of the vessel, creating a new channel for the blood. The length of the channel grows, resulting in closing off access to other arteries, which in turn leads to heart attack, strokes, abdominal pain, and nerve damage.

Etiology

Aortic dissection is most common in men ages 50 to 60. Common risk factors include:

- Family history
- Smoking
- Heart disease
- Blunt trauma to the chest

■ Genetic disorders, such as Marfan syndrome or Ehlers-Danlos syndrome
■ Insertion of a catheter

Symptoms of acute thoracic aortic dissection are often sudden and include severe pain, often described as a very sharp or tearing pain in the chest or in the back between the shoulder blades. The pain may radiate to the shoulder, neck, arm, jaw, abdomen, or hips, and the location may change as the aortic dissection progresses. Other associated symptoms may include dizziness, oliguria or hematuria, elevated blood pressure.

Clinical Pearl	Chest pain that is severe, sudden, and at maximal intensity at the time of onset should raise suspicion for aortic dissection.

Clinical Pearl	Painless aortic dissection presenting with neurologic symptoms may be easily missed if the history, physical examination, and review of imaging studies are not conducted with dissection in the differential, especially in elderly patients.

Aortic dissections are classified by the type (DeBakey System I–III) and the involvement (Stanford System Types A and B) of the dissection. The goal of treatment is to stop the progression of the dissection. Type A dissection is usually treated surgically and Type B dissections can be treated either medically or surgically. Indications for operative intervention in acute Type B include rupture, impending rupture, ischemia of viscera, uncontrolled pain, and progression of the dissection despite medical management.

Open surgical repairs carry a much higher risk of complications. A newer procedure, thoracic endovascular aortic repair (TEVAR), in the treatment of Type B dissections is associated with reductions in morbidity and mortality in the treatment of complicated dissections (Apostolakis, Baikoussis, & Georgiopoulos, 2010).

Treatment

Medical Treatment

As soon as the diagnosis of aortic dissection is made, medical therapy should be initiated including for those patients that are surgical candidates. The main goal is to decrease the blood pressure in order to decrease the force of the myocardial contractility and minimize spread of the dissection. Pain and blood pressure control to a target systolic pressure of

100 to 110 mmHg can be achieved using morphine sulfate and IV beta blockers (metoprolol, propranolol, or labetalol) or in combination with vasodilating drugs such as sodium nitroprusside (Nienaber & Eagle, 2003).

Pain management is always difficult in persons with aortic dissection although good pain management will promote overall patient comfort and reduce the sympathetic drive, which increases blood pressure and heart rate. Pain should be treated with adequate analgesics; opiates are the preferred agents for pain.

Surgical Treatment

In descending dissection, the role of epidural analgesia is controversial because of its potential to cause or mask spinal damage (Hebballi & Swanevelder, 2009). Postoperative care includes administering medications (beta blockers, vasodilators) to control heart rate and blood pressure, prevent hypotension to prevent graft occlusion, and reduce pressure on the repaired aorta. Expect to give adequate analgesia (such as morphine sulfate) as needed for pain control.

ACUTE PERICARDITIS

When the pericardium becomes inflamed, the amount of fluid between the two layers increases, squeezing the heart and restricting its movement. Pericarditis can be caused by a virus, bacteria, idiopathic causes, or postinfarction.

The pericardium is a two layered sac that contains the heart, the fibrous pericardium, and the serous pericardium. The serous pericardium is divided into two layers, the parietal and the visceral pericardium, which is part of the epicardium. Located between the visceral and parietal layers of the pericardium is the pericardial cavity. The pericardial cavity contains approximately 20 mL of plasma-like fluid, and can accommodate another 120 mL of fluid without causing significant hemodynamic changes. The fluid serves as a lubricant to prevent friction in the heart. Inflammation of the pericardial sac and increased fluid in the pericardial cavity can lead to pericardial effusion. Since space is limited, excessive fluid build up affects the heart's ability to pump, leading to decreased cardiac output and stroke volume.

The incidence of acute pericarditis is unknown; up to 5% of visits to ED for non-acute MI chest pain may be related to pericarditis (Tingle, Molina, & Calvert, 2007).

Pericardial disease is the most common cardiovascular manifestation of AIDS, occurring in up to 20% of patients with HIV/AIDS. Approximately 20% of uremic patients requiring chronic dialysis develop pericarditis, but that number is decreasing because of effective dialysis and renal transplantation (Tingle et al., 2007).

Etiology

The classic findings are chest pain, pericardial friction rub heard best over the sternal border, and ECG changes. Sudden onset, and nonradiating, sharp pain occur with inspiration or coughing. The pain may also be over the anterior chest or the back; it may be relieved when the patient sits upright.

A potentially lethal complication of pericarditis is cardiac tamponade. It is reported in about 15% of patients with idiopathic pericarditis but in as many as 60% of those with neoplastic, tuberculosis, or purulent pericarditis (Tingle et al., 2007). The presence of systemic hypotension, tachycardia, JVD, and pulsus paradoxus indicates cardiac tamponade. The accumulation of pericardial fluid increases the pressure so that it exceeds that in the right side of the heart, collapsing the right atrium and ventricle and diminishing cardiac output. This requires prompt medical attention.

Treatment

Basic care for patients with pericarditis is rest, and oxygen and cardiac monitoring. Appropriate diagnostic studies should rule out other life-threatening conditions such as aortic dissection. An enlarging cardiac effusion that is left untreated can ultimately become cardiac tamponade; if the patient becomes hemodynamically unstable, an emergent pericardial window or pericardiocentesis is performed.

If a patient has pericarditis, anticoagulant therapy or thrombolytics are not contraindicated unless they develop a pericardial effusion or the effusion increases in size. The 2008 ESC guidelines recommend the use of an NSAID (Level B, Class 1) as the primary treatment of pain in acute pericarditis.

Clinical Pearl	Steroids are indicated in patients who are refractory to NSAIDs and colchicine.

NSAIDs and corticosteroids should be avoided in acute MI pericarditis, because they may interfere with ventricular healing, remodeling, or both.

THORACOTOMY

Thoracotomy has been and is still recognized as one of the most painful surgical procedures. A thoracotomy can produce both nociceptive and neuropathic pain. The pain can be worsened by coughing, breathing, and movement. Failure to adequately manage incisional or pleural pain can lead to hypoventilation, putting the patient at much higher risk for complications such as atelectasis, pneumonia, and chronic pain syndrome.

Etiology

Thoracotomy pain is generally severe, intense, and possibly could last for a few weeks. After surgery the presence of chest tubes or drains can further aggravate the patient's pain. Patients often complain of neuropathic pain around the wound incision site or along a dermatome where the affected nerve has been injured. It is commonly described as a burning, shooting, numbness or electric shock-like sensation. Some of the other descriptors patients use to describe their nociceptive pain are aching, constant, dull, and sharp.

Treatment

The choice of analgesic technique needs to be individualized for each patient. The Procedure Specific Pain Management (PROSPECT) for surgical pain is a web-based program developed with graded evidence-based recommendations in order to provide best outcomes on various surgical procedures including thoracotomy. Thoracic epidural analgesia has been considered the "gold" standard of analgesia for thoracotomy (Joshi et al., 2008).

In a systematic review various regional techniques were evaluated comparing them to one another and to systemic opioid analgesia in adult thoracotomy. Thoracic epidural analgesia with local anesthetic plus opioid or continuous paravertebral block with local anesthetic is recommended (Joshi et al., 2008). When these techniques are not possible, intrathecal opioid or intercostal nerve blocks are recommended, although the patient will usually require additional systemic analgesia supporting PROSPECT recommendations. The epidural catheter is placed pre- or intra-operatively at the level corresponding to the center of the dermatomal distribution of the incision.

Patients are evaluated preoperatively for individual risk and selection of the most appropriate analgesic method. Regional analgesic techniques are preferred over traditional methods (Table 14.1). Pain that is not managed with these methods can be supplemented with additional analgesia based upon the patient's level of reported pain:

- *Mild pain:* +NSAID/COX 2 or acetaminophen
- *Moderate:* +NSAID/COX 2 or acetaminophen + weak opioid
- *Severe:* IV PCA strong opioid + NSAID/COX 2 or acetaminophen

The site of the thoracotomy incision is determined based upon the type of surgery or procedure necessary. The posterolateral approach for thoracotomy has been associated with greater tissue damage and a higher incidence of nerve injury, resulting in development of chronic pain; it is not the recommended surgical approach (Ryu, Lee, Kim, & Bahk, 2011).

Table 14.1 ■ *Guidelines for NSAID Use in Acute Pericarditis*

Medication	Dosing	Frequency	Comments
Ibuprofen (Advil, Motrin)	300–800 mg	bid or tid	
Naproxen (Aleve)	250–500 mg	tid	
Indomethacin (Indocin)	25–50 mg	bid	Avoid in the elderly
Aspirin	325–650 mg	tid	Preferred in patients with recent MI
Adjunctive Agents			
Colchicine (Colcrys)	0.5 mg	bid	May be used in combination with or as alternative to NSAIDs; long-term colchicine may be used for recurrent pericarditis
Prednisone	Up to 1.5 mg/kg/ day × 3–4 weeks		May be added in patients with severe symptoms of acute pericarditis and suspected connective tissue disease. Corticosteroid use reserved for refractory or recurrent cases (ESC, 2008)

The incidence of postthoracotomy pain syndrome has been reported to be 30%–70% (Liu & Kehlet, 2009). Patients often report a continuous dysesthetic burning and aching in the general area of the incision that persists at least 2 months after thoracotomy. Multiple risk factors have been identified in the open versus thoracoscopic approach, including increased acute pain, not using thoracic epidural analgesia with local anesthetics, and resultant intercostal nerve injury. It is inconclusive that pre-emptive analgesia prevents chronic postoperative thoracotomy pain (Ryu et al., 2011; Wildgaard, Ravn, & Kehlet, 2009; Bong, Samuel, Ng, & Ip-Yam, 2005).

Newer surgical techniques including limited or muscle-sparing thoracotomy, video-assisted thoracoscopic surgery (VATS), and robotic surgery may lessen the degree of chronic postthoracotomy pain. A systematic review favored VATS over thoracotomy, reporting lower analgesia requirements and a shorter length of hospital stay (Sedrakyan, van der Meulen, Lewsey, & Treasure, 2004). Aggressive pain management and surgical technique may be useful in reducing development of chronic pain.

CARDIAC CATHETERIZATION

Cardiac catheterization is done to confirm and define the extent of coronary artery disease, evaluate cardiac function, and perform interventional procedures to treat coronary artery disease and other cardiac disorders. Angioplasty is considered the gold standard of care. The major advantage is that it avoids a major surgical procedure, scar, and long postoperative recovery period.

Right heart catheterization is usually done via femoral venous access but alternate venous access sites can be used, including the internal jugular veins, subclavian vein, or brachial veins. Once the superior or inferior vena cava is reached, the catheter is advanced through the right atrium, right ventricle, and into the pulmonary artery. Pressures are recorded and O_2 saturations obtained when indicated. Contrast dye can be injected for imaging of the right atrium, right ventricle, or pulmonary artery. Cardiac output is determined using the thermodilution technique. In some procedures, such as catheter-based mitral valve repair or closure of a patent foramen ovale, the left atrium is accessed via transseptal puncture through the atrial septum.

A sheath is generally cannulated into the femoral artery under fluoroscopy. Procedural sedation and analgesia are given for the procedure. Once the procedure is over, the sheath will be removed. Bleeding times are assessed prior to removal. The sheath removal is usually uncomfortable for the patient and some may even report it as painful. Patient education on what is to be expected may assist in allaying their fears. Clinical judgment is utilized in determining the best analgesic method for the patient—IV opioid analgesia and/or a short acting local anesthetic injected around the site in order to reduce pain and avoid a vagal reaction as the sheath is being pulled (refer to Chapter 7). In a Cochrane Review of four studies that looked at pain relief in sheath pull, one of the studies compared IV pain regimens and subcutaneous levobupivacaine appeared to reduce the pain experienced during femoral sheath removal although the amount of the reduction was small (Wensley, Kent, & McAleer, 2008). Overall, the

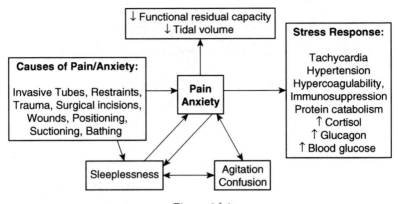

Figure 14.1

review concluded that some patients may benefit from routine pain relief using levobupivacaine or IV pain regimens. Clinicians should use clinical judgment as to who may benefit from pain relief and what is appropriate including patient preference.

Pressure is applied to the area for a minimum of 30 minutes. The patient lies flat and the leg must remain straight for at least 6 hours. Some patients may require an anxiolytic for anxiety.

Case Study

Sarah is a 32-year-old female who presents to the ED with chest pain of 4 hours duration. Sarah reported that her pain was sharp and worsened on inspiration. It had a sudden onset, did not radiate, and was not associated with any shortness of breath. It was relieved slightly when she sat up and leaned forward. Sarah had no cardiac risk factors and no past medical conditions except for a recent "flu-like" illness last month.

On clinical examination, she was afebrile and, except for a soft pericardial friction rub, she had no other positive findings. ECG and chest X-ray were unremarkable. She had mild leukocytosis and moderately elevated C-reactive protein (CRP).

On the basis of her clinical findings, recent viral infection, and low risk for ischemic heart disease, she was diagnosed with viral pericarditis.

Questions to Consider

1. Why was her pain relieved when she was sitting up and leaning forward?
2. What is recommended to relieve her pain?
3. Are steroids indicated in Sarah's case?

REFERENCES

Amr, Y. M., Yousef, A. A., Alzeftawy, A. E., Messbah, W. I., & Saber, A. M. (2010). Effect of pre-incisional epidural fentanyl and bupivacaine on post thoracotomy pain and pulmonary function. *The Annals of Thoracic Surgery, 89,* 381–386.

Apostolakis, E., Baikoussis, N. G., & Georgiopoulos, M. (2010). Acute type-B aortic dissection: The treatment strategy Hellenic. *Journal of Cardiology, 51,* 338–347.

Baumann, M. H., Strange, C., Heffner, J. E., Light, R., Kirby, T. J., Klein, J., . . ., Sahn, SA (2001). Management of spontaneous pneumothorax: An American College of Chest Physicians Delphi consensus statement. *Chest, 119*(2), 590–602.

Bong, C. L., Samuel, M., Ng, J. M., & Ip-Yam, C. (2005). Effects of preemptive epidural analgesia on post-thoracotomy pain. *Journal of Cardiothoracic and Vascular Anesthesia, 19,* 786–793.

Brims, F. J., Davies, H. E., & Lee, Y. C. (2010). Respiratory chest pain: Diagnosis and treatment. *The Medical clinics of North America, 94,* 217–232.

Cabello, J. B., Burls, A., Emparanza, J. I., Bayliss, S., & Quinn, T. (2010). Oxygen therapy for acute myocardial infarction. *Cochrane Database of Systematic Reviews,* (6), CD007160. doi:10.1002/14651858.CD007160.pub2

Chaikof E. L., Mutrie, C., Kasirajan, K., Milner, R., Chen, E. P., Veeraswamy, R. K., . . ., Salam, A. A. (2009). Endovascular repair for diverse pathologies of the thoracic aorta: An initial decade of experience. *Journal of the American College Of Surgeons, 208*(5), 802–816.

Fysh, E. T., Smith, N. A., & Lee, Y. C. (2010). Optimal chest drain size: The rise of the small-bore pleural catheter. *Seminars in respiratory and critical care medicine, 31*(6), 760–768.

Gerner, P. (2008). Postthoracotomy pain management problems. *Anesthesiology Clinics, 26*(2), 355–367.

Hebballi, R., & Swanevelder, J. (2009). Diagnosis and management of aortic dissection. *Continuing Education in Anaesthesia, Critical Care & Pain, 9*(1), 14–18.

Joshi, G. P., Bonnet, F., Shah, R., Wilkinson, R. C., Camu, F., Fischer, B., . . ., Kehlet, H. (2008). A systematic review of randomized trials evaluating regional techniques for postthoracotomy analgesia. *Anesthesia and Analgesia, 107,* 1026–1040. doi:10.1213/01.ane.0000333274.63501.ff

Karmakar, M. K., & Ho, A. M. (2004). Postthoracotomy pain syndrome. *Thoracic Surgery Clinics, 14*(3), 345–352.

Kehlet, H., Wilkinson, R. C., Fischer, H. B., & Camu, F. (2007). PROSPECT: Evidence-based, procedure-specific postoperative pain management. *Best Practice & Research Clinical Anaesthesiology, 21,* 149–159.

Koehler, R. P., & Keenan, R. J. (2006). Management of postthoracotomy pain: Acute and chronic. *Thoracic Surgery Clinics, 16*(3), 287–297.

Kushner, F. G., Hand, M., Smith, S. C. Jr., King, S. B. III, Anderson, J. L., Antman, E. M., . . ., Williams, D. O. (2009). Focused updates: ACC/AHA guidelines for the management of patients with ST-elevation myocardial infarction and ACC/AHA/SCAI guidelines on percutaneous coronary intervention: a report of the American College of Cardiology Foundation/American Heart Association Task Force on Practice Guidelines. *Circulation, 120*(22), 2271–2306.

Lange, R. A., & Hillis, L. D. (2004). Acute pericarditis. *The New England Journal of Medicine, 351,* 2195–2202.

Leeper, B. (2007). Advanced cardiovascular concepts. In M. Chulay, & S. M. Burns (Eds.). *AACN Essentials of progressive care nursing* (pp. 447–475). New York, NY: McGraw Hill.

Leeper, B. (2007). Cardiovascular concepts. In M. Chulay, & S. M. Burns (Eds.). *AACN Essentials of progressive care nursing* (pp. 221–251). New York, NY: McGraw Hill.

McGettigan, M. D., & Henry, D. (2006). Cardiovascular risk and inhibition of cyclooxygenase: A systematic review of the observational studies of selective and nonselective inhibitors of cyclooxygenase 2. *Journal of the American Medical Association, 296*(13), 1633–1644. doi:10.1001/jama.296.13.jrv60011

Meine, T. J., Roe, M. T., Chen, A. Y., Patel, M. R., Washam, J. B., Ohman, E. M., . . ., Peterson, E. D. (2005). Association of IV morphine use and outcomes in acute coronary syndromes: Results from the CRUSADE Quality Improvement Initiative. *American Heart Journal, 149,* 1043–1049.

Nienaber, C. A., & Eagle, K. A. (2003). Aortic dissection: New frontiers in diagnosis and management part II: Therapeutic management and follow-up. *Circulation, 108,* 772–778.

Owen, A. R., & Gibson, M. R. (2004). Pulmonary embolism: advances in diagnosis and treatment. *Care of the Critically Ill, 20,* 79–84.

PROSPECT Working Group. (2011). Retrieved May 16, 2011, from http://www.postoppain.org

Roumie, C. L., Mitchel, E. F. Jr., Kaltenbach, L., Arbogast, P. G., Gideon, P., & Griffin, M. R. (2008). Nonaspirin NSAIDs, cyclooxygenase 2 inhibitors, and the risk for stroke. *Stroke, 39,* 2037–2045.

Ryu, H. G., Lee, C. J., Kim, Y. T., & Bahk, J. H. (2011). Preemptive low-dose epidural ketamine for preventing chronic postthoracotomy pain: A prospective, double-blinded, randomized clinical trial. *The Clinical Journal of Pain, 27*(4), 304–308.

Sedrakyan, A., van der Meulen, J., Lewsey, J., & Treasure, T. (2004). Video assisted thoracic surgery for treatment of pneumothorax and lung resections: Systematic review of randomized clinical trials. *British Medical Journal, 329*(7473), 1008.

Strebel, B. M., & Ross, S. (2007). Chronic post-thoracotomy pain syndrome. *Canadian Medical Association journal, 177*(9), 1027.

Tingle, L. E., Molina, D., & Calvert, C. W. (2007). Acute pericarditis. *American Family Physician, 76*(10), 1509–1514.

Torbicki, A., Perrier, A., Konstantinides, S., Agnelli, G., Galiè, N., Pruszczyk, P., . . ., Bassand, J. P. (2008). Guidelines on the diagnosis and management of acute pulmonary embolism: The Task Force for the Diagnosis and Management of Acute Pulmonary Embolism of the European Society of Cardiology (ESC). *European Heart Journal, 29*(18), 2276–2315. doi:10.1093/eurheartj/ehn310

Wildgaard, K., Ravn, J., & Kehlet, H. (2009). Chronic post-thoracotomy pain: A critical review of pathogenic mechanisms and strategies for prevention. *European Journal of Cardio-Thoracic Surgery, 36*(1), 170–180.

15

Managing Patient Pain in the Medical Intensive Care Unit

Critically ill patients are challenged by many perils because of the seriousness of their illness. Patients often experience pain, fear, and loss of control. Patients are generally confined to bed, are attached to various pieces of equipment, and often are intubated and ventilated. The ICU environment and the patient's critical illness create responses of anxiety, confusion, agitation, pain, and sleeplessness. Without accurate assessment of these distressing patient responses, management strategies cannot occur. The nurse must be attuned to the environment and the patient, and must continuously assess for factors from the simple to the complex, such as changes in blood pressure, pain behaviors, or challenging ventilatory issues.

Pain is not an exception and often a bigger challenge because of the patient's inability to communicate, which makes it difficult for the clinician to determine if pain is present. Inadequately treated pain and anxiety lead to a stress response that can increase the patient's mortality in the ICU setting. Pain that follows major thoracic or abdominal surgery can lead to abnormalities in pulmonary function and gas exchange. This can involve a decreased functional residual capacity and tidal volume leading to atelectasis, hypoxemia, and respiratory infection. This exacerbates the stress response, which increases levels of cortisol, glucagon, blood glucose, the rate of gluconeogenesis, hypercoagulability, protein catabolism, and increases sympathetic nervous system activity.

As a result, the myocardium can be affected and the increased sympathetic activity may result in myocardial ischemia or infarction in the cardiac-compromised patient. Simply controlling pain and analgesia can provide vital protection from these adverse events.

ABDOMINAL PAIN

Abdominal pain can be life threatening. In the critically ill patient, abdominal pain can be a primary diagnosis or the patient may develop abdominal pain as a secondary problem. Because of the patient's underlying comorbidities and diagnosis, identifying and managing these complications can be challenging.

Etiology

Abdominal pain can originate from the abdomen itself, the mesentery, peritoneum, abdominal wall muscle, or skin or subcutaneous tissue, or it can be referred from organs or structures outside the abdominal cavity. Abdominal pain can be classified as visceral, somatic, or referred.

Visceral pain originates from the stimulation of nerve fibers within the abdomen this is usually the earliest sign of abdominal pathology. Pain is usually felt in the midline, epigastric, or umbilical areas and is poorly localized, diffuse pain. This is related to the limited number of nerve endings in the abdomen and afferent nerve fibers that enter the spinal cord at multiple levels.

Visceral pain is described as dull, aching, and cramping. If hollow organs are involved, the pain is described as cramping, colicky, dull, and intermittent. Solid organs usually produce dull but constant pain. Vague pain often triggers the sympathetic nervous system and produces nausea, vomiting, diaphoresis, and tachycardia.

Somatic pain is produced when the peritoneum nerve fibers are stimulated. This type of pain is more localized and the patient is able to pinpoint the area. The parietal nerve fibers travel along specific peripheral nerves that enter the spinal cord and directly correspond with the dermatomes between T6 and L1. Parietal pain is described as sharp, intense, and constant. Patients typically lie in a fetal position to relax the peritoneum and reduce pain.

Clinical Pearl   *Visceral pain* results from gut distension and stretching or spasm of the muscle fibers. Carried by sympathetic nerve fibers, it is experienced as dull, vague, poorly localized pain in the mid zones of the abdomen.

Somatic pain results when the parietal peritoneum is inflamed or irritated. Carried by sensory fibers in somatic nerves, it is better defined, more localized, and greater in intensity. It is associated with localized tenderness and spasm of the muscle groups supplied by the same dermatome.

Referred pain is experienced at a site other than the actual site of injury or illness but in the somatic zones supplied by the same or adjacent segments of the spinal cord. This pain is well localized in the skin or deeper tissue.

Abdominal organs are not sensitive to tearing, except for the aorta. Stretching or distension of the organ, the fibrous capsule of some solid organs, and the peritoneum will stimulate nerve fibers and produce pain. Rapid distension usually produces significant pain, while a gradual distension related to a chronic condition may be associated with little pain.

If blood flow to an organ is obstructed, the tissue becomes ischemic. Metabolites and waste products build up within the tissue and organ, which stimulate pain receptors. As ischemia progresses, the pain usually worsens in intensity.

Signs of an Acute Abdomen

Pain is usually the principal and presenting feature of an acute abdomen. The initial evaluation of a patient with an acute abdomen begins with a comprehensive history and physical examination. Many factors may impact the ability to gather the appropriate information to diagnose the patient:

- The patient is unable to provide a good history.
- Physical examination is impacted by the primary diagnosis, sedation, and/or analgesia.
- Imaging studies may be limited because of severity of underlying disease.
- Symptoms of acute abdomen as secondary diagnosis may be vague.

Physical Examination

A complete, comprehensive history and physical exam are the principal diagnostic aids to identify conditions that require immediate surgical intervention, further monitoring, or only medical intervention. The physical examination itself provides critical information for making the diagnosis, determining the severity of the condition, assessing operative risk, and making a sound management plan.

The major components of an abdominal exam include: inspection, auscultation, percussion, and palpation in this specified order. If the physical findings are inconclusive, the patient should be re-examined frequently until a diagnosis can be made and/or proper management of the patient determined (Table 15.1).

| *Clinical Pearl* | Patients with visceral pain are unable to lie still. Patients with peritonitis prefer to stay immobile. |

Table 15.1 ▦ *Assessing and Differentiating Acute Abdominal Pain*

RUQ	RLQ	Epigastric	Pelvic
Hepatitis	Appendicitis	PUD	UTI
Cholecystitis	Colon Ischemia	Gastritis	Prostatitis
Cholangitis	Colon Perforation	Pancreatitis	Bladder outlet obstruction
Liver abscess	Colon Carcinoma	GERD	PID
Subdiaphrag- matic abscess	Incarcerated inguinal hernia	Cardiac (MI, pericarditis, etc.)	Uterine pathology
	Nephrolithiasis		
	IBD		
	Salpingitis		
	Ectopic pregnancy		
	Ovarian pathology		

LUQ	LLQ	Periumbilical	Diffuse
Splenic infarct	Diverticulitis	Pancreatitis	Gastroenteritis
Splenic abscess	Incarcerated inguinal hernia	Obstruction	Ischemia
Gastritis/PUD	Colon ischemia	Early appendicitis	Obstruction
Abdominal abscess	Colon perforation	Small bowel pathology	DKA
	Colon carcinoma	Gastroenteritis	IBS
	Ectopic pregnancy	Aortic aneurysm	Adrenal insufficiency
	Ovarian pathology	Mesenteric bleeding	

Although in the past ED physicians did not treat acute abdominal pain with analgesics for fear of altering or obscuring the diagnosis, current literature favors the use of opioids judiciously in such patients. In a Cochrane systematic review, six adult studies were reviewed and no differences were found between the opioid and control groups in changes in the physical examination, errors in treatment or diagnosis, or morbidity (Manterola, Vial, Moraga, & Astudillo, 2011). They did note significant reductions in pain intensity and improved patient comfort for those receiving opioids.

Treatment

Since there are many causes of acute abdominal pain, a systematic approach is imperative in order to narrow the differential diagnosis. The clinician must have an acute understanding of the mechanisms of pain generation as well as be familiar with the presentations of various disease processes that may cause abdominal pain. Recognizing the critical signs in the history and physical assessment and the imaging and laboratory findings helps to determine a serious underlying disease process warranting an expedited evaluation and treatment.

Fentanyl or one of its analogues can be a useful agent in this situation due to the combination of potency and short half-life.

GASTROINTESTINAL BLEEDING

Upper gastrointestinal bleeding (UGIB) represents a substantial clinical and economic burden, with reported incidences ranging from 48 to 160 cases per 100,000 adults per year, and mortality generally from 10% to 14% (Barkun, et al., 2010).

Etiology

In the critically ill patient, the two major causes of upper GI bleeding include peptic ulcer disease and stress-related mucosal damage. Bleeding from the upper GI tract is five times more common than from the lower GI tract (Proctor, 2003). Other common causes of lower GI bleeding are diverticular disease, carcinoma of the colon, inflammatory bowel disease, and colonic polyps.

Critically ill patients at high risk for GI bleeding include those who require mechanical ventilation, as well as those who are coagulopathic and/or experience a neurological event.

Stress-related mucosal disease (SRMD) is a frequent complication in critically ill patients. Stress ulceration is a form of hemorrhagic gastritis that may occur following trauma or critical illness. SRMD results from physiological stress that causes damage to the gastric mucosa; it is a major cause of morbidity and mortality in critically ill patients in the ICU. The morbidity due to SRMD can increase the length of stay in the ICU. Mortality rates range from 50% to 77% in critically ill patients who develop stress-related mucosal bleeding during hospitalization, which can be as much as four times higher than it is in ICU patients without this complication (Sesler, 2007). Patients generally die from other associated conditions and not directly from the bleeding itself.

More than 75% of patients in the ICU will have gastroduodenal lesions by endoscopy (Proctor, 2003). The patients who are at highest risk for developing clinically significant GI bleeding are intubated patients; those who have multi-system organ failure, coagulopathy, sepsis, or extensive burns; or those who have experienced head trauma or neurosurgery.

The occurrence of GI bleeding has declined, which is probably the result of improved medical management of mucosal blood flow.

Critically ill patients are at risk of GI bleeding mainly from gastric or duodenal ulcers. Increased gastric acidity and a decrease in the gastric mucosal barrier are believed to be the cause. The longer the gastric pH remains below 4 the greater the risk of hemorrhage. Patients most at risk include critically ill patients requiring mechanical ventilation long than 48 hours, coagulopathic patient, and patients with a history of GI bleeding, experiencing organ failure, or with hypotension/shock.

Patient presentation will depend upon the amount of blood the patient has lost. Acute upper GI bleeding may present with either hematemesis or melena or both. Intensive monitoring of blood pressure, pulse, and evidence of ongoing bleeding is required. Agitation, pallor, hypotension, and tachycardia may indicate shock requiring immediate volume replacement. Lab tests can help determine the extent of bleeding but the hemoglobin and hematocrit are poor indicators of severity of blood loss. It can take as long as 48 hours for the hemoglobin and hematocrit to equilibrate.

Treatment

Controlling the bleeding is necessary in order to reduce mortality. The patient must be hemodynamically stable before undergoing an endoscopy. Most patients are able to be medically managed with early identification and interventions. The reduction of gastric acidity and identification of at-risk patients with prophylactic interventions minimizes their risk as follows:

- Fluid resuscitation
- Control of bleeding
- Monitoring for complications and further bleeding
- Pain control without use of aspirin or NSAIDs. Use acetaminophen for mild pain; for moderate and severe pain, use opioid analgesia
- Acid suppression therapy (Table 15.2)
- Surgery may be necessary for patients whose bleeding cannot be controlled.

Table 15.2 ▦ *Acid Suppression Therapy*

Histamine 2-receptor antagonists *(Adjustments in dosing for creatinine clearance less than 30 mL/min)*	
Cimetidine (Tagamet)	50 mg/hr IV continuous infusion 300 mg PO, naso-gastric tube every 6 hr
Famotidine (Pepcid, Pepcid AC)	1.7 mg/hr IV continuous infusion 20 mg PO, naso-gastric tube, IV every 12 hr
Sucrose-aluminum complex	
Sucralfate (Carafate)	1 g PO, naso-gastric tube every 6 hr Use with caution in severe renal impairment
Proton pump inhibitors	
Esomeprazole (Nexium, Nexium IV)	40 mg IV, PO, naso-gastric tube every day
Lansoprazole (Prevacid, Prevacid SoluTab)	15 or 30 mg IV, PO, naso-gastric tube every day
Omeprazole (Losec, Prilosec)	Initially, two 40 mg doses PO, naso-gastric tube given at least 6–8 hr apart, then 20–40 mg daily PO, naso-gastric tube
Pantoprazole (Protonix, Protonix IV)	40 mg PO, IV, naso-gastric tube every day

BOWEL OBSTRUCTION

Bowel obstruction is a common cause for hospitalization for abdominal pain. Intestinal transit can be affected by either mechanical or functional obstruction. Mechanical obstruction can be affected when the lumen of the bowel is blocked due to incarceration, strangulation, or neoplasm. Functional obstructions also known as paralytic ileus are blockages in the intestinal flow resulting from impaired motility. It can be caused by tumor infiltration or malignancy, previous gastric surgery, and other neurological disorders. Ileus, fecal impaction, dehydration, and constipating medications are all likely to contribute to the development of bowel obstruction.

The patient usually presents with nausea, vomiting, cramp-like abdominal pain and the inability to pass stool. In patients with mechanical obstruction, bowel sounds are low-pitched, tinkling, and hyperactive proximal to the obstruction site and hypoactive or active distal to the obstruction. As with functional obstruction, bowel sounds are low-pitched, hypoactive, or absent.

Small bowel obstruction is usually a mechanical obstruction. Patients will complain of cramp-like abdominal pain and distension, projectile vomiting, and nausea. Abdominal pain comes in waves and is severe in nature. The higher the obstruction, the more extreme the pain.

Treatment

The management of intestinal obstruction includes supportive care and treatment of the underlying problem. Determination of treatment ranges from conservative medical management to surgical intervention. *Partial small bowel obstructions* may be resolved medically without surgical intervention. Treatment options include managing pain, decompression of the intestine to relieve abdominal distension, and controlling nausea with antiemetics. IV fluid and electrolytes replacement are ordered depending on the results of lab tests as well as the overall condition of the patient. The choice of surgical intervention is determined based upon the nature and location of the obstruction. In cases of vascular insufficiency, perforation, or strangulation, surgical intervention is urgent.

In *large bowel obstruction*, surgery is generally performed for malignant tumors, perforation, and diverticula. Many of these surgical cases result in a colostomy.

Parenteral opioids such as morphine, fentanyl, or dilaudid are indicated for relief of pain (see Chapter 7). Often significant pain relief can simply be obtained by bowel decompression alone.

ACUTE MESENTERIC ISCHEMIA

Acute mesenteric ischemia is uncommon but is a catastrophic surgical emergency. Delays in diagnosis and treatment of acute mesenteric ischemia, partly a result of its relative infrequency and its nonspecific clinical presentation, have contributed to an unacceptably high mortality rate estimated at 60%–80% (Oldenburg, Lau, Rodenberg, Edmonds, & Burger, 2004). Early diagnosis and prompt aggressive treatment are associated with improved survival.

The classic presentation for mesenteric ischemia is usually in a patient older than 50 years of age who presents with sudden onset of abdominal pain, which may be associated with nausea, vomiting, and diarrhea. The abdominal pain will initially be severe and diffuse without localization. The unique characteristic of acute mesenteric ischemia is that the abdominal pain is out of proportion to examination. The abdomen is soft with no guarding or rebound, although the patient is screaming and writhing in pain. As the bowel becomes infarcted, the patient will develop abdominal distension with guarding, rebound, and absence of bowel sounds.

MESENTERIC ARTERY EMBOLUS

The prognosis is poor with a 70% mortality rate (Schermerhorn, Giles, Hamdan, Wyers, & Pomposelli, 2009). Risk factors for mesenteric artery embolus include arrhythmias (atrial fibrillation being the most common), postmyocardial infarction with mural thrombi, valvular heart disease, and structural heart defects (such as right to left shunts).

MESENTERIC ARTERY THROMBOSIS

Mesenteric artery thrombosis accounts for 25% to 30% of mesenteric ischemia cases and possibly carries the worst prognosis with a mortality of 90% (Schermerhorn et al., 2009). Risk factors include systemic atherosclerosis and older age.

MESENTERIC VEIN THROMBOSIS (MVT)

MVT is the least common cause of mesenteric ischemia involving 10% of cases with a mortality of 20% to 50% (Oldenburg et al., 2004). MVT risk factors include hypercoagulable states (Factor V Ledien, protein C deficiency, etc.), recent surgery, malignancy, and cirrhosis. In addition, up to 50% of patients will have a history of deep vein thrombosis.

NONOCCLUSIVE ISCHEMIA

Nonocclusive ischemia accounts for 20% to 30% of cases with mortality rates ranging from 50% to 90% (Oldenburg et al., 2004). This type of mesenteric ischemia occurs in low flow states in the absence of an arterial or venous occlusion. Any condition associated with decreased cardiac output can cause nonocclusive ischemia including cardiogenic shock, congestive heart failure, and arrhythmias. Sepsis, hypotensive states, and drugs inducing mesenteric vasoconstriction (digoxin, cocaine, alpha-agonists, beta-blockers) can also be causes.

Treatment

Treatment must be initiated early in patients suspected of having mesenteric ischemia. Immediate surgery is necessary in all cases except nonocclusive mesenteric ischemia. Initial management of patients suspected of having bowel ischemia include aggressive fluid resuscitation and administration of empiric broad spectrum antibiotics (Herbert & Steele, 2007). Continuous monitoring of vital signs is critical and central venous pressure monitoring may be required to guide IV fluid treatment, especially in patients with a history of cardiac disease. An IV bolus of unfractionated heparin is given followed by heparin infusion to prevent further thrombosis within the mesenteric vessels (Herbert & Steele, 2007). Additional management depends on the underlying cause of ischemia. Opioid analgesia is the treatment of choice for pain management (morphine, hydromorphone, and fentanyl; see Chapter 7). Postoperatively, the use of PCA should be considered if the patient meets the institution's criteria.

PANCREATITIS

Most incidences of acute pancreatitis are mild and reversible, but necrotizing pancreatitis has mortality as high as 50% (Holcomb, 2007). Even without necrosis, the mortality is as high as 9% in the United States (Despins, Kivlahan, & Cox, 2005; Nathens et al., 2004). Inflammation of the pancreas can be defined as acute, chronic, or relapsing and associated with gallstones or alcoholism. The pancreas provides many hormones and enzymes that perform essential functions, and, as a result, acute pancreatitis can cause serious complications that affect the entire body.

Acute pancreatitis causes a blockage of enzymes, which builds up levels in the pancreas, causing auto-digestion. The damage to the pancreas and the surrounding tissues releases inflammatory mediators and the patient develops an inflammatory response causing symptoms of shock (Holcomb, 2007).

The pancreatic duct becomes blocked, preventing the release of pancreatic enzymes into the small bowel. The enzymes continue to be produced and cause inflammation of the pancreas.

In the chronic phase it may lead to malabsorption syndromes and diabetes (Holcomb, 2007).

The two most common causes for acute pancreatitis are alcoholism and cholecystitis. Other less common factors include peptic ulcer disease, some medications, surgical trauma, and vascular disease.

Patients with pancreatitis often present with steady dull upper abdominal pain of variable intensity radiating to the back, flanks, or lower abdomen. The patient is distressed and anxious, the abdomen tender and guarded, but the bowel sounds are faint or absent. In severe cases there may be third spacing of fluids and inflammatory exudates within the abdominal cavity. Diffuse symmetrical crackles throughout both lung fields and deteriorating O_2 saturation suggest developing adult respiratory distress syndrome (ARDS). Cullen's sign (periumbilical discoloration) and Grey-Turner sign (discoloration of the flank) may occur in necrotizing pancreatitis. Most patients have only edematous pancreatitis and require only supportive care, fluid/electrolytes, and pain management, and fully recover in 3 to 5 days. Those less likely to recover may be predicted by the presence of more than two of the prognostic criteria of Ranson's or Modified Glasgow Criteria. Most patients who die of pancreatitis die from sepsis. Antibiotic prophylaxis in high-risk patients has been shown to reduce mortality (Villatoro, 2006).

Treatment

The main goals of acute pancreatitis medical management are fluid resuscitation, minimizing pancreatic function, pain management, electrolyte balance, and adequate oxygenation and ventilation.

Patients with pancreatitis have tremendous visceral pain. Acceptable pain relief is one of the most important treatment goals of pancreatitis. There are a few pain concepts that should be considered on an individual basis; i.e., use of nonsteroidal analgesia and/or opioids. Some recent studies have used thoracic epidural analgesia. Some patients may require high doses of analgesia, particularly those that have tolerance. Patients need to be monitored closely for sedation and respiratory depression.

Medications commonly used to control pain and inflammation in adults with pancreatitis include:

Drug	Dose	Frequency	Comments
acetaminophen	1000 mg IV every 6 hr ATC/PRN	Maximum 4000 mg per day	May dose every 4 hr Use IV if patient NPO Decrease dosing in patients with liver dysfunction
NSAIDs		Caution in patients at risk for bleeding	

(continued)

Drug	Dose	Frequency	Comments
ibuprofen	400–800 mg IV every 6 hr ATC/PRN	Maximum 5200 mg per day	
ketoralac	30 mg IM/IV every 6 hr 15 mg IM/IV every 6 hr	No more than 5 days ≥65 yr or <110 lb, or with renal impairment	Caution in patients with bleeding risk

PERITONITIS

Peritonitis is inflammation of the peritoneum that may be caused by bacteria carried in the bloodstream from perforation or rupture of the GI tract. Peritonitis carries a great risk of septicemia.

Patients with peritonitis present with either acute or insidious onset of abdominal pain. The pain described is visceral in nature, dull and poorly localized with progression to severe and more localized pain. If the infection is not contained, such as from a perforation or intestinal ischemia, then the pain becomes diffuse.

Upon physical examination, patients with peritonitis most often appear unwell and in acute distress. Diffuse abdominal pain is felt. The pain tends to become constant, localized, and more intense near the site of the inflammation. An acutely ill patient tends to lie very still because any movement causes excruciating pain. They will lie with their knees bent to decrease strain on the tender peritoneum. The affected area becomes extremely tender and distended, and the muscles become rigid. Usually, nausea and vomiting occur and bowel sounds decrease. Fever, tachycardia, and leukocytosis are evident. On abdominal examination, patients demonstrate tenderness to palpation. In most patients, the point of maximal tenderness or referred rebound tenderness lies approximately over the pathologic process.

Types of Peritonitis

Primary: Caused by the spread of an infection from the blood and lymph nodes to the peritoneum. Usually occurs in people who have an accumulation of fluid in their abdomens (ascites or with peritoneal dialysis). The fluid that accumulates creates a good environment for the growth of bacteria.

Secondary: Caused by the entry of bacteria or enzymes into the peritoneum from the GI or biliary tract. This is usually caused by a perforation of an ulcer or intestine. Also, it can occur from abdominal trauma resulting in perforation or hemorrhage in the abdominal cavity.

Treatment

The general aim for peritonitis is treating the underlying condition. Often, emergency exploratory surgery is needed, especially when appendicitis, perforation, or diverticulitis may be the cause of the infection. If a definitive diagnosis of pelvic inflammatory disease or pancreatitis can be made, surgery is not generally necessary. Peritonitis from any cause is treated with broad spectrum antibiotics until the culture results are available. With primary peritonitis, antibiotics are the therapy. A Cochrane Review of 36 studies found that intra-peritoneal antibiotics are superior to IV antibiotics and no other single intervention was found to be superior (Wiggins, Craig, Johnson, & Strippoli, 2008). Other therapies include IV fluids, nasogastric tube, and antiemetics. Pain is managed using an IV opioid analgesic (morphine, hydromorphone, and fentanyl) since the patient is NPO (see Chapter 7). Assisting the patient in finding a comfortable position may also decrease pain.

ABDOMINAL COMPARTMENT SYNDROME (ACS)

Abdominal compartment syndrome (ACS) occurs as a result of an insult that causes a sustained increase in intra-abdominal pressure that affects tissue perfusion, causing organ ischemia. If left untreated, organ failure and ultimately death can result.

The normal pressure within the abdominal cavity is 5–7 mmHg in a critically ill adult. A sustained intra-abdominal pressure (IAP) greater than 20 mmHg that is associated with new organ dysfunction/failure is defined as ACS. The abdominal cavity responds to a volume increase of any of its contents with an increase in intra-abdominal pressure. An elevated intra-abdominal pressure may greatly affect the physiology and organ function because the abdominal compliance limit has been met.

All critically ill patients can develop ACS. Identifying the patient with intra-abdominal hypertension is critical and it has been recommended that all patients be screened upon admission to the ICU and in the presence of new or progressive organ failure (WSACS, 2007, Grade 1B evidence). Patients who are at higher risk are those who have had a trauma, damage control surgery associated with the compressive effect of intra-abdominal packing, coagulopathic disorders, bowel edema, and fascial or skin closure (Morken & West, 2001). Massive fluid resuscitation has been considered a major contributor to the development of ACS in critically ill patients (Papavramidis, Marinis, Pliakos, Kesisoglou, & Papavramidou, 2011). These patients have increased vascular permeability and massive fluid resuscitation leads to third spacing of fluid causing ascites, bowel edema, and engorgement of the mesenteric vessels and the lymphatic system, causing a decreased venous return.

The clinical presentation of ACS is not only evident within the abdomen but can exhibit signs of dysfunction in all systems including the pulmonary, cardiovascular, renal, GI, and neurological systems. The most common symptoms are:

- Increased airway pressures
- Decreased tidal volume
- Hypoxia
- Increased CVP
- Decreased cardiac output
- Oliguria
- Increase in abdominal tenseness and girth

Treatment

Recognition of early signs and symptoms is the best way of preventing the adverse outcomes of ACS, requiring monitoring the IAP of all high-risk patients early and trending with the vital signs and other hemodynamic parameters. Medical interventions usually are the first-line treatment before surgical decompression unless the IAP warrants urgent treatment. Different medical treatments have been recommended to decrease IAP based upon the following mechanisms (Gallagher, 2010; Malbrain & De laet, 2009).

Improvement of Abdominal Wall Compliance
- Use of sedation and analgesia
- Addition of neuromuscular blockade if sedation and analgesia are ineffective (WSACS, 2007; Grade 2C)
- Negative fluid balance
- Maintaining the head of the bed at less than 20 degrees or placing the patient in a reverse Trendelenburg position (Cheatham et al., 2009; Vasquez, Berg-Copas, & Wetta-Hall, 2007; De Keulenaer, De Waele, Powell, & Malbrain, 2009).

Evacuation of Intraluminal Contents
- Nasogastric and/or rectal drainage, enemas

Evacuation of Abdominal Fluid Collections (WSACS, 2007; Grade 2C)

- Ascites drainage (Sugrue, 2005)
- CT- or ultrasound (US)-guided aspiration of abscess/hematoma

Fluid Resuscitation (WSACS, 2007; Grade 1B)

- Avoid over resuscitation (WSACS, 2007; Grade 1B)
- Albumin with diuretics
- Colloids instead of crystalloids
- Dobutamine
- Dialysis or CVVH with ultrafiltration

Surgical decompression is used for ACS that reaches Grade IV with low cardiac output and/or an increase in peak airway pressures or IAH that is refractory to treatment. Surgical decompression is considered a life-saving intervention. When surgical decompression is done, the abdomen is left open until it can be closed. The surgeon may use a KCI Vac Pac or an Ioban dressing until the abdomen is ready to be closed.

Ensuring analgesia is paramount. Adequate pain medication should be administered, especially after abdominal surgery; even repositioning the patient may induce abdominal pain and muscle contractions, leading to falsely elevated IAP readings. Pain, agitation, ventilator asynchrony, and accessory muscle use during breathing may lead to increased abdominal muscle tone or increased abdominal wall compliance. Use of sedation and analgesia can reduce muscle tone, thereby decreasing IAP. In patients with capillary leak and abdominal wall edema, control of pain and agitation are usually not sufficient and the use of neuromuscular blockade should be considered. The recommendations on pain from WSACS (2007) are inconclusive due to the lack of prospective trials. Treating patients for pain and sedating them is still prudent.

CEREBRAL VASCULAR ACCIDENT

The brain is dependent upon the blood to deliver oxygen and other critical nutrients to maintain the viability of brain tissue. The blood supply can be altered via embolism, thrombosis, ischemia, hemorrhage, or spasm of the blood vessel, resulting in a cerebral vascular accident (CVA) or stroke. Stroke results from the interruption of the blood supply to the brain, which causes damage to a portion of brain tissue that can lead to a myriad of consequences such as weakness, numbness, paralysis, and speech difficulties that can impact a stroke survivor. Functionally, 17% of stroke survivors still have difficulty performing the basic activities of their daily lives (Centers for Disease Control and Prevention [CDC], 2010a).

Each year, 795,000 people experience a stroke. Approximately 610,000 of these are first attacks, and 185,000 are recurrent attacks. Of all strokes, 87% are ischemic, 10% are intracerebral hemorrhage, and 3% are subarachnoid hemorrhage strokes (Lloyd-Jones et al., 2009).

Pain after stroke is a symptom that often goes unnoticed. Some think that because a person has had a stroke that the person is unable to feel pain because he or she is unable to move an area of the body—that is simply not the case. Stroke patients may also experience pain from rigidity and reduced mobility, or from pre-existing conditions, such as osteoarthritis, which should be differentiated when making the diagnosis.

Shoulder Pain

Shoulder pain affects up to 72% of patients after a stroke and always occurs on the affected side, resulting in prolonged stiffness, loss of movement, and often severe pain. Hemiplegic shoulder pain may contribute to poor functional recovery of the arm and hand, depression, and sleeplessness (Lindsay et al., 2008). Shoulder subluxation is a common problem in hemiplegic patients although not all patients who have subluxation experience pain. During the initial flaccid stage of hemiplegia, the involved extremity must be adequately supported or the weight of the arm will result in shoulder subluxation. Improper positioning in the bed, lack of support while the patient is in the upright position, or pulling on the affected arm when transferring the patient all contribute to subluxation.

Lo et al. (2003) give the following distribution of types of shoulder pain;

- 50% adhesive capsulitis
- 44% shoulder subluxation
- 22% rotator cuff tears
- 16% having shoulder-hand syndrome/complex regional pain syndrome (CRPS)

Treatment

- *Analgesia:* Mild painkillers such as acetaminophen and/or anti-inflammatory drugs are often adequate. Consider round-the-clock dosing and before therapies that are known to cause pain, especially if the patient is unable to report pain. Stronger analgesics can be used as needed.
- Physical therapy consult as soon as possible.
- Detailed education on managing and protecting the affected limb from trauma for all team and family members (Evidence Level B).
- No blood draws, IVs, name bands on affected side.

■ Correct positioning and handling; good movement, positioning, and alignment, including shoulder care (Evidence Level B).

■ Support affected arm at all times; never pull on a limb during a transfer or positioning (Evidence Level B).

■ Avoid the use of overhead pulleys (Evidence Level A; Ottawa Panel et al., 2006).

Neuropathic Pain

A serious consequence of stroke is the development of severe burning pain on the side of the body affected by the stroke known as central post-stroke pain (CPSP). CPSP is also referred to as thalamic pain, neurogenic pain, or central pain syndrome, and occurs most frequently following strokes on the right side of the brain, which affect the left side of the body. Central pain is a result of the stroke and not from damaged nerves. The exact etiology of post-stroke pain is unknown, although it has been suggested that CPSP can arise from a chemical imbalance between glutamate and gamma-aminobutyric acid (GABA; Misrah, Kalita, & Kumar, 2008). By correcting the imbalance, pain relief is possible. Although the brain has been damaged, pain is still able to be felt even though pain is not being sensed.

The exact prevalence of CPSP is not known but estimated to be 1%–8%. Pain onset generally begins within 1–3 months after stroke in 63% of patients, 3 and 6 months in 19% of patients, and more than 6 months after stroke in 19% of patients (Misrah et al., 2008).

CPSP is characterized by constant or intermittent, moderate or severe pain, which is worsened by touch, movement, emotions, and changes in temperature. Common pain descriptors are stabbing, aching, dull and burning, shooting/lancinating. Pain may be unilateral or may only affect small areas. Symptoms may also exacerbated by stress and reduced by relaxation.

Treatment

Medication	Dosing
1. *First-line treatment:*	
gabapentin	1200–3600 mg/day
pregabalin (Level A)	150–600 mg twice a day
amitriptyline (Level B)	25–150 mg/day
2. *Second-/third-line treatment:*	
tramadol (Level A)	200–400 mm/day
opioids (Level B)	Not for chronic therapy
3. lamotrigine (Level B)	200 mg/day
4. *Combination therapy ([Level A]:* Gabapentin combined with opioids or TCA) is recommended for patients who show partial response to drugs administered alone.	

Spasticity and Contractures Post-Stroke

Some degree of spasticity is found in almost every patient with hemiplegia and usually occurs in the first 3 months following stroke. This can make normal movement impossible causing painful muscular spasms. Spasticity affects a patient's quality of life, decreasing function and activity. Left untreated, spasticity can lead to contracture although not all spasticity needs to be treated, a determination which needs to be made by the health care team.

The pathophysiology of spasticity is not completely understood, although it is thought to be associated with an interruption of descending inhibitory nerve signals along the spinal cord and brain, which causes an imbalance between inhibition and excitation.

Spasticity can cause an array of problems that can impact the patient's overall quality of life and function, such as causing pain, joint deformity, macerated skin, difficulty performing activities of daily living, ambulating, muscle tightness or stiffness, muscle spasms, or fatigue, and puts the patient at increased risk for falls.

Treatment

1. *Preventive Measures:* Early mobilization and return to self-care, skin care.
2. *Physical and Occupational Therapy:* Early physical therapy aims to prevent or reduce contractures and should begin as soon as the patient is able. It involves passive stretching performed to the affected joint, moving it in all possible positions without ever forcing the joint.
3. *Positioning/Orthotics:* Including taping, splints/orthotics, sitting (especially upper extremities), bed.
4. *Analgesia:* Pain from damage to muscle or other soft tissue that make movement, especially of the arms or legs, difficult or uncontrollable. This type of pain can usually be treated with some mild pain reliever such as aspirin, acetaminophen, or ibuprofen. Caution should be used for patients at risk for bleeding or patients who have experienced a cerebral bleed. Opioids may be tried but often have mixed results. Other medications may include amitriptyline, lamotrigine, and gabapentin.
5. *Oral Medications:* Oral medicines that may be prescribed for generalized spasticity include the following.

Table 15.3 ▨ *Anti-Spasticity Medications*

Medication	Mechanism of Action	Starting Dose	Maximum Dose	Side Effects
baclofen	GABA analogue; inhibits muscle stretch flex	5 mg 3 times a day	80 mg in 4 divided doses	Sedation, seizures, confusions, fatigue, ataxia
tizanidine	Alpha adrenergic agonist	2–4 mg	Daily dose should not exceed 36 mg	Drowsiness, sedation
dantrolene	Reduces calcium flux across the SR skeletal muscle	25 mg daily	100 mg 4 times a day	Muscle weakness, dizziness, hepatotoxicity
diazepam	GABA A receptor blocker	2 to 10 mg, 3 or 4 times per day		Sedation, cognitive dysfunction
gabapentin	GABA analogue	100 mg 3 times a day	600–800 mg 4 times a day	Sedation, dizziness, ataxia

Long-Term Treatments

6. *Injectable medications (Botulinum toxins and phenol)*: If spasticity affects only one or two specific parts of the body, injections of botulinum toxin (Botox) may be given directly into the muscle. The muscle relaxing effects usually last for about 3 months and do not interfere with nerve sensation.

7. *Surgical Intervention:* In severe cases of contractures, surgery to release tendons may be carried out. Advances in drug treatment have reduced the need for surgical treatment.

8. *Regional Spasticity:* Intrathecal drug therapy can be administered directly into subarachnoid space of the CNS with a programmable pump. Intrathecal baclofen, morphine sulphate (Duramorph), fentanyl are used. Use of this therapy has been found to improve walking speed and functional mobility without impairing uninvolved extremity. Fewer systemic side effects occur because the drug is not circulating in the blood stream.

Case Study

Jake Anderson, a 46-year-old male with a 15-year history of alcohol abuse, was admitted to the ICU with a 3-day complaint of severe upper abdominal pain, vomiting, and fevers.

Medical History: Negative
Surgical History: Negative
Medications: None
Allergies: NKDA
Social History: Homeless, heavy alcohol use, smokes 2 packs per day, no drug use
Vital Signs: T: 38.4, HR: 125, BP: 90/65, R: 26, O_2 sat: 93% room air
General: Appears ill, pale; restless and moaning in pain
Pain: Patient reports his pain intensity at 8–9/10. Pain radiates into his back. He describes it as excruciating.
CV: Tachycardia, normal heart sounds, pulses normal
Lungs: Clear
Abdomen: Mildly distended, moderately tympanic epigastrium, with voluntary guarding. Bluish discoloration around the umbilicus and bluish discoloration of the flank

Questions to Consider

1. What is your differential diagnosis?
2. What are the patient's risk factors?
3. What are the top three initial treatments you would expect to be implemented?
4. What would be the appropriate analgesia regimen for this patient? Do you have any concerns given his medical history?

REFERENCES

Apostolakis, E., Baikoussis, N. G., & Georgiopoulos, M. (2010). Acute type-B aortic dissection: The treatment strategy hellenic. *Journal of Cardiology, 51,* 338–347.

Barkun, A. N., Bardou, M., Kuipers, E. J., Sung, J., Hunt, R. H., Martel, M., & Sinclair, P. (2010). Clinical Guidelines: International consensus recommendations on the management of patients with nonvariceal upper gastrointestinal bleeding for the international consensus upper gastrointestinal bleeding conference group. *Annals of Internal Medicine, 152,* 101–113. doi:10.1059/0003-4819-152-2-201001190-00009.

Cheatham, M. L., De Waele, J. J., De Laet, I., De Keulenaer, B., Widder, S., Kirkpatrick, A. W., . . . Puig, S. (2009). The impact of body position on intra-abdominal pressure measurement: A multicenter analysis. *Critical Care Medicine, 37*(7), 2187–2190.

Cheatham, M. L., Malbrain, M. L. N. G., Kirkpatrick, A., Sugrue, M., Parr, M., De Waele, J., . . . Wilmer, A. (2007). Results from the conference of experts on intra-abdominal hypertension and abdominal compartment syndrome. Part II: Recommendations. *Intensive Care Medicine, 33,* 951–962.

De Keulenaer, B. L., De Waele, J. J., Powell, B., & Malbrain, M. L. (2009). What is normal intra-abdominal pressure and how is it affected by positioning, body mass and positive end-expiratory pressure? *Intensive Care Medicine, 35*(6), 969–976.

Despins, L. A., Kivlahan, C., & Cox, K. R. (2005). Acute pancreatitis: Diagnosis and treatment of a potentially fatal condition. *American Journal of Nursing, 105*(11), 54–57.

Gallagher, J. J. (2010). Intra-abdominal hypertension: Detecting and managing a lethal complication of critical illness. *AACN Advanced Critical Care, 21*(2), 205–217.

Herbert, G. S., & Steele, S. R. (2007). Acute and chronic mesenteric ischemia. *Surgery Clinics of North America, 87*(5), 1115–1134.

Holcomb, S. S. (2007). Stopping the destruction of acute pancreatitis. *Nursing, 37*(6), 42–47.

Leeper, B. (2007). Advanced cardiovascular concepts. In M. Chulay & S. M. Burns (Eds.), *AACN Essentials of progressive care nursing* (pp. 447–475). New York, NY: McGraw Hill.

Leeper, B. (2007). Cardiovascular concepts. In M. Chulay & S. M. Burns (Eds.), *AACN Essentials of progressive care nursing* (pp. 221–251). New York, NY: McGraw Hill.

Lindsay, P., Bayley, M., Hellings, C., Hill, M., Woodbury, E., & Phillips, S. (2008). Selected topics in stroke management. Shoulder pain assessment and treatment. Canadian best practice recommendations for stroke care. *Canadian Medical Association Journal, 179*(12 Suppl), E70–E72.

Lloyd-Jones, D., Adams, R., Carnethon, M., De Simone, G., Ferguson, T. B., Flegal, K., . . ., Hong, Y. (2009). Heart disease and stroke statistics 2009 update: A report from the American Heart Association statistics committee and stroke statistics subcommittee. *Circulation, 119,* 480–486.

Lo, S., Chen, S., Lin, H., Jim, Y., Meng, N., & Kao, M. (2003). Arthrographic and clinical findings in patients with hemiplegic shoulder pain. *Archives Physical Medicine and Rehabilitation, 84,* 1786–1791.

Malbrain, M. L. N. G., & De laet, I. E. (2009). Intra-abdominal hypertension: Evolving concepts. *Clinics in Chest Medicine, 30,* 45–70.

Manterola, C., Vial, M., Moraga, J., & Astudillo, P. (2011). Analgesia in patients with acute abdominal pain. *Cochrane Database of Systematic Reviews,* Issue 1. Art. No.: CD005660. doi:10.1002/14651858.CD005660.pub3.

Misrah, U. K., Kalita, J., & Kumar, B. J. (2008). Spasticity is particularly in the affected arm, prolonged stiffness & contracture. *Pain 9*(12), 11186–11122.

Morken, J., & West, M. A. (2001). Abdominal compartment syndrome in the intensive care unit. *Current Opinion in Critical Care, 7,* 268–274.

Nathens, A.B., Curtis, J. R., Beale, R. J., Cook, D. J., Moreno, R. P., Romand, J.- A., . . ., Waldmann, C. S. (2004). Management of the critically ill patient with severe acute pancreatitis. *Critical Care Medicine, 32,* 2524–2536.

Oldenburg, W. A., Lau, L. L., Rodenberg, T. J., Edmonds, H. J., & Burger, C. D. (2004). Acute mesenteric ischemia: A clinical review. *Archives of Internal Medicine, 164*(10), 1054–1062.

Papavramidis, T. S., Marinis, A. D., Pliakos, I., Kesisoglou, I., & Papavramidou, N. (2011). Abdominal compartment syndrome—Intra-abdominal hypertension: Defining, diagnosing, and managing. *Journal of Emergency Trauma Shock, 4*, 279–291.

Proctor, D. D. (2003). Critical issues in digestive diseases. *Clinics in Chest Medicine, 24*, 623–632.

Roger, V. L., Go, A. S., Lloyd-Jones, D. M., Adams, R. J., Berry, J. D., Brown, T. M., . . ., Wylie-Rosett, J. (2011). Heart disease and stroke statistics—2011 update: A report from the American Heart Association. *Circulation, 123*, e18–e209. doi:10.1161/CIR.0b013e3182009701.

Schermerhorn, M. L., Giles, K. A., Hamdan, A. D., Wyers, M. C., & Pomposelli, F. B. (2009). Mesenteric revascularization: Management and outcomes in the United States, 1988–2006. *Journal of Vascular Surgery, 50*, 341–348.

Sesler, J. M. (2007). Stress-related mucosal disease in the intensive care unit: An update on prophylaxis. *AACN Advanced Critical Care, 18*(2), 119–128.

Sugrue, M. (2005). Abdominal compartment syndrome. *Current Opinion in Critical Care, 11*, 333–338.

Vasquez, D. G., Berg-Copas, G. M., & Wetta-Hall, R. (2007). Influence of semi-recumbent position on intra-abdominal pressure as measured by bladder pressure. *The Journal of Surgical Research, 139*(2), 2802–85.

Wiggins, K. J., Craig, J. C., Johnson, D. W., & Strippoli, G. F.M. (2008). Treatment for peritoneal dialysis-associated peritonitis. *Cochrane Database of Systematic Reviews, Issue 1*. Art. No.: CD005284. doi:10.1002/14651858.CD005284.pub2.

16

Managing Patients Seeking Pain Relief in the Emergency Department

Pain as a presenting complaint accounts for two-thirds of all emergency department (ED) visits. Pain management in the ED has evolved over the years and continues to change with improved recognition, assessment, and treatment. Although awareness of pain has increased, patients continue to be undertreated or fail to be treated, or there is a delay in the treatment of pain.

The most common problem in the ED is oligoanalgesia. Oligoanalgesia is inadequate use of methods to relieve pain. One of the first studies addressing the issue of oligoanalgesia in the ED was a retrospective study by Wilson and Pendleton (1989), who were the first to coin the term. In the study, 198 patients were evaluated; 56% of patients received no analgesic medications while waiting in the ED; 69% waited for more than one hour before receiving analgesia, and 42% waited for more than two hours. Of those receiving analgesics, 32% received less than adequate doses of analgesic. Todd et al. (2007) conducted a study looking at current ED pain management practices at 20 U.S. and Canadian hospitals. The results showed that only 60% of patients received analgesics after an average wait time of 90 minutes. Seventy-four percent of patients were discharged in moderate to severe pain.

Documentation of pain scores in a consistent manner is an important mechanism for identifying unrelieved pain. In 2003, Eder, Sloan, and Todd evaluated the documentation of pain in the ED by physicians and nurses by retrospective study. Initial pain assessments were present in 94% of the charts, but use of a pain scale in only 23%. Prior to administration of analgesics, 39% had pain documentation and a pain scale was used 19% of the time. Nurses were two times more likely to document reassessment of pain than physicians (30% vs. 16%). In Guéant et al.'s (2011) multisite study of 50 EDs, patients' pain intensity was assessed by the visual analogue scale. A total of 11,760 patients were included; approximately 50% of the patients reported pain on admission, 90% were assessed for pain, and 44% reported severe pain. Forty-eight percent of patients were reassessed; 27%

of them still had pain and 8% reported severe pain on discharge. Delays in pain management were significantly related to the ED's volume, lack of triage nurses, patients' disorders, and initial pain intensity.

There is extensive research that reports that patients of racial minorities are being underevaluated and undertreated in the ED for their pain. A study conducted by Pletcher, Kertesz, Kohn, and Gonzales from 1995 to 2005 tried to determine whether there were any racial or ethnic disparities in prescribing opioids in the ED (Pletcher, Kertesz, Kohn, & Gonzales, 2008). The results indicated that Caucasians were more likely to receive an opioid pain medication (31%) than African American (23%), Hispanic (24%), or Asian/ Other (28%) patients. Disparities were more pronounced in patients with severe pain, long bone fractures, and nephrolithiasis. In another prospective study by Bijur, Bérard, Esses, Calderon, and Gallagher (2008) of patients with long bone fractures showed that 74% of Hispanic, 66% of African American, and 69% of Caucasians received opioid analgesics. Furthermore, there were no significant differences in the time to administer medication, analgesic dosages, routes of the analgesics given, or changes in pain.

Lack of time is a barrier in the nurse's ability to provide adequate pain management. ED volumes are growing, there is a growing nursing shortage, more institutions are fiscally restrained, and as workloads for all health practitioners increase, nurses need to prioritize care in order to provide safe patient care. Hwang, Richardson, Sonuyi, and Morrison (2006) suggested that, during periods of high ED volume, staff were less likely to be responsive to reports of pain especially in those patients that are the most vulnerable and unable to speak for themselves.

Pines and Hollander (2007) conducted a retrospective study evaluating the impact of ED crowding on patients with severe pain. Results showed that 49% of the patients received pain medication and of those patients who received analgesia, 59% experienced delays in treatment from triage and 20% experienced delays from time of room placement. Fosnocht and Swanson's (2007) study evaluated the ability of a triage pain protocol to improve frequency and time to delivery of analgesia for musculoskeletal injuries in the ED. The researchers showed that the time to medication administration was reduced from 76 minutes to 40 minutes after the implementation of the protocol and the number of patients receiving analgesia increased from 45% to 70%.

Nursing and medical schools have not emphasized pain education. Many health care providers have received little education in pain management. The Joint Commission, as a basis for accreditation, has mandated hospitals to recognize pain as the "fifth vital sign" although pain still remains undertreated. Knowledge deficits related to pain and analgesia are significant. With an emphasized focus on the recognition of pain, more nursing schools have placed increased importance on pain and have included it in their curriculum.Deficits in nurses' knowledge about pain and its management are also cited in the literature as contributing to oligoanalgesia. Jastrzab et al. (2003) used a questionnaire to determine the level of knowledge about analgesia among 272 nurses in a teaching hospital. Emergency nurses scored 61% on average. The researchers also noted that younger, less-experienced nurses were more knowledgeable than their more-experienced colleagues. This could reflect the current focus on recognition of pain in nursing schools.

Stalnikowicz, Mahami, Kaspi, and Brezis (2007) identified some factors that play a role in inadequate pain:

- A pre-occupation with the diagnosis and treatment of the underlying medical problem
- Concerns about masking symptoms
- Fears about contributing to or causing addiction
- Caregiver underestimation of pain experienced by the patient
- Cultural differences in pain expression
- Poor communication among patients, health care professionals, and caregivers
- Reluctance of patients to complain of pain or demand pain treatment
- A pain-free interval after acute traumatic injuries
- Inadequate training in the recognition and management of pain

In 2010, the American Society for Pain Management Nursing (ASPMN) and the Emergency Nurses Association (ENA), in collaboration with the American College of Emergency Physicians (ACEP) and the American Pain Society (APS), developed a position statement entitled "Optimizing the Treatment of Pain in Patients with Acute Presentations," addressing patients who present with acute pain. Their efforts support a collaborative responsibility between the physician and the nurse. Recommendations were made to improve pain in all health care settings. The basic principles support:

1. Comprehensive pain assessment including patients' self-reports. Recognize those populations at high risk.
2. Acknowledge cultural differences in pain expression.
3. Utilize evidence-based pain management assessment and management practices.
4. Analgesic management should begin as soon as possible when indicated and not wait until a definitive diagnosis is made.
5. Patients with addictive disease have special needs that must be addressed to ensure adequate and safe delivery of analgesia. Those with

addictive behaviors and repeated visits should be given the appropriate referral.

6. Aberrant behaviors do not equate with addictive disease and may indicate undertreatment of pain.

7. Health care settings should have appropriate pharmacologic agents and nonpharmacologic interventions readily available.

8. The development and adoption of analgesic protocols are encouraged. Protocols should be physician/nurse developed and nurse initiated.

9. Discharge instructions with an individualized pain treatment plan, including medication safety considerations.

10. Nursing and physician leadership is critical in promoting best practice treatment and referral for patients with a report of pain.

11. Clinician education and resources support optimal pain management.

12. Research and education are encouraged to support evidence-based analgesic practices.

WOUND MANAGEMENT

Traumatic wounds account for over 12 million ED visits a year in the United States, making them one of the most common reasons for an ED visit (Pfaff & Moore, 2007). The ultimate goal of wound management is to achieve rapid healing with optimal functional and aesthetic results (Hollander, Singer, Valentine, et al., 2001; Singer & Dagum, 2008).

Anatomy of the Skin

The skin is the largest organ in the body serving as a protective barrier from bacteria and trauma. Other important functions include temperature regulation, excretion, sensation, and metabolism of vitamin D.

The skin's characteristics vary throughout the body.

The skin is made up of the following layers:

Epidermis: The epidermis is the thin outer layer of the skin and consists of three parts:

▪ *Stratum corneum*: This layer consists of fully mature keratinocytes, which contain fibrous proteins. The outermost layer continuously sheds. The stratum corneum prevents the entry of most foreign substances as well as the loss of fluid from the body.

▪ *Keratinocytes (squamous cells)*: This layer, just beneath the stratum corneum, contains living keratinocytes (squamous cells), which mature and form the stratum corneum.

▓ *Basal layer*: The basal layer is the deepest layer of the epidermis, containing basal cells. Basal cells continually divide, forming new keratinocytes that replace the cells that are shed from the skin's surface.

Dermis: The dermis is the middle layer of the skin. Its main role is to regulate temperature and to supply the epidermis with nutrient-saturated blood. It is made up of fibroblasts, which produce collagen connective tissues and which give elasticity and support to the skin. The dermis contains the hair follicles, nerve endings, and pressure receptors. It also serves as the first defense against disease.

Subcutaneous: The subcutaneous layer or superficial fascia is not technically a layer of skin. It consists of a network of collagen and fat cells, which helps conserve the body's heat and protects the body from injury by acting as a shock absorber.

TYPES OF WOUNDS

There are acute and chronic wounds. Chronic wounds are defined as wounds that fail to progress over a period of 30 days (Hartoch et al., 2007).

Lacerations/Incisions

Injury occurs when tissue is cut or torn with a sharp object or as a result of blunt trauma resulting in tissue tearing. Incision is similar to laceration except wound ends are smooth and even. These types of wounds may penetrate the top layers of skin and spread deep into the dermis and surrounding structures.

These wounds include deep wounds of the hand or foot, full-thickness lacerations, lacerations involving nerves, arteries, bones, joints, and crush injuries.

Treatment
▓ Provide adequate pain control. Local anesthetic is administered prior to wound closure.
▓ Evaluate and explore the wound for severity, involvement of nerves, tendons, ligaments, blood vessels, and/or bones.
▓ Control bleeding.
▓ Cleanse the tissue of any blood clots or foreign material, remove necrotic tissue, and irrigate.
▓ Approximate wound edges.
▓ Apply sterile dressings.
▓ Immobilization is recommended for complex extremity wounds.

Abrasions

This is an injury to the skin where layers of tissue are removed as a result of the skin rubbing against a hard surface. The abrasion may be superficial or may involve multiple layers of skin. Pain is in proportion to the degree of injury. Foreign bodies such as dirt and gravel may be embedded into the affected area. If the area is not cleaned it may result in permanent tattooing.

Treatment

- Provide adequate analgesia prior to cleaning the affected area. Topical lidocaine, local anesthetic, or regional anesthetic should be used for abrasions of small to moderate size; for extensive abrasions, parenteral opioids or procedural sedation should be employed.
- Nonsurgical, moist dressings and a topical antibiotic are applied to protect the wound and aid healing.

Avulsions

An avulsion results from an injury that removes all the layers of skin, exposing fat or muscle. In partial avulsions, the tissue is elevated but remains attached to the body; the torn tissue is still well-vascularized and viable. In total avulsion, the tissue is completely torn from the body. If the torn tissue is nonviable, it is often excised and the wound is closed using a skin graft or local flap.

Treatment

- Provide adequate analgesia. Avoid local anesthetics with epinephrine due to their vasoconstriction abilities, which can compromise blood flow to the affected tissue.
- Inspect the tissue, clean and gently irrigate the area and control bleeding. Debride nonviable tissue.
- The flap is reattached to its anatomical position with a few sutures. Plastic surgery maybe an option for extensive injuries.

Abscesses

Abscesses develop as a result of pus that is unable to drain through the skin from an injury that has closed, allowing pus to accumulate.

Treatment

- Provide adequate analgesia or procedural sedation for patients experiencing severe pain.
- Local anesthetic can be used on the perimeter of the abscess to decrease or dull pain.

■ An incision is performed to the tense area of the abscess to allow drainage.
■ Packing is placed within the cavity of the abscess to prevent re-accumulation of pus.
■ Antibiotics may be given.

Puncture Wounds

Puncture wounds are deep wounds made by a sharp object such as a bullet, nail, or a jagged piece of metal or wood, the latter occurs especially to the foot. Puncture wounds have a rather high risk of infection particularly when the feet are involved.

Treatment
■ Provide adequate analgesia and examine the wound.
■ Remove debris, debride, and irrigate the wound.
■ Apply a sterile dressing. Some wounds may require packing.
■ Medication and follow-up treatment; e.g., tetanus immunization, antibiotics.

Crush Injuries/Crush Syndrome

Crush injuries occur as a result of a crushing and compressive force powerful enough to interfere with the normal metabolic function of the injured tissue.

Causes of Crush Syndrome
■ Collapse of a structure onto a body area
■ Compressive trauma to a body area
■ Prolonged compression in a chronic situation

Most often associated with severe fractures, the skin may remain intact. The area may be painful, swollen, deformed with little or no external bleeding although internal bleeding may be severe.

May Lead to
■ Rhabdomyolysis
■ Electrolyte abnormalities
■ Acid-base abnormalities
■ Hypovolemia
■ Acute renal failure

Early signs of crush syndrome are paralysis and sensory loss to the injured area, rigor of the joint distal to the injured muscles, pain, swelling, sensory changes, and weakness; may have pulses present and warm skin.

Treatment

Crush injuries can create injuries as minor as a laceration that heals in a few days or as severe as a traumatic amputation. Treatment is focused on saving the life first and salvaging the affected extremity or body part when possible.

▓ Pain management for the relief of pain and to promote mobilization.

▓ Aggressive and appropriate reversal of fluid deficits as indicated.

▓ Lab values (including CK, renal function, etc.).

▓ If signs and symptoms of rhabdomyolosis are found, treatment is initiated to prevent renal failure.

▓ Tetanus prophylaxis and antibiotics should be given to treat infection.

▓ Consult specialist for management of fractures.

Compartment Syndrome

Compartment syndrome occurs as a result of compressive forces within a closed space. Tissue pressure increases the capillary hydrostatic pressure, resulting in ischemia to muscle.

Moreover, muscle cell edema begins. If there is ischemia greater than 6 hours it leads to tissue hypoxia and cell death. Direct soft tissue trauma adds to edema and ischemia. Signs indicating compartment syndrome are known as the "5 Ps": pain, paresthesia, pallor, pressure, pulselessness.

Treatment

▓ Initiate medical management while surgical procedure is being arranged. If done in the ED, provide anesthesia or procedural sedation and analgesia for pain management (see Table 16.1).

▓ Measure compartment pressure

▓ Remove any constrictive casts or dressings and assess for improvement.

▓ Clinical signs and symptoms may indicate the need for an emergency fasciotomy. Early fasciotomy can preserve the limb.

Bites

Bites can occur from animals and humans; both types of bites are high risk for developing infection or transmitting disease. Facial bites are generally closed immediately but those on the hands, arms, legs, and torso are managed in a variety of ways.

Treatment

▓ Anesthetize and inspect affected areas for other damage to tendons, muscles, etc.

Table 16.1 ■ *Common Medications for Procedural Sedation*

Medication	Usual Dose (mg)	Usual Dose Range	Onset	Duration
fentanyl	1.0–3.0 mcg/kg	25–200 mcg	1 min	10–15 min
lorazepam	0.5–2 mg	1–6 mg	5–20 min	6–8 hrs
morphine	0.03–0.15 mg/kg	2–10 mg	1–2 min	30–60 min
midazolam	0.5–1 mg	1–5 mg	1–3 min	15–30 min
meperidine	0.5–1.0 mg/kg	25–100 mg	1–2 min	20–40 min
valium		2–10 mg		

■ Irrigate, remove debris, and debride nonviable areas.
■ Medication and follow-up treatment (tetanus immunization, antibiotics, rabies prophylaxis).
■ Closing of the bite is determined by the practitioner.
■ Cover area with a dry sterile dressing. The wound needs to be monitored for development of an infection.

WOUND HEALING

Trauma or injury results in tissue damage. After the injury, a pattern of local reactions and systemic changes occur. Most tissues in the body heal by going through the three phases: inflammatory, proliferative, and remodeling/maturation phases. These steps produce a scar in the place of a wound (Baum & Arpey, 2005).

■ The *inflammatory phase* occurs in response to an injury. The blood vessels in the wound contract and a clot is formed. Once hemostasis has been achieved, blood vessels then dilate to allow cells (antibodies, white blood cells, growth factors, enzymes, and nutrients) to reach the wounded area. Characteristic signs of inflammation can be seen: erythema, heat, edema, and pain.

■ After the inflammatory stage, the *proliferative stage* lasts about 3 weeks depending on the severity of the wound. Granulation occurs; fibroblasts make collagen to fill in the wound. New blood vessels form. The wound gradually contracts and is covered by a layer of skin.

■ *Remodeling/maturation*, the final phase, occurs once the wound has closed. This stage may last up to 2 years. New collagen forms, which increase the tensile strength of the scar tissue that is only 80% as strong as original tissue (Dealey, 2005).

Types of Healing

Wound healing is divided into repair by first, second, and third intention.

▪ First intention occurs when tissue is cleanly cut and re-approximated; healing occurs without complication.

▪ Secondary intention healing occurs in open wounds. When the wound edges are not approximated, it heals with formation of granulation tissue (i.e., skin ulceration, abscess cavities, punctures, and animal bites).

▪ Third intention occurs when a wound is allowed to heal open for a few days and then closed as if it were by first intention. Wounds are left open initially because of contamination.

WOUND ANESTHESIA

The research is clear that there are many procedures that are painful and distressing to patients. So health care professionals must place more focus on ensuring that procedural pain is managed. Evaluation of a wound and suture placement can be pretty painful. The area must be adequately anesthetized in order to perform these procedures properly. There are many pharmacologic agents and nerve-block techniques available to help minimize painful procedures. If adequate pain control is not attained, the patient should be taken to the operating room for general anesthesia.

Pain control should be provided prior to wound preparation to enable better preparation and treatment. Patients are then more relaxed and willing to cooperate without excessive anxiety and pain. The sensory, motor, and vascular examination should be performed prior to the administration of local or regional anesthetic.

Local anesthetics (LAs) work by temporarily blocking nerve conduction and the sensation of sharp pain, but the sensation of pressure is still felt although dulled. LAs can be administered topically, by infiltration directly into the area to be anesthetized or into the area of the peripheral nerves supplying the area to be anesthetized, and by IV.

Dosing of all LAs varies with procedure, degree of anesthesia needed, vascularity of tissue, duration of anesthesia required, and the physical condition of the patient. The smallest dose and concentration required to produce the desired effect should be used.

There are two classes of LAs, amides and esters. Both classes work by reversibly blocking sodium channels and inhibiting the propagation of nerve impulses (Heavner, 2007) (Table 16.2). The amides include prilocaine, lidocaine, bupivacaine, and mepivacaine. The esters include

Table 16.2 ▨ *Local Anesthetics for Wounds*

Agent	Concentration	Infiltration	Duration of Block
lidocaine	1%, 2%	Immediate	30–60 min
lidocaine with epidural	1%	Immediate	60–120 min
bupivacaine	0.25%, 0.5%	Slower	240–480 min
topical	Dependent	5–15 min	20–30 min

procaine and tetracaine. A way to remember the difference between the two classes of the drugs is that there are two "i"s in the amides.

Most LAs have a vasodilatory effect. Epinepherine (1:100,000) is often added to LAs before administration. Adding epinephrine to the LA increases the duration of anesthesia, provides wound hemostasis, and slows systemic absorption. Because vasoconstriction can cause tissue ischemia and necrosis, epinephrine should be avoided in the digits, pinna, nose, penis, and avulsed flaps with poor blood supply.

Injecting LA can be painful. The pH of LA solutions is acidic, depending upon the agent, additives, and buffers. The addition of sodium bicarbonate to the LA shortens the onset of action by raising tissue pH, reducing the pain of injection (Crystal, McArthur, & Harrison, 2007; Cepeda, Tzortzopoulou, & Thackrey, 2009). Other effective means of reducing pain of infiltration include use of a 27- to 30-gauge needle, slow injection, warming the solution to body temperature, and injecting through the margins of a wound rather than through intact skin surrounding the wound (Zilinsky Bar-Meir, Zaslansky, Mendes, Winkler, & Orenstein, 2005; Crystal et al., 2007).

Adverse reactions to local anesthetics are mostly related to the preservatives or the epinephrine in the solution, and true allergic reactions are extremely rare (Phillips, Yates, & Deshazo, 2007). In patients with true allergies to local anesthetics, two nontraditional agents can be used for wound repair via local injection: diphenhydramine and benzyl alcohol (Bartfield, Jandreau, & Raccio-Robak, 1998; Bartfield, May-Wheeling, Raccio-Robak, & Lai, 2001).

LOCAL ANESTHETIC TOXICITY (LAST)

Although it is rare for patients to experience serious side effects or complications of LAs, adverse events do occur. The ability of the health care professional to recognize signs and symptoms as early as possible to avoid a potential untoward outcome is essential.

There are many factors that play a role in the severity of LAST, such as the individual's risk factors, concurrent medications, location and technique of block, specific local anesthetic compound, total local anesthetic dose, timeliness of detection, and adequacy of treatment (Neal et al., 2010).

Bupivacaine is more likely than lidocaine to precipitate cardiovascular system (CVS) toxicity and central nervous system (CNS) toxicity simultaneously and risk is also increased in pregnancy. Patients who may be at higher risk are those with ischemic heart disease, metabolic or respiratory acidosis, severe cardiac dysfunction, advanced age, conduction abnormalities, metabolic disease, heart failure, and liver disease, and who are taking medications that inhibit sodium channels.

In 2010, the American Society of Regional Anesthesia (ASRA) published the Practice Advisory on Local Anesthetic Systemic Toxicity. The Advisory's focus is on prevention, although no single intervention can fully eliminate all risk. Some of the Practice Advisory's (2010) recommendations follow:

- Use of the lowest effective dose of LA.
- Use incremental dosing, pausing between injections.
- Avoid intravascular injection; aspirate prior to injection.
- If possible, use epinephrine with LA.

Diligent patient monitoring can minimize the risk to the patient and prevent LAST. Patient assessment is a key component while patients are receiving local anesthetic. Baseline physical assessment, vital signs, and neurological status must be conducted prior to the administration of the local anesthetic, followed by ongoing assessment for signs and symptoms of LAST. Patients should be educated to report any signs and symptoms of LAST to the health care professional.

Symptoms of LAST are dependent on plasma concentration of the local anesthetic drug. They are categorized into CNS and CVS signs and symptoms. The CNS is generally more common and occurs with a lesser plasma concentration. It is possible for CVS collapse to occur without preceding CNS warning signs.

Treatment for CNS toxicity is supportive, including maintaining a patent airway, monitoring vital signs, administering IV fluids, and giving antiseizure medications. Intralipid is currently recommended to prevent the development of CVS toxicity associated with LAST. The pharmacokinetics of lipid emulsion therapy in the treatment of LAST has not been fully explained but it likely involves increasing metabolism, distribution, or partitioning of the local anesthetic away from receptors into lipid within tissues (Burch, McAllister, & Meyer, 2011).

Table 16.3 ■ *Signs and Symptoms of LAST in Order of Increasing Plasma Concentrations*

Central Nervous System	Cardiovascular System
• Disorientation • Metallic taste • Tingling (numbness) and (circum-oral numbness) • Lightheadedness • Tinnitus (ringing in ear), auditory/visual hallucinations • Muscular twitching/spasms • Unconsciousness • Seizures • Coma • Respiratory arrest	• Hypertension and tachycardia • Decreased cardiac output due to negative inotropic effect of local anesthetic • Hypotension due to vascular bed vasodilatation • Sinus bradycardia • Ventricular arrhythmias (torsade de pointes common) • Cardiovascular collapse

The ASRA Practice Advisory (2010) also made the following ACLS modifications in the event of a cardiac event:

■ If epinephrine is used, small initial doses are preferred. Giving epinephrine may enhance dysrhythmias induced by local anesthetic; therefore, it is recommended to avoid high doses of epinephrine and use smaller doses for treating hypotension.
■ Vasopressin is not recommended.
■ Avoid calcium channel blockers and beta adrenergic receptor blockers.
■ If ventricular arrhythmias develop, amiodarone is preferred; treatment with local anesthetics such as lidocaine or procainamide is not recommended.

TOPICAL ANESTHESIA

Topical anesthetics provide effective, short term analgesia for uncomplicated lacerations and may potentially eliminate the need for LA infiltration. They do not distort wound edges, which may occur with subcutaneous infiltration. Topical anesthetics may cause ischemia where there is only a single blood supply (e.g., fingers, toes, nose, pinna of ear, or penis) or mucous membranes because of its vasoconstrictive properties. There are three categories of topical anesthetic based upon their use: mucous membranes, nonintact skin, and intact skin. Topical anesthetics come in liquids or gels. A zone of blanching around the wound indicates anesthesia. Five percent of wounds anesthetized with a topical anesthetic will require supplemental infiltration (Hirschmann, 2008). EMLA cream is rarely used to anesthetize wounds due to the prolonged onset of action of approximately 1 hour.

Liposome Encapsulated Lidocaine (LMX4) Lidocaine 4%

▪ *Indications:* Produce surface anesthesia of the skin prior to venous cannulation, venipuncture, or dermal procedures
▪ *Onset:* Apply thick layer (2 g to 2.5 g) of cream with an occlusive dressing. Leave on for 60 minutes for effect.
▪ *Side Effects*: Irritation, redness, itching, burning, rash, methemglobinenia.

LET (4% Lidocaine, 1:2,000 Epinephrine, and 0.5% Tetracaine)

▪ *Indications*: Uncomplicated facial and scalp lacerations
▪ *Onset:* 1 to 3 mL swabbed directly to the wound bed and edges, then applied as a LET-soaked sterile gauze or cotton for 20 to 30 minutes and removed before the procedure. Not for nose, pinna of ear, penis, and digits; avoid mucous membranes, vasoconstriction.
▪ *Duration*: Not established.
▪ *Efficacy:* Similar to TAC for face and scalp lacerations; less effective on extremities.
▪ *Side Effects*: No severe adverse effects reported.

EMLA (Eutectic Mixture of Local Anesthetics) Lidocaine 2.5% and Prilocaine 2.5%

▪ *Indications*: Used on intact skin to relieve the pain associated with venipuncture, arterial puncture, port access, skin grafting procedures, and other superficial skin procedures.
▪ Thick layer (1 to 2 g per 10 cm^2) applied to intact skin to create a dense sensory loss (Pasero & McCaffery, 2011).
▪ *Onset*: Must be left on for 1 to 2 hours prior to procedure and cover with occlusive dressing.
▪ *Duration:* 0.5 to 2 hours.
▪ *Efficacy:* Variable, depending on duration of application.
▪ *Side Effects*: Contact dermatitis, methemoglobinemia (very rare).

DIRECT WOUND INFILTRATION

Direct infiltration is the most common technique used in the ED and works on most minor wounds. It requires multiple contiguous injections of anesthetic along the length of the wound edges. The following is recommended to minimize discomfort from anesthetic infiltration:

- Use thinnest needle possible.
- Minimize the number of skin punctures.
- Perform subsequent needle stick through already anesthetized skin.
- Inject into the subdermis rather than the dermis; raising a wheal is painful.
- Anesthetic injected slowly over 10 seconds is less painful and more comfortable.

DIGITAL BLOCKS

The most common nerve block used in the ED is the digital block. It can be used when the nerve supply to the wound is superficial and the skin is sensitive. This technique is recommended for the digits, palms, and soles, as well as nail removal, nail-bed repair, paronychia, and removal of foreign bodies. Digital block does not alter the wound or affect approximation. This technique provides anesthesia to the entire digit and is an excellent block for lacerations of the fingers or toes, drainage of paronychia, finger or toenail removal or repair, and reduction of fractured or dislocated fingers or toes (Kang, 2007).

BIER BLOCK

Intravenous regional blocks (Bier blocks) can be performed on injuries that are distal to the elbow or the knee. The extremity is purposefully exsanguinated and application of a tourniquet is applied. A large volume of diluted lidocaine is injected into a vein. The lidocaine diffuses to local nerves to produce a neural blockade. The Bier block provides surgical-level anesthesia for up to 60 minutes without the risks of general anesthesia. It is an excellent block for large complex lacerations or fracture reductions (Mohr, 2006).

It is important to assess neurovascular status in the involved limb before the block to prevent masking a primary traumatic neurovascular injury. The major safety concern is that lidocaine only is recommended for use in the event the tourniquet is opened prematurely. The other local anesthetics each reach toxic levels resulting in seizure and/or cardiac arrest compared to lidocaine since they are limited by body weight.

MODERATE SEDATION

Some patients, due to the extent of their injuries or the level of their anxiety and pain, may require the use of moderate sedation in order to be treated. The ED may use moderate sedation for a number of reasons, including the repair of complex lacerations, reduction of fractures and casting, wound care, and abscess incision and drainage. The Joint Commission (2008) defines moderate sedation/analgesia as a "drug-induced depression of consciousness" during which individuals respond purposefully to verbal commands either alone or accompanied by light tactile stimulation. No interventions are required to maintain a patent airway, and spontaneous ventilation is adequate. The patient must be closely and continuously monitored to prevent progression to a deeper sedated state.

Appropriate patient selection and assessment prior to drug administration are essential in order to provide safe patient care during and after sedation. Pre-sedation selection includes the recognition of risk factors that may place the patient at increased risk of complication such as patients with high levels of anxiety or those with pre-existing comorbidities that may put them at increased risk.

The American Society of Anesthesiologists (ASA) developed a Physical Status Classification System to determine the risk for complications among patients undergoing anesthesia (Table 16.4). Patients in Classes 1 and 2 are considered good candidates for moderate sedation procedures; those in Classes 3 and Class 4 carry higher risks but are not excluded based upon their score.

The nurse performs a complete pre-procedure health history assessment (NPO status, patient education, discharge instructions, insertion

Table 16.4 ▪ *American Society of Anesthesiology/ASA Classification*

	ASA Classification
ASA Physical Status 1	A normal healthy patient
ASA Physical Status 2	A patient with mild systemic disease
ASA Physical Status 3	A patient with severe systemic disease
ASA Physical Status 4	A patient with severe systemic disease that is a constant threat to life
ASA Physical Status 5	A moribund patient who is not expected to survive without the operation
ASA Physical Status 6	A declared brain-dead patient whose organs are being removed for donor purposes

of IV). The procedural area must be equipped prior to the procedure with emergency equipment, medications, and supplies.

At the end of the sedation period, the patient will continue to be monitored until the patient reaches his/her pre-sedation level of consciousness and functioning. The procedural monitoring nurse accompanies the patient to the recovery area and will give a concise report to the nurse assuming care of the patient (respiratory, circulatory, and neurologic function of the patient before and during the procedure, measures to control the patient's pain, and the time and effectiveness of pain medications). Other important items to include are the total amount of mediations received and reversal agent administration, if given. Post-procedure patients are typically monitored by recording vital signs and other parameters every 15 minutes in the procedure area or a recovery area. The recovery period lasts from the conclusion of the operative procedure until the patient has returned to baseline and discharge criteria are met.

RENAL AND URETERAL CALCULI

Overview

Nephrolithiasis is the most common cause of sudden onset of persistent flank pain. Over 1 million ED visits are made annually for renal colic and urinary stone disease in the United States (Sterrett, Moore, & Nakada, 2009). The average lifetime risk of stone formation has been reported in the range of 5% to 10% (Türk, Knoll, Petrik, & Sarica, 2010). In the United States, the prevalence is highest in Caucasian men and women with a 3:1 male-to-female ratio occurring in the third to fifth decades of life (Worcester & Coe, 2008). Fifty-five percent of those with recurrent stones have a family history of urolithiasis, and having a history increases the risk of stones (Teichman, 2004). African Americans have a higher incidence of infected renal calculi than Caucasians.

Nephrolithiasis has a higher prevalence in hot, arid, or dry climates such as the mountains, desert, or tropical areas. An increased incidence has been noted in the southeastern United States, prompting the term "stone belt" for this region of the country (Worcester & Coe, 2008).

Pathophysiology

Renal calculi form from a collection of crystals that build in the urine when there is a high enough concentration of certain compounds. The development of stones is multifactorial. There are different types of renal calculi and determining the type of stone will decide the cause. Calcium stones are the most common type, making up 80% of all renal calculi. Some risk factors include increased urinary excretion of a specific solute, hyperparathyroidism, low urine volume, inflammatory bowel disease, and result of small bowel resection. Uric acid stones accounts for 10% of renal calculi. Patients may also develop gout. Risk factors may include elevated levels of uric acid in the urine and acidic urine with a pH less than 5.5. Struvite stones account for 10% of renal calculi. These stones are often associated with infection from urea-splitting organisms, which include *Proteus* and *Klebsiella* (Manthey, Nicks, n.d.). These stones are particularly large and usually have to be removed by surgery. The risk of urosepsis is high as long as the stones remain. Cystine stones are rare and account for less than 1% of all renal calculi. This is a result of an autosomal recessive disorder that results in abnormal intestinal and renal tubular absorption of the amino acids cystine, ornithine, lysine, and arginine called cystinuria.

Certain medications are also associated with an increased risk of stone formation including antacids, medications to treat glaucoma, sodium- and calcium-containing medications, vitamins C and D, and protease inhibitors. These medications can lead to higher levels of minerals that promote calculi formation.

Clinical Presentation

Patients classically present with sudden-onset of flank pain, often radiating to the ipsilateral abdomen and groin. The pain typically comes in waves and stops when the ureter relaxes or the patient passes the stone into the bladder. The patient's pain is so severe that it is unrelieved by position changes and the patient may writhe in agony. The pain is caused by distension of the renal pelvis and upper ureter as well as by peristalsis of the ureter. The site of referred pain depends on the position of the stone in the collecting system (Vasavada, Comiter, & Raz, 2001). Flank tenderness can be elicited upon exam.

There may be associated nausea and vomiting. A small percentage of patients with renal colic do not have hematuria. Fever is not part of the presentation of uncomplicated renal calculi; if present, suspect infection. Abdominal examination usually is unremarkable. Bowel sounds may be hypoactive, a reflection of mild ileus, which is not uncommon in patients with severe, acute pain. In patients older than 60 years with no prior history of renal stones, the patient needs to be examined for abdominal aortic aneurysm. Differential diagnoses may be often confused with renal colic due to the presentation of the patient's discomfort (Table 16.5).

Most kidney stones pass out of the body without any intervention by a physician. Cases that cause lasting symptoms or other complications

Table 16.5 ■ *Renal Calculi: Differential Diagnosis*

Stone Location	Common Symptom	Differential Diagnosis
Kidney	• Vague flank pain • Hematuria	Right- sided pain • Cholecystitis Left-sided pain • Acute pancreatitis • Peptic ulcer disease • Gastritis
Proximal ureter	• Renal colic • Flank pain • Upper abdominal pain	
Middle section of ureter	• Renal colic • Anterior abdominal pain • Flank pain	Right-sided pain • Appendicitis Left-sided pain • Acute diverticulitis
Distal ureter	• Renal colic • Dysuria • Urinary frequency • Anterior abdominal pain • Diarrhea and tenesmus • Flank pain • Radiatingpain into the groin, testicle, or labia	• Cystitis • Urethritis • Pelvic inflammatory disease • Ovarian cyst rupture • Torsion • Menstrual pain

may be treated by various techniques, most of which do not involve major surgery.

Diagnostic Testing

Imaging Studies
■ Computed tomography (CT) without contrast
■ Intravenous pyelography
■ Tomography
■ KUB films and directed ultrasonography
■ Helical CT

Laboratory Examinations

- Urinalysis
- Blood urea nitrogen (BUN)
- Creatinine
- Blood uric acid (BUA)
- Complete blood count (CBC)
- Urine culture
- Stone analysis

Treatment Options

First line treatment for acute renal calculi is conservative management (hydration, analgesia, and antiemetics). Antibiotics are to be given for those who have evidence of infection. Patients presenting with typical symptoms should receive rapid analgesic therapy without delays in treatment for confirmatory testing with urinalysis or imaging studies (Safdar et al., 2006).

In patients with acute renal colic, nonsteroidal anti-inflammatory drugs (NSAIDs) should be the drug treatment of choice. In a Cochrane Review of 20 clinical trials comparing any opioid with any NSAID via various routes of administration, the combination of opioid and NSAID resulted in the greatest reduction of patient pain reports. It was also noted that there was significantly less vomiting in patients treated with NSAIDs. Patients who received opioids, in particular meperidine, had a much higher incidence of vomiting. Patients who received NSAIDs also were considerably less likely to receive rescue medication (Holdgate & Pollock, 2004).

Ketorolac works at the peripheral site of pain production rather than on the central nervous system and has fewer adverse effects. The major disadvantage of an NSAID is that it can affect renal function in patients with already reduced renal function. The GI effects of prolonged NSAID use are also well known. Dosage should be adjusted for patients 65 years or older, for patients under 50 kg (110 lbs) of body weight, and for patients with moderately elevated serum creatinine.

Ketoralac

- IV preferred or IM, 30 mg every 6 hours (maximum 120 mg in a 24-hour period). Not to exceed more than 5 days.
- Switching from parenteral to oral therapy, the first oral dose is 20 mg, followed by 10 mg PO every 4–6 hours (maximum 40 mg in a 24-hour period).

- Greater than 65 years of age, weight less than 50 kg, or renal impairment: 15 mg IV every 6 hours. Not to exceed more than 5 days.
- Weight less than 50 kg: Switching from parenteral to oral therapy, 10 mg every 4–6 hours (maximum 40 mg in a 24-hour period).

For patients in the outpatient setting oral NSAIDs (ibuprophen, cyclo-oxygenase-2 inhibitors, and meloxicam) are generally used by practitioners. A new intranasal ketorolac has become available and may be useful for outpatients.

The pain associated with ureteral stones has been conventionally managed with narcotics. In severe cases of renal colic it is recommended to use an NSAID with an opioid. NSAIDs used in conjunction with narcotics are thought to decrease pain by diminishing ureterospasm and renal capsular pressure. A prospective, double-blinded, randomized controlled study looked at 130 patients for the efficacy of IV ketorolac, morphine, and both drugs in combination in reducing pain in acute renal colic (Safdar et al., 2006). The combination of morphine and ketorolac was superior in pain relief compared to the other combinations as well as the requirement for rescue analgesia (Safdar et al., 2006).

For people with ureteral stones that are expected to pass, the European Association of Urology recommends the use of rectal or oral diclofenac sodium for reducing the inflammatory process and the risk of recurrent pain (European Association of Urology, 2008). This recommendation came from a small double-blind, placebo-controlled trial that found oral diclofenac was effective, especially during the first 4 days, and reduced the number of hospital re-admissions.

IV hydration is given to correct any fluid deficit related to nausea, vomiting, or for limited oral intake. IV boluses will not force stone passage or manage the patient's pain (Springhart et al., 2006).

Nausea and vomiting occur in at least 50% of patients. Nausea is caused by the common innervation pathway of the renal pelvis, stomach, and intestines through the celiac axis and vagal nerve afferents. Nausea is also compounded by the effects of opioid analgesics. Metoclopramide has been specifically studied for its antiemetic effect for the treatment of renal colic. The antiemetic effect comes from blocking the dopamine receptors in the central nervous system. The usual dose in adults is 10 mg IV or IM every 4–6 hours as needed. Metoclopramide is not available as a suppository and has been associated with movement disorders such as extra-pyramidal reactions; tardive dyskinesia it is a cumulative effect with long-term use. Ondansetron is a serotonin (5-HTP) receptor antagonist. It is thought to affect both peripheral and central nerves by reducing the activity of the vagus nerve and blocks the serotonin receptors in the chemoreceptor trigger zone. The usual dose is 4 mg slow IV push (over 2–5 minutes) or 4 mg IM.

Other Treatment Options

- Dissolution agents
- Extracorporeal shock wave lithotripsy (ESWL)
- Ureteroscopic stone extraction
- Percutaneous nephrolitotomy (PCNL)
- Open stone surgery

BACK PAIN

Back pain is a common complaint that affects up to 90% of the general population at some time in their lives (Della-Giustina, 1999). Patients are often seen in the ED with acute back pain because of lack of accessibility to their primary care practitioner. Back pain is such a common complaint and not generally associated with significant pathology, although potentially life- or neurologically threatening diseases may be overlooked.

In 2008, the Agency for Healthcare Research and Quality (AHRQ) reported 7.3 million ED visits at U.S. hospitals were attributed to back problems. Of all the ED visits, 46.9% had back problems listed as a principal diagnosis. ED visits and inpatient stays for patients with any diagnosis of back problems increased with age, with the highest rate being for patients 85 years and older. The rate of ED visits for patients with a principal diagnosis of back problems was highest for 18 to 44 year olds and were the most likely to require just ED care for back pain; men were the least likely to need ED care. The overall costs for inpatient stays related to a principal diagnosis of back problems was over $9.5 billion, making it the ninth most expensive condition treated in U.S. hospitals (Owens, Woeltje, & Mutter, 2011).

Back pain can be divided into three types: acute, subacute, and chronic pain. Acute pain is back pain that lasts less than 6 weeks and approximately 60% of patients will return to function within a month. Subacute pain lasts 6 to 12 weeks, and 90% of those patients return to function within 3 months. Chronic pain lasts 12 weeks or longer; this type of pain is less likely to resolve over time.

The most common diagnosis for back pain is nonspecified spinal pain. Patients will present with localized pain and minimal or no physical findings; the origin of the pain is generally unknown. Radicular back pain presents with symptoms of radiating pain that is dermatomal or runs along the affected nerve root as a result of nerve compression and/or irritation. The most serious and concerning type of back pain is a result of a serious spinal condition. Only 20% of patients with back pain have a true cause found (Ross, 2006). The healthcare practitioner needs to determine the cause of back pain to rule out serious illness by ruling out the "red flags."

Obtain a comprehensive clinical history and focused assessment with consideration of age, duration of pain, history of trauma, location and radiation of pain, systemic complaints, history of cancer, neurologic deficits, psychological and social risks, and functional pain (Hayes, Huckstadt, & Daggett, 2006). Focus on identifying and eliminating red flags or historical factors that should raise the clinician's suspicion for more serious etiology (Table 16.6). Radiographic films are not part of the initial evaluation.

American College of Physicians and the American Pain Society Practice Recommendations for the Diagnosis and Treatment of Low Back Pain

These guidelines were developed as a collaborative with the American College of Physicians (ACP) and the American Pain Society Practice (APS) to standardize treatment for the diagnosis and treatment of low back pain. The guidelines are specific for patients with nonspecific low back pain, back pain associated with radiculopathy or spinal stenosis, and back pain associated with another specific spinal cause. Eighty-five percent of patients who present to primary care have low back pain (Chou, Huffman, American Pain Society, & American College of Physicians, 2007a, 2007b). Spinal stenosis and herniated disc are present in about 3% and 4%, respectively, of patients with lower back pain, cancer 0.7%, compression fracture 4%, spinal infection 0.01%, ankylosing spondylitis 0.3% to 5%, and cauda equina syndrome 0.04% (Chou et al., 2007a, 2007b).

Health care practitioners should conduct a focused history and physical examination that include an assessment of psychosocial risk factors, which may be indicative of predicting risk for chronic back pain. Include duration of symptoms, risk factors for serious conditions, symptoms suggestive of radiculopathy or spinal stenosis, and presence and severity of neurologic deficit.

- *Initial Assessment*: Medical history or physical examination findings may indicate serious underlying condition such as fracture, tumor, infection or cauda equina syndrome.

Table 16.6 ■ *Red Flags for Acute Low Back Pain With Potential Etiology*

Red Flags	Etiology
Historical Red Flags	
Age <18>50	Congenital, tumor
Major trauma	Fracture
Minor trauma in elderly	Fracture
History of cancer	Tumor
Fever and chills	Infection
Weight loss	Tumor, infection
Injection drug use	Infection
Immunocompromised	Infection
Night pain	Tumor, infection
Unremitting pain, even when supine	Tumor, infection
Incontinence	Epidural compression
Saddle anesthesia	Epidural compression
Severe or rapidly progressive neurologic deficit	Epidural compression
Physical Red Flags	
Fever	Infection
Unexpected anal sphincter laxity	Epidural compression
Perianal/perineal sensory loss	Epidural compression
Major motor weakness	Single or multiple nerve root compression

■ *Focused Physical Examination:* General observation of the patient for level of function, range of motion testing, a regional back exam, neuromuscular examination and testing for nerve root compromise.

■ *Neurologic Examination:* Assess for evidence of nerve root impairment, peripheral neuropathy, or spinal cord dysfunction. Emphasize gait examination, ankle and knee reflexes, ankle and great toe dorsiflexion strength, straight leg raising test, and distribution of sensory complaints.

Routine imaging or other diagnostic testing is not recommended in patients with nonspecific low back pain. Patients with low back pain with severe or progressive neurologic deficits or when serious underlying conditions are suspected such as vertebral infection, cauda equina syndrome, or cancer with impending spinal cord compression because of delayed diagnosis and treatment are associated with poorer outcomes (Chou et al., 2007a, 2007b).

For patients with persistent low back pain and those with signs or symptoms of radiculopathy or spinal stenosis, obtain an MRI or CT only if they are potential candidates for surgery or epidural steroid injection. The evidence does not suggest that routine imaging affects treatment decisions or improves outcomes (Modic et al., 2005).

Provide patients with evidence-based information on low back pain and provide information about effective self-care options.

Use of medications with proven benefits should be utilized. Assess severity of baseline pain and functional deficits, potential benefits, risks, and relative lack of long-term efficacy and safety data before initiating therapy.

Utilize non-parmacologic therapy for acute low back pain when self-care options have not improved. Spinal manipulation administered by providers with appropriate training has some short-term benefits (Modic et al., 2005).

Patients with low back pain have been treated with various medications that have risk benefits associated with their use (acetaminophen, NSAIDs, muscle relaxants, opioid analgesics, and oral corticosteroids). First-line medication options such as acetaminophen or NSAIDs can be effective.

Medication Recommendations

The evidence supports the effectiveness of acetaminophen, NSAIDs, and muscle relaxants for use in acute low back pain. Additional information regarding specific medications is presented in Chapters 6 to 9.

Acetaminophen

Acetaminophen is the most widely used over-the-counter medication in a class of medications called analgesics and antipyretics. Acetaminophen is also known as paracetamol and N-acetyl-p-aminophenol (APAP). It has analgesic and antipyretic effects that are similar to aspirin although it has a weak anti-inflammatory effect. In acute low back pain, studies indicate no clear difference was seen in pain relief between acetaminophen and NSAIDs (van Tulder, Scholten, Koes, & Deyo, 2000, 2006, 2008).

Although the exact site and mechanism of analgesic action is not clearly defined, acetaminophen appears to produce analgesia by elevation of the pain threshold. The potential mechanism may involve inhibition of the nitric oxide pathway mediated by a variety of neurotransmitter receptors.

Acetaminophen is available in various forms. The oral dose for adults is 325 to 650 mg every 4 to 6 hours. The maximum daily dose is 4 g. Onset of analgesia is less than 1 hour after oral administration of acetaminophen, and its half-life is approximately 2 hours. Acetaminophen is metabolized by the liver and doses that exceed the maximum dose may result in severe liver damage. Guidelines recommend acetaminophen as a first line treatment analgesic for acute low back pain.

NSAIDs

In 2008, a Cochrane Review of 65 studies (11,237 patients) in which NSAIDs were given for low back pain, with or without sciatica, showed the drugs are more effective than placebo. NSAIDs have significantly more side effects compared to acetaminophen. There is no specific type of NSAIDs that is more effective (Roelofs, Deyo, Koes, Scholten, & van Tulder, 2008). The selective COX-2 inhibitors showed fewer side effects compared to traditional NSAIDs in the randomized control trials, although recent studies have shown that COX-2 inhibitors are associated with increased cardiovascular risks in specific patient populations (Roelofs et al., 2008).

The findings support guidelines that suggest NSAIDs be used only after acetaminophen has been tried since there are fewer side effects with acetaminophen. The 65 studies compared NSAIDs to placebo, acetaminophen, muscle relaxants, other drugs, non-drug treatments, and other NSAIDs. There was no significant difference if the patients were suffering from sciatica. For chronic pain, NSAIDs also significantly reduced pain but had significantly more side effects. Seven of the studies compared one or more types of NSAIDs with acetaminophen; researchers found moderate evidence that the two forms of medication are equivalent in reducing acute low back pain, moderate evidence that NSAIDs are no more effective than other drugs for acute low back pain, and strong evidence that various types of NSAIDs, including the COX-2 inhibitors, are equally effective for acute low back pain (Roelofs et al., 2008).

Patients often take these medications intermittently, and an effective level of the anti-inflammatory properties is not sustained. Patients should be advised to take the medications on a round-the-clock schedule in order to maximize the analgesic and anti-inflammatory effects. The major adverse reactions to NSAIDs include GI bleeding and renal damage. NSAIDs also have been shown to slow bone and tissue healing (Roelofs et al., 2008). Prolonged use should be avoided to minimize the associated risks.

Muscle Relaxants

Muscle relaxants are often prescribed in the management of acute low back pain. They have been shown to be more effective when they are used in conjunction with NSAIDs (Beebe, Barkin, & Barkin, 2005; van Tulder, Touray, Furlan, Solway, & Bouter, 2003). Non-benzodiazepine muscle relaxants such ascyclobenzaprine, carisoprodol, and methocarbamol are preferable only for a short period of time, generally 2 weeks (Beebe et al., 2005). The most frequently reported side effect of muscle relaxants is sedation and it is usually recommended to take the medication at bedtime to avoid this side effect.

Opioid Analgesics

Opioids in patients with acute low back pain should be considered as a second-line option or for short-term use if necessary for patients with sciatica. There is no evidence to support the use of one opioid versus another (Chou, Clark, & Helfand, 2003). In a 2006 Cochrane Review, there was no significant advantage of opioid use in symptom relief or return to work when compared with NSAIDs or acetaminophen (van Tulder et al., 2006).

Oral Steroids

No studies support the use of oral steroids in patients with acute low back pain.

LOW BACK PAIN

Acute back pain usually resolves within 6–8 weeks regardless of treatment options used (D'Arcy, 2011). The goal of treatment in this population is to prevent immobility and to provide acceptable analgesia while the condition resolves.

Signs and Symptoms

- Localized asymmetrical pain in the lumbar or sacral paraspinous muscles.
- Pain may be described as an ache or spasm.
- Radiating pain into buttock or thigh worsened upon activity and relieved with rest.
- Sensory loss, weakness, or reflex changes.

Diagnostic Criteria

- If no red flags are found during the clinical history and physical assessment, no other testing is required (Chou et al., 2007).
- If pain continues longer than 4–6 weeks, then imaging studies are recommended.

Treatment Options

- Conservative treatment including application of heat by heating pads or heated blankets is recommended for short-term relief of acute low back pain. There is insufficient evidence to recommend the application of cold packs (French, Cameron, Walker, Reggars, & Esterman, 2006).

■ Activity as tolerated.

■ Pain medications, such as acetaminophen or NSAIDs if no contraindication is identified and/or muscle relaxants. Opioids should be considered as a second line option.

■ Follow-up care with primary physician.

SPINAL INFECTIONS (DISCITIS, SPINAL EPIDURAL ABSCESS, VERTEBRAL OSTEOMYELITIS, AND POST-SURGICAL WOUND INFECTIONS)

Spinal epidural abscess is caused by an infection that forms in the space around the dura, the casing that surrounds the spinal cord and nerve root. These pockets of purulent fluid may surround the spinal cord and/or the nerve roots exerting enough pressure to affect neurological function. Epidural abscesses usually occur in the thoracic or lumbar regions. An infection forms as a result of an underlying infection or it may occur remotely from dental abscess, decubiti, or endocarditis. Damage to the cord occurs either by direct compression, vein thrombosis, arterial interruption, or toxins. Epidural abscess is common in IV drug users, but may also occur after trauma, spinal surgery, or spontaneously. At least half of the patients have diabetes or HIV.

Risk factors for developing spinal infection include conditions that compromise the immune system, such as:

■ Advanced age

■ IV drug use

■ HIV infection

■ Long-term systemic usage of steroids

■ Diabetes mellitus

■ Organ transplantation

■ Malnutrition

■ Cancer

Surgical risk factors include an operation of long duration, high blood loss, use of instrumentation, and multiple or revision surgeries at the same site.

Signs and Symptoms

■ Saddle anesthesia or a sensory level, diminished rectal tone, and evidence of motor weakness

■ Unrelenting pain at rest

■ Asymmetry, paravertebral swelling and tender vertebrae

- Fever
- Paresthesia or mild weakness.

Diagnostic Criteria

- Lab work including erythrocyte sedimentation rate (ESR), C-reactive protein (CRP) levels, WBC and blood cultures. If red flags or concern for infection, tumor or rheumatologic etiology.
- MRI

Treatment Options

- Surgical decompression of the spinal cord for increasing neurological deficit, persistent severe pain, or increasing temperature and WBC.
- Debridement of wound infection
- Broad spectrum antibiotics for infection

EPIDURAL COMPRESSION SYNDROME (SPINAL CORD COMPRESSION, CAUDA EQUINA)

Epidural compression syndrome arises from pressure being exerted on the central cord or cauda equina from a space-occupying lesion. This is considered a medical emergency because of the catastrophic neurologic loss that can develop if it is not recognized and treated promptly. Early recognition of patients who present with mild symptoms is vital to minimize the greatest neurological impairment. Outcomes of these patients largely depend on their neurologic deficits at the time of presentation.

Symptoms

- Bowel incontinence
- Urinary retention with overflow incontinence or increased urinary frequency
- Saddle anesthesia with decreased anal sphincter tone
- Major motor weakness in the legs (and arms if a cervical lesion) with loss of deep tendon reflexes
- Anesthesia or hyperthesia in the legs, thorax, and arms depending on the location of the lesion

Etiology

- Large central disc herniation
- Spinal canal hematoma

- Spinal canal abscess
- Metastatic tumor
- Primary tumor
- Traumatic compression

Treatment and Evaluation

- IV dexamethasone; high-dose systemic corticosteroids
- Emergent MRI of cervical, thoracic, lumbo-sacral spine
- Consultation with specialist

MUSCULOSKELETAL INJURIES

Trauma to the musculoskeletal system may represent a threat to life, place a limb at risk, and potentially interfere with return to full function. In 2004, an estimated 57.2 million musculoskeletal injury visits to physician offices, EDs, outpatient clinics, and hospitals were reported (Academy of Orthopedic Surgeons, 2008).

Musculoskeletal injuries may be blunt or penetrating. They may involve bone, soft tissue, muscles, nerves, and/or blood vessels. Injuries include fractures and/or dislocations of the bone or joint, sprains, strains, ligament or tendon tears, and neurovascular compromise. Injuries to the bones may also be associated with other injuries to the nerves, arteries, veins, or soft tissue. Disruption in the skin can result in a disturbance in fluid and electrolyte levels, or temperature control. Any skin surface wound with loss of skin integrity provides an entry for microorganisms. This can lead to infection, especially if necrotic tissue is present.

The following terms are used to describe soft tissue injuries.

- *Abrasion*: An epidermal and dermal injury caused by friction, rubbing, or a scraping motion
- *Avulsion:* A full thickness skin loss or resultant flap in which the wound edges cannot be approximated
- *Degloving:* A serious type of avulsion injury resulting from high-energy shearing forces that tear large areas of skin and subcutaneous tissue away from the underlying vascular supply
- *Contusion:* Disruption of small blood vessels and extravasation of blood into the skin and/or mucous membranes that do not interrupt the skin integrity
- *Laceration*: Open wound from external forces causing a tearing or splitting of the skin, involving the dermis, epidermis, or underlying structures
- *Puncture:* Wound with a narrow opening that can penetrate deeply into the skin. Puncture wounds bleed minimally and tend to trap foreign

material that can lead to infection. Animal and human bites can be considered puncture wounds and should be treated as contaminated wounds.

Musculoskeletal injuries are classified into two categories:

A *sprain* is an injury to ligament tissue frequently caused by a pull or twist, resulting in joint instability. Ligaments connect bone to bone and maintain joint stability. The severity of the injury depends on whether the ligament tear is partial or complete. More than one ligament may be torn, which would also increase the severity of the injury. On the other hand, a *strain* is a stretching, partial tearing, or complete tearing of a muscle or tendon. Tendons connect muscle to bone and, depending on the severity of the tear, can cause extreme joint immobility.

Strain

Strains are generally identified according to severity:

- *Mild*: Pain and stiffness lasting for several days.
- *Moderate*: Partial muscle tears result in extensive pain, edema, and ecchymosis. The pain may last for 1–3 weeks.
- *Severe*: Ruptured muscle creates significant internal bleeding, edema, and ecchymosis around the muscle. A completely torn muscle often requires surgical intervention.

Sprains

Sprains result from a trauma that throws a joint out of position or even ruptures supporting ligaments. Pain, bruising, and inflammation are common to all three categories of sprains given below. You may feel a tear or pop in the joint. Sprains happen most often in the ankle. Repeated sprains can lead to ankle arthritis, a loose ankle, or tendon injury.

Sprains are classified according to the severity of the injury.

- *Mild*: There is a minor tear or excessive stretching to the ligament. The area is painful, especially upon movement.
- *Moderate*: The fibers in the ligament tear although there is no rupture. The joint is swollen, tender, ecchymotic and painful, especially upon movement.
- *Severe*: There maybe one or more completely torn ligaments. The joint is painful, and the patient may be unable to actively move the joint or bear weight. The patient may report that the affected joint feels like it "gives in."

FRACTURES

Fractures involve a disruption in the continuity of the bone resulting from a strong force that that is applied to a bone. A *complete* fracture is a total break of the bone, whereas in an *incomplete* fracture there is not a complete separation of the bone but a hairline crack in the bone. *Open* fractures are also known as a compound fracture. The broken bone protrudes out through the skin. These types of fractures are at high risk of infection because of the compromised integrity of the skin (Table 16.7).

Table 16.7 ■ *Types of Fractures*

Transverse Fracture	Complete break at a right angle to the long axis
Spiral Fracture	Produced by a rotational force
Oblique Fracture	Angular stress on the long axis
Comminuted	Indicates a pattern with more than two fragments
Greenstick Fracture	Incomplete fracture with opposite cortex intact
Torus Fracture	Buckles or is compacted
Displaced Fracture	Complete separation of the bone fragments
Nondisplaced Fracture	Occurs when a plane of cleavage exists in a bone without separation or displacement
Stress Fracture	Due to repetitive forces. Common in sports/running
Secondary/Pathologic	Fracture due to disease that has weakened the bone (neoplasm, osteoporosis, etc.)
Impacted	Complete. One end of the break is driven to the other end

JOINT DISLOCATIONS

Dislocation of the joint occurs when the two articular surfaces of the bone are not in contact with each other; it often is a result of sudden impact to the joint. The dislocated joint may be visibly deformed, swollen, with intense pain upon movement. Dislocations are considered an orthopedic emergency due to the potential for neurologic or circulatory compromise. Irreversible damage exists the longer it is untreated.

Assessment

■ Comprehensive history
■ Physical examination

- Inspection of injured area
- Active and passive range of motion proximal and distal to joint
- Palpation for tenderness or deformity
- Neurovascular assessment
- *5 Ps:* Evaluate neurovascular status of the injured area. Any patient that experiences trauma is at risk for neurovascular injuries and tissue ischemia. Use the 5 Ps to evaluate the limbs circulation, sensation, and motor function: Pain, Pallor, Pulses, Paresthesia, and Paralysis.

Diagnosis

- Radiographs obtained as indicated. Radiographs are a very important diagnostic aid but should not be used as the sole resource for diagnosis.
- MRI may be used to confirm diagnosis, determine the extent of injury, differentiate between partial tear and complete tear, and look at other associated injuries.

Treatment

Sprains and Strains

- Rest, ice, compression, elevation (RICE)
  - Elastic bandage wrap (Ace) if comfortable
  - Jones compression dressing for more severe injuries
- Anti-inflammatory medications
- Orthosis (splint) for pain relief and stability
- Air cast-type devices provide effective stability and pain relief
- Crutches and crutch gait training
- Orthopedic consult if indicated

Fractures

Fracture

- Prepare patient for reduction of fracture or dislocation.
- Neurologic and vascular status before and after reduction.
- Immobilization of fractures and dislocated joints that have been reduced.
- Application of ice and elevation in an effort to minimize swelling. Swelling intensifies pain and delays immobilization (casting).
- Analgesics are given as needed.

Open Fracture

- Achievement of hemostasis through direct pressure.

■ Initial management of open wound is irrigation and debridement of wound and administration of antibiotics.
■ Analgesics are given as needed.

Pain Control

The pain from sprains and strains is often equivalent to pain from a fracture. Pain may be caused by the injury itself, continued movement of an unstable fracture, muscle spasm, surrounding soft-tissue injury, nerve injury, or muscle ischemia. It is important to assess the level of pain and continually reassess after each intervention to determine the effectiveness of the treatment and/ or intervention. The goal is to reduce the patient's pain to a tolerable level. Never underestimate the basics—splinting, elevation and application of heat or cold—to help reduce pain. Patients who have experienced major injuries and have altered mental status may still be experiencing pain although they may not be able to respond.

Complications

Complications associated with musculoskeletal injuries:
■ Hemorrhage
■ Instability
■ Loss of tissue
■ Simple laceration and contamination
■ Interruption of blood supply
■ Nerve damage
■ Chronic pain
■ Long-term disability

HEADACHES

Headaches are a recurrent and very common complaint in medicine. There is great cost incurred to society due to loss of work, decreased productivity, etc. The percentage of the adult population worldwide with an active headache disorder is 47% for headache in general, 10% for migraine, 38% for tension-type headache, and 3% for chronic headache (Jensen & Stovner, 2008). In the United States, headaches account for 2.2% of all ED visits (Goldstein, Camargo, Pelletier, & Edlow, 2006). According to the American Academy of Neurology, migraine is a neurobiologic disorder that occurs in 18% of women and 6% of men, although it may be undiagnosed or undertreated.

When a patient presents to the ED with a headache, it is up to the physician to determine what type of headache the patient is presenting.

Ninety percent of patients presenting to the ED will have a primary headache (Martin, 2011). Physicians should exclude serious problems, such as a subarachnoid hemorrhage. Using a comprehensive medical history can rule out serious causes of headache or may reveal red flags that require further investigation.

Types of Headaches

The National Headache Society recognizes two general groups of headache—primary and secondary (National Headache Foundation, 1996). Primary headaches are typically recurrent without known pathology or cause. Secondary headaches are associated with a recognized disease or disorder.

The International Headache Society (IHS) then further classifies each group into types.

Primary headaches are classified into four types:

- Migraine
- Tension-type headache
- Cluster headache
- Other primary headaches

Secondary headaches are classified into eight types:

- Headache attributed to head and/or neck trauma
- Headache attributed to cranial or cervical vascular disorder
- Headache attributed to nonvascular intracranial disorder
- Headache attributed to a substance or its withdrawal
- Headache attributed to infection
- Headache attributed to disorder of homeostasis
- Headache or facial pain attributed to disorder of the cranium, neck, eyes, ears, nose, sinuses, teeth, mouth, or other facial or cranial structures
- Headache attributed to psychiatric disorder

Diagnostic Considerations

The cause or type of most headaches can be determined by a careful history and physical examination. It is essential that the clinician recognize the warning signals that raise "red flags" and prompt further diagnostic testing. In the absence of worrisome features in the history or examination, the task is then to diagnose the primary disorder based upon the clinical presentation. A study by Goldstein et al. (2006) showed that 14% of headache patients who presented to EDs have neuroimaging, 5.5% had organic pathology, and 2% had lumbar puncture, and abnormal in 11% of cases. If unusual features are present or the patient does not respond to therapy, the diagnosis should be questioned and the likelihood of

Table 16.8 ▓ *Red Flags of a Secondary Headache ("SNOOP")*

Systemic symptoms or illness	Fever, altered level of consciousness, anti-coagulation, pregnancy, cancer, HIV
Neurologic symptoms	Papilledema, asymmetric cranial nerve function, asymmetric motor function, nuchal
	Rigidity, visual disturbance other than aura, dysphasia, abnormal cerebellar function
Onset sudden	Abrupt, split-second, seconds to minutes, rapid onset of headache
Older	New headache onset in an older patient or a progressively worsening headache in a middle-aged patient (more than 50 years of age)
Progression pattern	Previous headache history; a major change in attack frequency, severity, or clinical features; a first headache or different headache unlike any experienced before

Adapted from Martin, V.T. (2004). Simplifying the diagnosis of migraine headache. *Advanced Studies in Medicine, 4*, pp. 200–207.

a secondary headache disorder should be considered; further diagnostic testing is necessary (Table 16.8).

Headache History

▓ Site
▓ Onset
▓ Severity
▓ Worst headache of life should be evaluated for sub-arachnoid hemorrhage (SAH)
▓ Increasing severity should lower threshold for intervention
▓ Quality
▓ Associated symptoms
▓ History of previous headaches
▓ Exacerbating and alleviating factors
▓ Efficacy of pain relief should not have any diagnostic significance attached to it

Physical Examination

- Vital signs
- Cognition
- Neurologic examination
- Cranial nerves
- Fundoscopy
- Visual fields

Headache "Red Flags"

- First or worst headache
- New onset headache in middle age or later
- New or progressive headache that lasts for days
- Precipitation of headache with Valsalva maneuvers
- Systemic symptoms such as myalgia, fever, malaise, weight loss, scalp tenderness, jaw claudication, stiff neck
- Focal symptoms, seizures, confusion, impaired consciousness, physical examination abnormalities
- The presence of associated neurologic signs or symptoms (e.g., diplopia, loss of sensation, weakness, ataxia)
- Headache developing after head injury or major trauma
- Persistent one-sided throbbing headache
- Atypical history or unusual character that does not fulfill the criteria for migraine
- Inadequate response to optimal therapy

Consultations

A neurologist, neuroophthalmologist, and/or neurosurgeon should be consulted as deemed clinically appropriate.

Laboratory Testing/Imaging Studies

Laboratory and/or imaging studies (CT or MRI) are determined by the individual presentation. For patients over 50 years old, erythrocyte sedimentation rate (ESR) and C-reactive protein (CRP) may be appropriate to rule out temporal arteritis.

Imaging studies are indicated for those with "red flag" findings and an abnormal neurologic exam. Imaging studies (CT scan or MRI) should precede a lumbar puncture to rule out a "thunder clap," atypical headache, mass, and/or increased intracranial pressure.

Other Therapeutic Treatment Considerations

- Minimize visual and auditory stimulation. Placing patient in a darkened, quiet room is helpful.
- Cool compresses to painful areas may be helpful to some patients.
- Provide antiemetics for nausea and vomiting such as metoclopramide, ondansetron, and prochlorperazine.
- Hospital admission for migraine may be indicated.
- Treatment of severe nausea, vomiting, and subsequent dehydration.
- Treatment of severe refractory migraine pain (i.e., status migrainosus).
- Detoxification from overuse of combination analgesics, ergots, or opioids.

Tension-Type Headache (TTH)

TTH is the most common type of headache. They can be intermittent, triggered by a precipitating condition such as stress, or chronic. TTH characteristics are based upon IHS diagnostic criteria; TTH must have at least two of the following criteria present:

- Pressing or tightening (nonpulsatile quality)
- Frontal-occipital location
- Bilateral, of mild/moderate intensity
- Not aggravated by physical activity

Treatment

- Rule out underlying serious pathology.
- Assess if patient is overusing medication, has drug dependence and depression.
- Pharmacologic:
  - Aspirin, acetaminophen, or NSAIDs are commonly effective.
  - Patients with persistent TTH may respond to analgesics. These should only be used on a short-term basis.
- Nonpharmacologic:
  - Hot or cold packs
  - Relaxation techniques

MIGRAINES (WITH AND WITHOUT AURAS)

Migraines are a disorder of the nervous system and occur more frequently in women than men. Approximately 60% of patients have a first-degree relative with a history of migraine (Ferrari, 2008). The risk of migraine is increased four-fold in relatives of people who have migraine (Evans, 2009).

The migraine starts when the nervous system is stimulated by an aggravating factor (stress, food, environmental, etc.) that produces chemical changes within the nervous system. The IHS defines a migraine as an occasional headache lasting 4–72 hours and includes two of the following:

- Unilateral location
- Throbbing
- Pain worsened with movement
- Moderate or severe pain intensity
- Must include nausea with vomiting or phonophobia and photophobia

Stages of Migraine

Prodrome

About 60% of people who experience migraines report prodrome symptoms that occur hours to days before headache onset. Most people who experience migraines can usually recognize the subtle clues that occur prior to a migraine. This is important for patients to plan appropriately and allow for more effective treatment. Most medications work best when taken early. Prodrome symptoms include:

- Food cravings
- Constipation or diarrhea
- Mood changes (depression, irritability)
- Heightened sensitivity to light, sound, and odors
- Lethargy or uncontrollable yawning

Aura

The migraine auras are neurological symptoms that may occur before a migraine although they may accompany the headache or occur in isolation. The aura if present develops over 5 to 20 minutes and can last up to 60 minutes. The aura can be visual, sensory, motor, or any combination. The aura is not harmful and results in no permanent damage but may be frightening for a patient who never experienced one before.

Headache Phase

This is the phase of the actual migraine itself that can last 24 to 72 hours. Migraines are not just limited to pain but a host of autonomic symptoms are associated with it.

Postdrome

Postdrome symptoms may persist for 24 to 48 hours after the headache has resolved. The patient may still continue to experience impaired functioning. They may experience the following:

- Feeling tired or irritable
- Feeling unusually refreshed or euphoric
- Muscle weakness or myalgia
- Anorexia or food cravings

Treatment

- Over-the-counter medications, including aspirin, acetaminophen/aspirin/caffeine, Midrin and NSAIDs
- Triptans
- Adjunctive therapy, including caffeine and metoclopramide
- IV dihydroergotamine (DHE) with metoclopramide for nausea
- Chlorpromazine or prochlorperazine
- Dexamethasone
- Intranasal lidocaine
- Ketorolac
- Opiates are not recommended as drugs of first choice

Abortive Therapy

The practitioner must make a decision on choice of medication based upon the individual characteristics such as intensity of headache, speed of onset of action of medication, associated symptoms, incapacitation and response of the patient. When the patient presents to the ED for an incapacitating migraine, the patient may have already taken medication for migraines. Migraines should be treated early and at onset, which improves the efficacy of treating the migraine. Utilizing simple analgesics such as aspirin, acetaminophen, and other NSAIDs may be effective in managing acute migraine if the severity of the headache is mild and there is no associated nausea or vomiting. More severe headaches will require more complex and specific medications. The use of abortive medications is limited to 2 to 3 days a week to prevent development of a rebound headache phenomenon.

Initiation of these abortive treatments at the onset of a migraine improves the efficacy of treating the migraine. If symptoms do not subside within 40 to 60 minutes, then migraine-specific agents should be added to the patient's current regimen.

Prochloperazine administered IV or IM has been shown to be significantly superior to metoclopramide in corresponding forms for the treatment of acute migraine headache pain, nausea, and vomiting (Aukerman,

Knutsen, & Miser, 2002; Kelly, Walcynski, & Gunn, 2009). In a recent randomized trial by Kostic, Gutierrez, Rieg, Moore, and Gendron (2010), 66 patients were given either prochlorperazine with diphenhydramine IV or sumatriptan SC. The results found that patients who received the prochlorperazine and diphenhydramine had greater reduction in their pain intensity than patients receiving sumatriptan.

The triptans, known as serotonin receptor agonists, are the treatment of choice for an acute migraine. Triptans are effective for mild, moderate, or severe migraine attacks that do not respond to NSAIDs or other analgesics (Aukerman et al., 2002). Various formulations of triptans are available for patients who need other routes of drug delivery. Triptans are usually well tolerated and therefore are good options for patients with nausea and vomiting. All triptans are most effective when taken early during a migraine and may be repeated in 2 hours as needed (maximum of 2 doses daily). SC sumatriptan has the quickest onset of action and is most effective compared to other triptan formulations (Silberstein, 2004). Triptans are contraindicated in patients with cardiovascular diseases (Aukerman, Knutsen, & Miser, 2004).

Dihydroergotamine (DHE) is a nonselective 5-HT1 receptor agonist that is often used for treating severe migraines and those that are not being controlled with commonly used medications. DHE has a low headache recurrence rate of less than 20% and demonstrates fewer adverse effects and a reduced incidence of rebound headaches than ergotamine (Silberstein & McCory, 2003). DHE is available in parenteral and nasal preparations. Chronic use of ergots is restricted because of their ability to cause peripheral vasoconstriction.

Medication Overuse Headache (MOH)

Bigal and Lipton (2009) identified that some patients progress from episodic migraines to chronic migraines. Medication overuse headache (MOH) is a secondary cause of chronic daily headache (CDH) as a result of the overuse of acute headache medication and has no relation to addiction of headache medications. Acute treatments of headaches can cause MOH. According to ICH, MOH headaches are experienced 15 or more days a month for at least 3 months and have developed or markedly worsened during medication overuse. Overuse is based upon the specific medication and appears to occur quicker with triptans than with other medications. Overuse makes headaches refractory to preventive medications but stopping them can result in withdrawal symptoms and a period of increased headache can occur, although improvement in headaches does not always occur. Since MOH is difficult to treat, outpatient detoxification maybe an option to terminate the headache cycle. Severe exacerbations of the patient's migraine during detoxification can occur. Withdrawal symptoms include severely exacerbated headaches accompanied by nausea, vomiting, agitation, restlessness, sleep disorder, and (rarely) seizures. Barbiturates, opioids, and benzodiazepines, unless replaced with long-acting derivatives, must be tapered to avoid a serious withdrawal syndrome (Silberstein, Lipton, & Saper, 2007).

CLUSTER HEADACHE (CH)

Cluster headache refers to a grouping or clustering of attacks. The incidence of CH is higher in men than in women. These headaches are quite debilitating and are often referred to as "suicide headaches" due to their severity. CH most commonly strikes 2 to 3 hours after falling asleep and generally recurs at the same time. It typically last for 30 to 45 minutes although it can last from only a few minutes to several hours. One to 4 headaches per day during the cluster cycle are common. Patients should be encouraged to avoid possible triggers such as smoking or alcohol consumption, especially during the cluster period. Treatment is both acute (abortive) and preventive (prophylactic). The goal of acute treatment is to stop or prevent the progression of a headache.

Symptoms

Symptoms are ipsilateral:
- Severe, unilateral, temporal and orbital (behind the eye) pain
- Swelling under or around the eye (may affect both eyes)
- Lacrimation and inflammation of the same eye
- Red eye
- Rhinorrhea or one-sided stuffy nose
- Red, flushed face

Abortive Therapy

- Oxygen 7–10 L/min
- Sumatriptan SC; contraindicated in patients with CV diseases (Law, Derry, & Moore, 2010)
- Zolmitriptan intranasal; contraindicated in patients with CV diseases (Law et al., 2010; Hedlund, Rapoport, Dodick, & Goadsby, 2009)
- Octreotide SC; Can be used in patients with CV diseases

- Dihydroergotamine IV; contraindicated in patients with CV diseases; cannot be used with triptans
- Intranasal lidocaine; used as adjunctive therapy not as a first line agent

Preventive Therapy

- Verapamil is the first-line maintenance medication due to its efficacy, safety, and reduced concern about drug interactions (Blau & Engel, 2004)
- Lithium
- Topiramate
- Valproic acid
- Clonidine
- Ergotamine
- Corticosteroid

Case Study

A 30-year-old male construction worker presents with headache in the middle of the night. He is agitated and pacing the cubicle. The headache assessment findings are as follows:

- *Site:* Unilateral pain around the left eye and forehead
- *Onset:* Headaches have been going on for a week and seem to occur at night, usually over 1 to 2 minutes.
- *Headaches:* Severe and usually only last about an hour
- *Severity:* Headache is 10/10 severity
- *Quality:* "Like a poker in my eye"
- *Associated Symptoms:* Left eye feels swollen, lacrimation, nasal congestion
- *History of Previous Headaches:* No
- *Exacerbating and Alleviating Factors:* Can't find relief: "Make it stop!"

Questions to Consider

1. What type of headache is this patient presenting with?
2. What abortive treatment would you recommend for this patient?
3. What prophylactic treatment would you recommend for this type of headache?

REFERENCES

American Academy of Orthopaedic Surgeons. (2008). Arthritis and joint pain. In *The burden of musculoskeletal disease in the United States: Prevalence, societal and economic cost.* Retrieved September 25, 2012, from http://www.boneandjointburden.org/[Context Link]

Ahovuo-Saloranta, A., Borisenko, O. V., Kovanen, N., Varonen, H., Rautakorpi, U. M., Williams, J. W. Jr., & Makela, M. (2008). Antibiotics for acute maxillary sinusitis. *Cochrane Database of Systematic Reviews, (2),* CD000243.

Aukerman, G., Knutsen, D., & Miser, W. F. (2002). Management of the acute migraine headache. *American Family Physician, 66,* 2123–2130.

Bartfield, J. M., Jandreau, S. W., & Raccio-Robak, N. (1998). Randomized trial of diphenhydramine versus benzyl alcohol with epinephrine as an alternative to lidocaine local anesthesia. *Annals of Emergency Medicine, 32,* 650.

Bartfield, J. M., May-Wheeling, H. E., Raccio-Robak, N., & Lai, S. Y. (2001). Benzyl alcohol with epinephrine as an alternative to lidocaine with epinephrine. *Journal of Emergency Medicine, 21,* 375.

Baum, C. L., & Arpey, C. J. (2005). Normal cutaneous wound healing: Clinical correlation with cellular and molecular events. *Dermatologic Surgery, 31*(6), 674–686.

Beebe, F. A., Barkin, R. L., & Barkin, S. (2005). A clinical and pharmacologic review of skeletal muscle relaxants for musculoskeletal conditions. *American Journal of Therapeutics, 12,* 151–171.

Bederson, J. B., Connolly, E. S., Jr., Batjer, H. H., Dacey, R. G., Dion, J. E., Diringer, M. N., . . . American Heart Association. (2009). Guidelines for the management of aneurysmal subarachnoid hemorrhage: A statement for healthcare professionals from a special writing group of the Stroke Council, American Heart Association. *Stroke, 40*(3), 994–1025.

Bijur, P., Bérard, A., Esses, D., Calderon, Y., & Gallagher, E. J. (2008). Race, ethnicity, and management of pain from long-bone fractures: A prospective study of two academic urban emergency departments. *Academy of Emergency Medicine,15,*589–597.

Blau, J. N., & Engel, H. O. (2004). Individualizing treatment with verapamil for cluster headache patients. *Headache: The Journal of Head and Face Pain, 44,* 1013–1018. doi: 10.1111/j.1526-4610.2004.04196.x.

Burch, M. S., McAllister, R. K., & Meyer, T. A. (2011). Treatment of local-anesthetic toxicity with lipid emulsion therapy. *American Journal of Health-System Pharmacy, 68*(2), 125–129.

Cepeda, S. M., Tzortzopoulou, A., Thackrey, M., Hudcova, J., Arora Gandhi, P., & Schumann, R. (2009). Adjusting the pH of lidocaine for reducing pain on injection. Cochrane Anaesthesia Group. *Cochrane Database of Systematic Reviews, 1.*

Chou, R., Clark, E., & Helfand, M. (2003). Comparative efficacy and safety of long-acting oral opioids for chronic non-cancer pain: Asystematic review. *Journal of Pain and Symptom Management, 26,* 1026–1048.

Chou, R., Huffman, L. H., American Pain Society, & American College of Physicians. (2007a). Medications for acute and chronic low back pain: A review of the evidence for an American Pain Society/American College of Physicians clinical practice guideline. *Annals of Internal Medicine, 147,* 505–514.

Chou, R., Huffman, L. H., American Pain Society, & American College of Physicians. (2007b). Nonpharmacologic therapies for acute and chronic low back pain: A review of the evidence for an American Pain Society/American College of Physicians clinical practice guideline. *Annals of Internal Medicine, 147*, 492–504.

Chou, R., Qaseem, A., Snow, V., Casey, D., Cross, J. T., Shekelle, P.,. . . American Pain Society Low Back Pain Guidelines Panel. (2007). Diagnosis and treatment of low back pain: a joint clinical practice guideline from the American College of Physicians and the American Pain Society. *Annals of Internal Medicine, 147*, 478–91.

Crystal, C. S., McArthur, T. J., & Harrison, B. (2007). Anesthetic and procedural sedation techniques for wound management. *Emergency Medicine Clinics of North America, 25*, 41–71.

Dealey, C. (2005). *The care of wounds. A guide for nurses* (3rd ed.). Oxford: Blackwell Publishing.

Della-Giustina, D. A. (1999). Emergency department evaluation and treatment of back pain. *Emergency Medicine Clinics of North America, 17*(4), 877–893.

Eder, S. C., Sloan, E. P., & Todd, K. (2003). Documentation of ED patient pain by nurses and physicians. *American Journal of Emergency Medicine, 21*, 253–257.

European Association of Urology (2008). *Guidelines on urolithiasis.* European Association of Urology. Retrieved from http://www.uroweb.org

Evans, R. W. (2009). Migraine: a question and answer review. *Medical Clinics of North America, 93*(2), 245–262.

Ferrari, M. D. (2008). Migraine genetics: A fascinating journey towards improved migraine therapy. *Headache: The Journal of Head and Face Pain, 48*, 697–700.

Fosnocht, D. E., & Swanson. E. R. (2007). Use of a triage pain protocol in the ED. *American Journal of Emergency Medicine, 25*(7), 791–793.

French, S. D., Cameron, M., Walker, B. F., Reggars, J. W., & Esterman, A. J. (2006). Superficial heat or cold for low back pain. *Cochrane Database of Systematic Reviews.*

Goldstein, J. N., Camargo, C. A. Jr., Pelletier, A. J., & Edlow, J. A. (2006). Headache in United States emergency departments: Demographics, work-up and frequency of pathological diagnoses. *Cephalalgia, 26*, 684–690.

Guéant, S., Taleb, A., Borel-Kühner, J., Cauterman, M., Raphael, M., Nathan, G., & Ricard-Hibon, A. (2011). Quality of pain management in the emergency department: Results of a multicentre prospective study. *European Journal of Anaesthesiology, 28*(2), 97–105.

Hartoch, R. S., McManus, J. G., Knapp, S., & Buettner, M. F. (2007). Emergency management of chronic wounds. *Emergency Medicine Clinics of North America, 25*, 203–221.

Hayes, K., Huckstadt, A., & Daggett, D. (2006). Acute low back pain in the emergency department. *Advanced Emergency Nursing Journal, 28*(3), 234–247.

Headache Classification Committee. (2004). *The international classification of headache disorders* (2nd ed.). *Cephalalgia, 24*, 1–160.

Heavner, J. E. (2007). Local anesthetics. *Current Opinionin Anaesthesiology, 20*, 336–342.

Hedlund, C., Rapoport, A. M., Dodick, D. W., & Goadsby, P. J. (2009). Zolmitriptan nasal spray in the acute treatment of cluster headache: A meta-analysis of two studies. *Headache: The Journal of Head and Face Pain, 49*, 1315–1323. doi: 10.1111/j.1526-4610.2009.01518.x.

Hirschmann, J. V. (2008). Topical and oral antibiotics in wound care. *Cutis, 82*(2, Suppl. 2), 18–20.

Hollander, J. E., Singer, A. J., Valentine, S. M., & Shofer, F. S. (2001). Risk factors for infection in patients with traumatic lacerations. *Academic Emergency Medicine, 8*(7), 716–720.

Holdgate, A., & Pollock, T. (2004). Nonsteroidal anti-inflammatory drugs (NSAIDs) versus opioids for acute renal colic. *Cochrane Database of Systematic Reviews,* (1), CD004137.

Hwang, P. H., & Getz, A. (2011). *Acute sinusitis and rhinosinusitis in adults.* UpToDate. Retrieved from http://www.uptodate.com. Accessed March 15, 2011.

Hwang, U., Richardson, L., Sonuyi, T. O., & Morrison, R. S. (2006). The effect of emergency department crowding on the management of pain in older adults with hip fracture. *Journal of the American Geriatrics Society, 54*(2), 270–275.

Institute for Clinical Systems Improvement (ICSI). (2009). *Diagnosis and treatment of headache.* Bloomington (MN): Institute for Clinical Systems Improvement (ICSI).

Jastrzab, G., Fairbrother, G., Kerr, S., & McInerney, M. (2003). Profiling the pain aware nurse, acute care nurses' attitudes and knowledge concerning adult pain management. *Australian Journal of Advanced Nursing, 21*(2), 27–33.

Jensen, R., & Stovner, L. J. (2008). Epidemiology and comorbidity of headache. *Lancet Neurology, 7,* 354–361.

Joint Commission. (2008). *Comprehensive accreditation manual for hospitals: The official handbook.* Oakbrook Terrace, IL: Joint Commission Resources.

Kang, S. N. (2007). Digital nerve blocks. *British Journal of Hospital Medicine (London), 68*(2), M30–M31.

Kelly, A. M., Walcynski, T., & Gunn, B. (2009). The relative efficacy of phenothiazines for the treatment of acute migraine: A meta-analysis. *Headache: The Journal of Head and Face Pain, 49*(9), 1324–1332. doi: 10.1111/j.1526-4610.2009.01465.x.

Kostic, M. A., Gutierrez, F. J., Rieg, T. S., Moore, T. S., & Gendron, R. T. (2010). A prospective, randomized trial of intravenous prochlorperazine versus subcutaneous sumatriptan in acute migraine therapy in the emergency department. *Annals of Emergency Medicine, 56*(1), 1–6. doi: 10.1016/j.annemergmed.2009.11.020.

Law, S., Derry, S., & Moore, R. A. (2010). Triptans for acute cluster headache. *Cochrane Database of Systematic Reviews,* 4, Art. No. CD008042.

Law, S., Derry, S., & Moore, R. A. (2010). Triptans for acute cluster headache. *Cochrane Database of Systematic Reviews,* (4). Art. No. CD008042. doi: 10.1002/14651858. CD008042.pub2

Martin, V. T. (2011). The diagnostic evaluation of secondary headache disorders. *Headache: The Journal of Head and Face Pain, 51,* 346–352. doi: 10.1111/j.1526-4610.2010.01841.x.

Matchar, D., Young, W. B., Rosenberg, J. H., Pietrzak, M. P., Silberstein, S. D., Lipton, R. B. . . . National Headache Foundation. (2002). Evidence-based guidelines for migraine headache in the primary care setting: Pharmacological management of acute attacks. Retrieved from Available at: http://www.aan.com/practice/guideline/index.cfm? fuseaction5home.welcome&Topics516&keywords5&Submit5Search1 Guidelines; 2000.

Migraine Therapy. (2008). *Headache: The Journal of Head and Face Pain, 48*, 697–700. doi: 10.1111/j.1526-4610.2008.01099.x.

Modic, M. T., Obuchowski, N. A., Ross, J. S., et al. (2005). Acute low back pain and radiculopathy. *Radiology, 237*, 597–604.

Mohr, B. (2006). Safety and effectiveness of intravenous regional anesthesia (Bier block) for outpatient management of forearm trauma. *CJEM, 8*, 247–250.

National Guidelines Clearinghouse. (2010). *Clinical practice guideline: Adult sinusitis.* National Guidelines Clearinghouse. Retrieved from http://guideline.gov/summary/summary.aspx?doc_id=12385. Accessed September 29, 2010.

Neal, J. M., Bernards, C. M., Butterworth, J. F., Di Gregorio, G., Drasner, K., Hejtmanek, M. R., . . . Weinberg, G. L. (2010). ASRA practice advisory on local anesthetic systemictoxicity. *Regional Anesthesia and Pain Medicine, 35*, 152–161.

Owens, P. L., Woeltje, M., & Mutter, R. (2011). *Emergency department visits and inpatient stays related to back problems, 2008.* HCUP Statistical Brief #105. Rockville, MD: Agency for Healthcare Research and Quality. Retrieved from http://www.hcup-us.ahrq.gov/reports/statbriefs/sb105.pdf

Pancioli, A. M. (2008). Hypertension management in neurologic emergencies. *Annals of Emergency Medicine,* 51(Suppl. 3), S24–S27.

Phillips, J. F., Yates, A. B., & Deshazo, R. D. (2007). Approach to patients with suspected hypersensitivity tolocal anesthetics. *American Journal of Medical Science, 334*, 190–196.

Pines, J. M., & Hollander, J. E. (2008). Emergency department crowding is associated with poor care for patients with severe pain, 03 October 2007. *Annals of Emergency Medicine, 51*(1), 1–5.

Pletcher, M. J., Kertesz, S. G., Kohn, A., & Gonzales, R. (2008). Trends in opioid prescribing by race/ethnicity for patients seeking care in US emergency departments. *JAMA, 299*, 70–78.

Roelofs, P. D. D. M., Deyo, R. A., Koes, B. W., Scholten, R. J. P. M., & van Tulder, M. W. (2008). Non-steroidal anti-inflammatory drugs for low back pain. *Cochrane Database of Systematic Reviews.*

Roelofs, P. D. D. M., Deyo, R. A., Koes, B. W., Scholten, R. J. P. M., & van Tulder, M. W. (2008). Non-steroidal anti-inflammatory drugs for low back pain. *The Cochrane Review,* 1. Chichester, England: John Wiley. Retrieved from http://www.thecochranelibrary.com

Safdar, B., Degutis, L. C., Landry, K., Vedere, S. R., Moscovitz, H. C., & D'Onofrio, G. (2006). Intravenous morphine plus ketorolac is superior to either drug alone for treatment of acute renal colic. *Annals of Emergency Medicine, 48*(2), 173–181, 181.e1.

Silberstein, S. D. (2004). Migraine. *Lancet, 363*, 381–391.

Silberstein, S. D., Lipton, R. B., & Saper J. R. (2007). Chronic daily headache including transformed migraine, chronic tension-type headache, and medication overuse headache. In S. D. Silberstein, R. B. Lipton, & D. W. Dodick (Eds.), *Wolff's headache and other head pain* (8th ed., pp. 315–378). New York, NY: Oxford University Press.

Singer, A.J., & Dagum, A. B. (2008). Review article current management of acute cutaneous wounds. *The New England Journal of Medicine, 359*, 1037–1046. Retrieved September 4, 2008, from DOI: 10.1056/NEJMra0707253

Springhart, W. P., Marguet, C. G., Sur, R. L., Norris, R. D., Delvecchio, F. C., Young, M. D., . . . Preminger, G. M. (2006). Forced versus minimal intravenous hydration in the management of acute renal colic: A randomized trial. *Journal of Endourology, 20*(10), 713–716.

Stalnikowicz, R., Mahamid, R., Kaspi, S., & Brezis, M. (2005). Undertreatment of acute pain in the emergency department: A challenge. *International Journal of Quality Health Care, 17*(2), 173–176.

Sterrett, S. P., Moore, N. W., & Nakada, S. Y. (2009). Emergency room follow-up trends in urolithiasis: Single-center report. *Urology, 73*(6), 1195–1197.

Teichman, J. M. H. (2004). Acute renal colic from ureteral calculus. *New England Journal of Medicine, 350*, 684–693.

Todd, K. H., Ducharme, J., Choiniere, M., Crandall, C. S., Fosnocht, D. E., Homel, P., . . . PEMI Study Group. (2007). Pain in the emergency department: results of the pain and emergency medicine initiative (PEMI) multicenter study. *The Journal of Pain, 8*(6), 460–466.doi: 10.1016/j.jpain.2006.12.005.

Türk, C., Knoll, T., Petrik, A., & Sarica, K. (2010). *EAU guidelines on urolithiasis.*Retrieved from http://www.uroweb.org/gls/pdf/Urolithiasis%202010.pdf

van Tulder, M. W., Scholten, R. J., Koes, B. W., & Deyo, R. A. (2000). Non-steroidal anti-inflammatory drugs for low back pain. *Cochrane Database of Systematic Reviews,* (2), CD000396.

van Tulder, M. W., Touray, T., Furlan, A. D., Solway, S., & Bouter, L. M. (2003). Muscle relaxants for non-specific low back pain. *Cochrane Database of Systematic Reviews,* (2), CD004252.

van Tulder, M. W., Touray, T., Furlan, A. D., Solway, S., & Bouter, L. M. (2003). Muscle relaxants for non-specific low-back pain. *Cochrane Database of Systematic Reviews,* (2). Art. No. CD004252. doi: 10.1002/14651858.CD004252.

Vasavada, A. N., Li, S., & Delp, S. L. (2001). Three-dimensional isometric strength of neck muscles in humans. *Spine, 26*(17), 1904–1909.

Wilson, J. E., & Pendleton, J. M. (1989). Oligoanalgesia in the emergency department. *American Journal of Emergency Medicine, 7*(6), 620–623.

Worcester, E. M., & Coe, F. L. (2008). Nephrolithiasis. *Primary Care, 35*(2), 369–391.

Zilinsky, I., Bar-Meir, E., Zaslansky, R., Mendes, D., Winkler, E., & Orenstein, A. (2005). Ten commandments for minimal pain during administration of local anesthetics. *Journal of Drugs in Dermatology, 4*, 212–216.

17

Managing Pain in the Patient Suffering Trauma

INTRODUCTION

Injury is the fifth leading cause of death in the United States, preceded only by heart disease, cancer, stroke, and chronic respiratory diseases (Xu, Kochanek, Murphy, & Tejada-Vera, 2010). Injury is a major public health problem and in the United States, and accounts for over 150,000 deaths and over 3 million nonfatal injuries per year. The leading causes of trauma are motor vehicle crashes, falls, and assaults. More than 2.8 million people are hospitalized with injury each year (Centers for Disease Control and Prevention [CDC], 2007). Most injuries are preventable with something as simple as a seatbelt or helmet. Among those age 65 and older, falls are the leading cause of injury-related deaths (CDC, 2007). In 2005, injuries accounted for $406 billion in medical costs and work loss costs (Finkelstein et al., 2006). Injury can be prevented and lives saved through education about the causes of injury and the implementation of injury prevention programs.

Trauma can be defined as injury to tissues and organs resulting from the transfer of energy from the environment to the patient's body. Injuries result from a type of energy that is beyond the body's ability to tolerate. The type and severity of injury depends on the affected body part, the amount and type of energy that was applied, as well as the mechanism of injury.

Pain is a significant co-morbidity of trauma. Unrelieved pain causes unnecessary suffering, and predisposes patients to complications and prolonged hospitalization. Research has shown that trauma patients often receive inadequate analgesia (Rupp & Delaney, 2004).

Trauma resuscitation is immediately intense once the patient arrives at a trauma center; it sets forth a cascade of events to provide the patient with much needed resources and often life-saving measures. The first of the three periods of trauma care is known as *resuscitation*. During this time the trauma team works to identify injuries and care priorities, and to re-establish hemodynamic stability. During this time analgesia should not be withheld unless there are circumstances that could hamper diagnosis of injuries, cause respiratory depression, or hemodynamic instability.

TRAUMA CARE

Pre-Hospital Resuscitation

Pre-hospital resuscitation begins where the trauma occurred. The patient receives immediate stabilization and transportation to the nearest facility. Stabilization occurs through physical assessment and intervention focused on ABC— airway, breathing, and circulation (Tintinalli, Kelen, & Stapczynski, 2000).

> *Clinical Pearl*   Trauma patients are often experiencing considerable pain while being clinically unstable.

Primary Survey

Once the patient arrives at the emergency department (ED), a rapid primary survey is performed to reveal any life-threatening injuries using the mnemonic ABCDE. This allows the practitioner to think in an ordered and prioritized manner:

- **A**irway maintenance with cervical spine protection
- **B**reathing and ventilation
- **C**irculation and hemorrhage control
- **D**isability and neurologic status
- **E**xposure/environmental control

Resuscitation Phase

While injuries are identified during the primary survey, resuscitation efforts are implemented simultaneously. Catheters, tubes, large bore IV catheters, or central lines may be placed in patients who are severely injured. Hypovolemia in these patients is not uncommon; infusions of crystalloids, colloids, and/or blood products are given to restore hemodynamic stability. Ongoing monitoring (vital signs, arterial blood gases, pulse oximetry, urinary output, body temperature, central venous pressure (CVP)) of patients can provide useful information to guide care.

Chest and pelvic x-rays are two essential studies that may change the course of treatment in patients with major blunt trauma. Other x-rays are not performed until the secondary survey. In patients with persistent hypotension and possible blunt trauma, a search for occult hemorrhage will include the focused assessment for the sonographic evaluation (FAST) or a diagnostic peritoneal lavage (DPL).

A final decision may be made to transfer the patient to a facility with more specialized care. Once the decision is made to transfer, communication between the physicians in both locations is imperative. The ongoing evaluation, re-evaluation and monitoring continues until the patient is safely transferred.

Secondary Survey

The secondary survey does not begin until the primary survey is completed, resuscitation has been initiated, re-evaluation of vital functions has been performed, and the patient's vital signs are beginning to return to normal.

The secondary survey involves the traditional history and physical examination. A good history is necessary; with patients under the influence of drugs or alcohol or who have a neurological injury, this often results in piecing the story together and obtaining the information from other sources. Essential elements can be described by a mnemonic AMPLE developed by Freeark and Baker:

- **A**llergies
- **M**edications currently used
- **P**ast medical history
- **L**ast meal
- **E**vents/environment related to injury

The patient will also undergo special testing and procedures (radiographic studies, peritoneal lavage, etc.).

Definitive Care/Operative Phase

Definitive care of the specific injuries identified in each anatomic area from the secondary survey occurs. Postoperatively, if indicated, the patient may be transferred to the critical care unit from the operating room.

HEAD TRAUMA

Head injuries are common and range from the minor bump on the head that usually warrants no investigation or treatment, to multiple trauma patients with associated head injury and depressed level of consciousness.

The National Head Injury Foundation defines brain injury as "a traumatic insult to the brain capable of producing physical, intellectual, emotional, social and vocational changes."

Traumatic brain injury (TBI) affects more than 1.4 million Americans annually (CDC, 2007). Mild traumatic brain injury (MTBI) accounts for approximately 75% of those injured. These injuries, defined as a blow or penetrating injury to the head that disrupts normal brain function, occur as a result of falls (28%), motor vehicle crashes (20%), being struck by or against a moving or stationary object (19%), and assaults (11%).

Head injuries occur when mechanical forces are transmitted to brain tissue. Identifying patients who have experienced an acute brain injury requires ongoing neurological examinations (Glasgow Coma Scale [GCS], CT scan, pupillary assessment). Patients may experience evidence of a TBI from the onset with subtle to severe symptoms, or the patient may develop symptoms hours later.

Performing serial neurologic examinations, including pupillary assessments, aids in identifying subtle changes in a patient's neurologic status. These subtle changes can indicate the presence of TBI and/or an acute deterioration in a patient's condition. The presence of TBI is confirmed with a CT scan and/or MRI. The CT scan can quickly aid in differentiating between a focal and diffuse brain injury.

TYPES OF HEAD INJURIES

Concussion

Concussion is the most common and least serious type of traumatic brain injury involving a transient loss of neurologic function and loss of consciousness. It can be caused by acceleration or deceleration forces, or by a direct blow. MTBI accounts for 75% of the total number of TBIs. Patients that are evaluated can be safely treated and discharged from the ED.

Etiology

The neurologic dysfunction from a concussion includes confusion, disorientation, and often a period of posttraumatic amnesia. Other symptoms can include a period of unconsciousness of less than 60 minutes, headache, dizziness, nausea, irritability, inability to concentrate, impaired memory, and fatigue. Amnesia, the hallmark sign of concussion, can be retrograde amnesia (loss of memories that were formed before the injury) or antero-grade amnesia (loss of memories formed postinjury) (Cantu, 2001, 2006). Length of fogginess postinjury is more indicative of severity then length of loss consciousness (Makdissi, 2010).

Since concussions may not include damage to the brain's structure, the condition of patients with uncomplicated concussions often either improves or stays the same. A deteriorating level of consciousness or symptoms of increased intracranial pressure (ICP) may mean that the patient has another problem, such as a more severe type of head injury.

Treatment

Mild TBIs are generally diagnosed after a series of cognitive and neurologic evaluations to assess alertness, attention, speech, memory, and reaction times. Physicians may also use brain imaging assessments such as CT scans and MRIs if there is suspicion of an intracranial hemorrhage. A concussion can usually be managed with plenty of rest and continued observation. Patients with severe concussive symptoms, although very rare, may be admitted; however, most patients are discharged home. Supportive care may include the use of non-narcotic analgesics (see Chapter 6) and anti-emetics. Prompt follow-up care and appropriate referral to a primary care physician, neurologist, or psychiatrist depending on the symptoms are required. Patient education on what to expect after MTBI is useful, as many patients will have symptoms for weeks after discharge.

Contusions

Contusions of the brain are bruises usually associated with more severe blunt trauma of local brain tissue. The area may lie directly under the site of the blow to the cranium or may be opposite to the site of impact (coup-contra-coup injury). The contusions can usually be seen acutely on CT scan as small petecchia in the brain parenchyma.

Etiology

- Confusion
- Neurologic deficit
- Personality changes
- Vision changes
- Speech changes

Epidural Hematoma

Epidural hematomas (EDHs) typically take place after a blow to the side of the head resulting in a fracture of the thin temporal bone overlying the middle meningeal artery. Bleeding occurs between the dura mater and skull. This causes rapid bleeding and reduction of oxygen to the tissues.

Etiology

The patient may awaken from this with a good level of consciousness only to lose consciousness later. If the bleeding is very severe, there is no awakening interval. Continued bleeding produces an enlarging epidural hematoma, associated symptoms such as severe and worsening headache, vomiting, and decreasing level of consciousness. Additional associated symptoms are ipsilateral dilated fixed pupil, signs of increasing intracranial pressure, unconsciousness, contralateral paralysis, and/or death.

Treatment

Open craniotomy for evacuation of the clot and control of bleeding is normally indicated for epidural hematoma. Conservative treatment may be indicated in some patients who meet all of the following criteria: clot volume <30 cm^3, maximum thickness <1.5 cm, and GCS <8 (Bullock et al., 2006). Prognosis after successful evacuation is better for epidural hematoma than subdural hematoma. Good outcomes are associated in most patients with epidural hematoma who undergo rapid CT scan and intervention.

Subdural Hematoma

Subdural hematomas are one type of focal brain injury occurring in approximately 30% of patients with TBI. An acute subdural hematoma occurs usually after a deceleration injury in which cerebral veins rupture because of either a linear or rotational shearing force (Davis, 2000). Rupture of these vessels causes bleeding into the subdural space. The bleeding may exert additional pressure onto the surrounding brain tissue, causing shifting of the tissue. As the size of the bleed increases, the effect on the brain increases resulting in a decline in neurologic status. If bleeding continues without intervention, the mortality rate increases. Subdural hematomas are most common in the elderly. Because the blood is under very low pressure, the hematoma builds slowly, causing signs and symptoms that develop over days to months. Often the head trauma can be so minor that it is not remembered. Patients who take anticoagulants are predisposed to subdural hematoma and intracerebral hemorrhage. Subdural venous bleeding is slow to accumulate, and gradual shifting of the brain occurs.

Etiology

Mild depression of consciousness, difficulty with cognitive function, and chronic headache may be the presenting picture. Acute deterioration may occur when the capacity to adapt for the expanding mass is exceeded. In many patients the symptoms of subdural hematoma wax and wane over hours or days. Besides the symptoms already mentioned—symptoms may include headache, depression of consciousness, confusion, and signs of focal cortical dysfunction (based on the region that is affected)—blood products in close proximity to the brain may also result in seizures.

Treatment

Open craniotomy for evacuation of acute subdural hematomas is indicated for any of the following: thickness >1 cm, midline shift >5 mm, or GCS drop by 2 or more points from the time of injury to hospitalization (Smith, Bauman, & Grady, n.d.). Some hematomas may eventually stabilize and reabsorb and become a chronic subdural hematoma. Frequent neurologic assessments are needed until stabilization of the clot is determined by serial head CT scans.

Basilar Skull Fracture

Basilar skull fracture is a fracture of the bones that form the base of the skull and results from severe blunt head trauma of significant force. The fracture commonly connects to the sinus cavities allowing fluid or air entry into the inside of the skull and may cause infection.

Etiology

The symptoms depend on the severity and distribution of the brain injury. Persistent localized pain usually suggests that a fracture is present. Fractures of the cranial vault may or may not produce swelling in the region of the fracture.

- *CSF otorrhea:* Cerebrospinal fluid leakage from the ears indicates a skull fracture. The patient is at risk for development of meningitis from the leakage tract.
- *CSF rhinorrhea:* Cerebrospinal fluid leaks from the nose.
- *Periorbital ecchymosis—"Raccoon eye's":* Ecchymosis around the eyes.

▦ *Battle's sign:* An ecchymotic discoloration over the mastoid bone behind the ear without skin or scalp contusion. It indicates periosteal bleeding, which drains toward the exterior from a basilar fracture and usually does not develop for several hours following the trauma.

Diffuse Axonal Injury

Diffuse axonal injury (DAI) is usually associated with severe head trauma and affects more than 2 million people every year. There are approximately 26,000 deaths per year associated with DAI and 20,000 to 45,000 surviving patients suffer neurobehavioral or physical impairments. More than 90% of patients that sustain DAI never regain consciousness and 10% who awaken are severely impaired.

Etiology

Contre-coup, also known as a shearing injury, can cause DAI. It causes damage to individual neurons and loss of connection to the neurons, which causes an overall breakdown in communication of the neurons (NINDS, 2011). The brain is injured so diffusely that there is generalized edema. Usually, there is no evidence of a structural lesion. In most cases, the patient presents unconscious, without focal deficits. Injury occurs immediately and is irreversible. Patients usually remain in a persistent vegetative state.

Treatment

Treatment of DAI is the same as for any severe TBI. Prevention of secondary brain injury is critical. Secondary brain injury refers to the changes that evolve over a period of time (from hours to days) after the primary brain injury. It includes an entire cascade of cellular, chemical, tissue, or blood vessel changes in the brain that contribute to further destruction of brain tissue. This injury has a poor prognosis and if the patient does recover, there will be deficits—personality changes, motor difficulties (poor coordination, paralysis, spasticity, etc.), changes in senses, sided neglect, spatial discernment, aphasia, dysphagia, and impaired ADL ability.

TREATMENT FOR SEVERE HEAD TRAUMA

The basics of TBI treatment have essentially remained unchanged over time. Ensuring maintenance of normal homeostasis and prevention and prompt treatment of secondary insults are critical components to care.

The injured brain is much more vulnerable to any insult than when the brain is unharmed. Basic care involves supporting the vital functions—airway, breathing, and circulation—and preventing further neurologic decline.

1. *Protect the airway and oxygenate:* Protection of the airway and ventilatory support are often needed in patients with severe TBI. Hypoxemia and hypotension are contributing factors to increased morbidity and mortality. Patients with GCS <9 and who are unable to maintain their airway or who remain hypoxemic despite supplemental O_2, require the airway secured by endotracheal intubation.

2. *Hyperventilation:* Hyperventilation has been the recommended treatment for reduction of intracranial pressure for many years and it has been assumed beneficial in all TBI patients. Level II evidence supports avoidance of prophylactic hyperventilation ($PaCO_2$ <30 mmHg) during the first 24 hours after severe TBI because it can compromise cerebral perfusion during a time when cerebral blood flow is already reduced (Brain Trauma Foundation, 2007). Hyperventilation may be necessary for brief periods when there is acute neurological deterioration or for longer periods if there is refractory intracranial hypertension.

3. *Correct hypovolemia and hypotension:* Hypotension (systolic blood pressure <90 mmHg) or hypoxia (apnea, cyanosis, or SaO_2 <90%) must be avoided, if possible, or corrected immediately in severe TBI patients.

   The mean arterial pressure (MAP) should be maintained above 90 mmHg through the infusion of fluids to maintain cerebral perfusion pressure (CPP) >70 mmHg (MAP − ICP = CPP; CPP 50 to 70).

   Level II evidence exists regarding hypotension, defined as a single observation of a systolic blood pressure of <90 mmHg, or hypoxia, defined as apnea/cyanosis in the field or a PaO_2 <60 mmHg by arterial blood gas analysis, to warrant the formation of guidelines stating that these values must be avoided, if possible, or rapidly corrected in severe head injury patients (Brain Trauma Foundation, 2007). A significant percentage of TBI patients have been found to be hypoxemic or hypotensive in the pre-hospital setting. Patients with severe head injury that are intubated in the pre-hospital setting appear to have better outcomes. Strong level II evidence suggests that raising the blood pressure in hypotensive, severe head injury patients improves outcome in proportion to the efficacy of the resuscitation (Brain Trauma Foundation, 2007).

4. *CT scan when appropriate:* A CT scan of the brain should be obtained based on the presence of injuries and/or neurological status. This will define the brain injury and determine the treatment—removal of an

intracranial mass, evacuation of epidural/subdural hematoma—and the degree of diffuse injury and cerebral swelling present.

5. *Neurosurgery if indicated.*

6. *Monitoring and management.* The patient who remains in a coma requires supportive treatment after the initial emergency treatment and management. In the comatose patient, the neurologic exam provides limited clinical information, although it can be supplemented by other measures.

Intracranial pressure (ICP) monitoring is a common measured indicator of cerebral status. The ventriculostomy is the gold standard of measuring ICP. A plastic tube is placed percutaneously into the cerebral ventricles. The ventriculostomy allows for management of intracranial hypertension via drainage of the CSF. Other measures that are commonly used are sedation, analgesics, pharmacologic paralysis, and IV mannitol.

Routine ICP monitoring is not indicated in patients with mild or moderate head injury. Comatose head injury patients with abnormal CT scans should undergo ICP monitoring. Current data support 20–25 mmHg as an upper threshold above which treatment to lower the ICP should generally be initiated. Interpretation and treatment of ICP based on threshold should be supported by frequent clinical examination and CPP trends.

Clinical Pearl	*Cushing's Triad-*: Signs of increased ICP
	• Widening pulse pressure; i.e., increased systolic/decreased diastolic blood pressure
	• Abnormal respiration pattern
	• Bradycardia

---

7. *Hyperosmolar therapy:* The guidelines currently recommend 20% mannitol (0.25 g/kg to 1 g/kg) infused over 20 minutes for trauma patients with elevated ICP or for patients with clinical signs of herniation and/or progressive neurological deterioration before ICP monitoring (Brain Injury Foundation, 2007). In an evidence-based review, higher dose mannitol is superior to conventional mannitol in improving mortality rates and clinical outcomes, although it is less effective than hypertonic saline for reducing ICP (Level I) (Meyer et al., 2010). Numerous case reports and small cohorts from studies with mixed patient populations have reported the efficacy of hypertonic saline bolus dosing to reduce TBI-induced intracranial hypertension in cases refractory to mannitol (Level I).

8. *Analgesics and sedatives:* Many medications have been utilized to treat pain and agitation in the TBI patient and to prevent or minimize damage associated with secondary injury by controlling intracranial pressure and cerebral oxygenation. Analgesics and sedatives reduce the metabolic demands placed on injured neurons by limiting nociceptive stimulation and reducing overall brain activity (Meyer et al., 2010).

Propofol

Propofol is a fast-acting, short-duration sedative that provides potentially neuroprotective effects (Level I evidence). Initiation of sedation should begin at 5 mcg/kg/min (0.3 mg/kg/hr). The infusion rate should be increased by increments of 5 to 10 mcg/kg/min (0.3 to 0.6 mg/kg/hr) until the desired level of sedation is achieved. A minimum period of 5 minutes between adjustments should be allowed for onset of peak drug effect. Most adult patients require maintenance rates of 5 to 50 mcg/kg/min (0.3 to 3 mg/kg/hr) or higher.

Propofol reduces ICP and the need for other ICP and sedative interventions when used in conjunction with morphine. A randomized control study by Kelly et al. (1999) compared propofol sedation to morphine for safety and efficacy. Propofol in combination with morphine reduced ICP and the need for neuromuscular blockades, benzodiazepines, pentobarbital, and drainage of cerebrospinal fluid (CSF) compared to using morphine alone. In patient follow up, there was no difference in patient outcomes.

Opioids

Patients with multiple traumas often have painful injuries that require analgesia and intubated patients require sedation. Short-acting sedatives and analgesics should be used to attain adequate sedation and analgesia without interfering with the ability to perform neurologic assessments.

Morphine has been the most commonly used opioid following a brain injury. The use of fentanyl and similar type medications are becoming popular due to their rapid onset and shorter duration of effect. Differing opinions exist on the effect of opioids on ICP and CPP; some studies have linked the use of opioids and brain injury to increases in ICP and CPP (Meyer et al., 2010).

- *Fentanyl:* 25–100 mcg IVP every 5–15 minutes
- *Hydromorphone:* 0.25–0.75 mg IVP every 5–15 minutes
- *Morphine:* 2–5 mg IVP every 5–15 minutes
- Repeat until pain is controlled then scheduled doses and PRN.

9. *Steroids:* Corticosteroids have been a common treatment for brain injury as they were thought to decrease intracranial pressure. In a Cochrane Review, one group received corticosteroids and another received standard care. In the first review of 20 studies and over 12,000 participants, the results were inconclusive. Another study completed at the same time as this review, called the CRASH study, showed an increase in the number of deaths in patients who received steroids than patients who received no treatment. The author concluded that steroids should no longer be the standard of care in patients with TBI (Alderson & Roberts, 2005; Brain Trauma Foundation, 2007).

10. *Optimize cerebral perfusion*: Cerebral perfusion pressure (CPP) is defined as: CPP = MAP − ICP. This represents the pressure driving cerebral blood flow (CBF) and oxygen delivery. Typically the brain regulates its blood flow to provide a constant flow regardless of blood pressure by altering the resistance of cerebral blood vessels. When brain trauma occurs, cerebral vascular resistance is usually increased, and the brain becomes vulnerable to changes in blood pressure. A CPP low enough to promote ischemia will initiate secondary cellular injury. Using fluids and vasopressors to aggressively raise CPP may cause pulmonary complications. Guidelines for the management of severe TBI cautions that a CPP above 70 mmHg and below 50 mmHg should be avoided (Brain Trauma Foundation et al., 2007). The guidelines further state that a threshold of 10 mmHg above the target threshold may be important to avoid dips below a critical level. A general threshold of 60 mmHg may be appropriate with further fine-tuning based on multimodality monitoring.

Brainstem Evaluation of the Patient With Head Trauma

The patient's level of consciousness is the most sensitive and reliable indicator of brain function. When the patient is initially examined, and on all subsequent exams, the level of consciousness is measured using clear terms. The most common coma scale used for measuring level of consciousness is the Glasgow Coma Scale (GCS) The GCS is used universally for assessing severity of brain injury and as a classification tool. It is particularly useful to monitor change in consciousness subsequent to injury. The scale is organized into three sections: eye opening, best motor response, and best verbal response. Scoring of the patient's response in each section helps to track the patient's clinical progress or deteriorization. The scoring range is from 3 to 15, with the lower score of 3 indicating a deep comatose state, and a score of 15 a fully alert individual. A score of 8 typically indicates a comatose state.

The examination focus is on determining brainstem function and includes evaluation of respiration, pupillary, vestibulo-ocular and motor response.

1. *Respiratory pattern*: Normal breathing progresses to hyperventilation ("central neurogenic hyperventilation") as the midbrain is compressed, and then to an irregular respiratory pattern or apnea as the medulla is compressed.

2. *Pupillary response*: Equally responsive pupils progress to mid-position without response to light as the upper midbrain is compressed.

3. *Oculocephalic reflex*: Also known as the "doll's eye reflex"; this is normally inhibited in the conscious person. Testing of the reflex involves keeping the eyes of the patient open and then rotating the head briskly from one side to the other (this test is avoided in patient with a suspected neck injury). If the brainstem is intact, the gaze deviates contralaterally and the patient looks away from rotation. With an injured brainstem, the eyes follow the direction of the head movement.

4. *Motor response*: Normal motor strength and tone progress to decorticate or decerebrate posturing as the midbrain is compressed. Decerebrate posturing manifests by leg and arm extension and toes point downward, occurring spontaneously or with noxious stimuli (Figure 17.1). This is suggestive of uncal or brain herniation.

   Decorticate posturing presents with the arms flexed, or bent inward on the chest, the hands clenched into fists, and the legs extended and feet turned inward (Figure 17. 2). This indicates possible damage to the cerebral hemispheres, thalamus, and the midbrain.

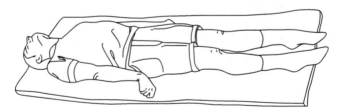

Figure 17.1 ■ Decerebrate posture.

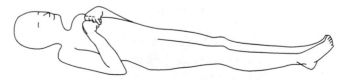

Figure 17.2 ■ Decorticate posture.

CHEST TRAUMA

Thoracic injuries remain common and are directly attributable for 20%–25% of all trauma deaths (Savetamal & Livingston, 2008). Chest injuries are associated with other injuries and pulmonary complications in more than one-third of cases and pneumonia in as many as 30% of cases. Rib fractures are the most commonly encountered injuries. In a review of over 7,000 patients seen in a Level I trauma center, 10% had rib fractures; of these, 94% had associated injuries and 12% died (Savetamal & Livingston, 2008).

Chest trauma is challenging as the injuries the patient can experience can be life threatening, worsen over time, or be benign. Health care professionals must use their astute assessment skills to identify injuries and anticipate potential injuries based upon the anatomical location and the mechanism of injury (penetrating or blunt injury).

> *Clinical Pearl:*   Cardiovascular, pulmonary, gastrointestinal, and hemostatic functions may all be negatively affected by poorly controlled pain.

Most thoracic injuries do not require major surgical intervention but can be managed with simple tube thoracostomy, mechanical ventilation, aggressive pain control, and other supportive care.

Mechanism of Injury

Penetrating thoracic injuries (e.g., stab wounds, gunshot wounds) primarily injure the peripheral lung, producing both a hemothorax and pneumothorax.

Blunt trauma can induce injury by three distinct mechanisms: a direct blow to the chest (e.g., rib fracture), deceleration injury (e.g., pulmonary or cardiac contusion and aortic tear), and compression injury (e.g., cardiac and diaphragm rupture).

Thoracic injuries can also be categorized according to the injury location on the chest wall, i.e., pulmonary and cardiovascular.

CHEST WALL

Rib Fractures

Rib fractures are the most common chest injury and present in approximately 10% of all traumatic injuries. Patients with one or two rib fractures have a 5% mortality rate and patients with seven or more fractures have a 29% mortality rate. The mechanism of injury is usually associated with age-related injuries:

- Sports/recreational injuries in adolescents
- Motor vehicle accidents/assaults in adults
- Falls in the geriatric population

The most common area affected is the fourth through ninth ribs. The break usually occurs at the point of impact and the posterior angle. The site of the break may be associated with other injuries:

- First and second rib fractures may indicate neck and great vessel injury (subclavian artery/vein, aortic injury).
- The most common associated injuries are pneumothorax, hemothorax, and pulmonary contusion (Wanek & Mayberry, 2004).
- Fractures of the ninth to 11th ribs are associated with intra-abdominal injury; lower left rib fractures have a 22% to 28% probability of splenic injury; lower right rib fractures have a 19% to 56% probability of liver injury (Wanek & Mayberry, 2004).
- Two or more rib fractures are associated with an increased incidence of internal injury.

Etiology

Physical findings include ecchymosis, local tenderness, and crepitus over the site of the fracture. If a pneumothorax is present, breath sounds may be decreased and resonance to percussion may be increased. Patients experience pain and guarding, resulting in decreased ventilations; pulmonary shunting may occur secondary to atelectasis and hypoxia. Chest wall pain increases with deep breathing, coughing, and movement.

Treatment

The primary treatment of rib fractures consists of pain management, which may be administered orally, parenterally, or epidurally, depending on the degree of discomfort and the number of ribs involved. In the ICU, parenteral analgesics or regional blocks are desirable. Generally, fractured ribs do not require any specific treatment. In patients with preexisting pulmonary disease, the restriction produced by fractured ribs can make the difference between normal gas exchange and severe respiratory failure (Jameel, 2010). Maintenance of adequate respiratory function is critical in the treatment of these patients.

Flail Chest

Flail chest is the rarest of all blunt chest wall injuries and the most serious as it is considered life-threatening. It is often associated with underlying pulmonary injury and seen most commonly in cases of significant injury.

Severe injury to the chest remains one of the leading causes of morbidity and mortality in both young and elderly trauma victims. The prevalence of flail chest among patients with chest wall injury is estimated to be between 5% and 13% (Wanek & Mayberry, 2004).

Etiology

Flail chest occurs when three or more ribs are fractured in two or more places and are no longer attached to the thoracic cage (Figure 17.3) A segment of the chest wall that is flail is unable to contribute to lung expansion. Large flail segments will involve a much greater proportion of the chest wall and may extend bilaterally or involve the sternum. In these cases, the disruption of normal pulmonary mechanics may require mechanical ventilation.

The main significance of a flail chest indicates the presence of an underlying pulmonary contusion. The severity and extent of the lung injury determines the clinical treatment. The management of flail chest consists of standard management of the rib fractures and the pulmonary contusions.

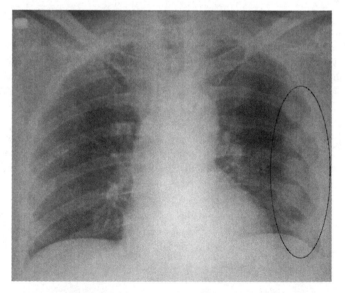

Figure 17.3 ■ Multiple rib fractures. *Source*: Smith, D. H., Meaney, D. F., & Shull, W. H. Diffuse axonal injury in head trauma. *Journal of Head Trauma and Rehabilitation, 18,* pp. 307–316.

Assessment

Flail chest is diagnosed upon physical examination. Visible signs of bruising or seatbelt imprints are noted on inspection, and crepitus is often felt on palpation. Patients will complain of pain on palpation of the chest wall or upon inspiration. A flail chest has paradoxical movement of a segment of the chest wall. During inspiration the intact or noninjured chest wall expands while the injured area is sucked in. During expiration, the opposite occurs. The physiological effects of an impaired chest wall lead to decreased tidal volume, impaired cough, and decreased vital capacity, which can lead to hypoventilation and atelectasis.

Treatment

In most cases it is the severity and extent of the lung injury that determines the clinical course and requirement for mechanical ventilation. Intubation and ventilator support is usually required for all patients with large flail segments, and any patient with underlying acute or chronic lung disease.

Management of chest wall injury is directed toward protecting the underlying lung and allowing adequate oxygenation, ventilation, and pulmonary toilet aimed at preventing the development of pneumonia.

Pain management is essential to promote pulmonary toilet and prevent the untoward effects of pain, i.e., splinting, atelectasis, and hypoventilation. In order to reduce morbidity and mortality, adequate pain relief is essential in chest trauma patients. Some patients may desaturate purely from inadequate pain management. Use of opioids may decrease respiratory drive, cause or worsen hypoxia, and cause hypotension; therefore, opioids should be used with caution in the presence of chest trauma. The use of optimal analgesia and aggressive chest physiotherapy should be applied to minimize the likelihood of respiratory failure and to ensure adequate ventilatory support.

PCA can be useful in cooperative patients with flail chest who are able to follow direction and push the button. NSAIDs may also serve as a useful adjuvant to opioids in providing pain relief. NSAIDs should not be used until all injuries are determined and there is no risk of bleeding. A thoracic pidural catheter delivering a continuous infusion of a local anesthetic agent (+/− an opioid) is the preferred mode of analgesia delivery in severe flail chest injury (Eastern Association for the Surgery of Trauma [EAST], 2006). This method provides complete analgesia allowing normal inspiration and coughing without the risks of respiratory depression. If the patient can cooperate, the epidural infusion can be advanced to an epidural PCA mode and the patient can give themselves additional medication on an as needed basis. Epidurals may be placed in the thoracic or high-lumbar positions. Nurses should request epidural analgesia as needed for patient comfort and maximum respiratory function.

PULMONARY

Pulmonary Contusion

Pulmonary contusion is a bruise of the lung associated with blunt trauma and other chest injuries such as rib fractures. Pulmonary contusion should be suspected in any patient who sustains significant, blunt chest impact.

Treatment

The treatment of pulmonary contusion is supportive, focusing on the respiratory distress it produces. Initial treatment should focus on any associated injuries with placement of chest tubes as needed and pain control for chest wall injuries. Supplemental oxygen to treat hypoxia, aggressive pulmonary toileting as needed, and postural positioning have been shown to improve outcomes (Wanek & Mayberry, 2004). Intubation without signs of impending respiratory failure is not indicated (EAST, 2006; Level II).

Most thoracic injuries do not require major surgical intervention but can be managed with simple tube thoracostomy, mechanical ventilation, aggressive pain control, and other supportive care (Wanek & Mayberry, 2004).

Trauma patients with pulmonary contusion should not be extremely fluid restricted, but should be resuscitated as necessary with isotonic crystalloid or colloid solution to maintain adequate tissue perfusion (EAST, 2006; Level II). Unnecessary fluid administration should be avoided.

THORACENTESIS

Thoracentesis is usually a simple uncomplicated procedure generally performed either for diagnostic/therapeutic purposes or during an emergency situation. It is a short-term procedure, although it may ultimately result in insertion of a chest tube.

Some clinicians use local anesthesia alone while others administer conscious sedation prior to beginning the procedure. Primary determination to use moderate sedation should be made upon patient's hemodynamic status with consideration of the patient's level of anxiety.

Pain occurs as a result of puncture of the skin and the parietal pleura, which is highly sensitive to pain. Contact with a rib surface will result in severe pain because of the abundant nociceptors on the periosteal surface

(Brims et al., 2010). The pain and discomfort generally resolve once the catheter is removed. Some may experience anxiety from anticipation of the procedure and any respiratory distress they may be experiencing. If the patient is hemodynamically stable, moderate sedation (IV midazolam or lorazepam) may be considered to minimize the patient's anxiety level. The area where the needle/catheter is going to be placed is anesthetized with a generous infiltration of lidocaine 1% or 2%. The skin, subcutaneous tissue, rib periosteum, intercostal muscle, and parietal pleura should all be well infiltrated with local anesthetic. Anesthetizing the deep part of the intercostal muscle and the parietal pleura is important, as puncture of these tissues generates the most pain.

Contraindications to thoracentesis are in patients who are:

- Coagulopathic
- Mechanically ventilated with risk of tension pneumothorax. Ultrasound guided thoracentesis may be beneficial in these situations (Goligher et al., 2011).
- Severe hemodynamic or respiratory compromise until the underlying condition can be stabilized.
- Cutaneous infections such as herpes zoster on the chest wall.

Other pain associated with thoracentesis may be related to drainage of fluid if it is drained too fast or if a large volume is drained. The patient may complain of chest pain that is an aching to a severe pleuritic pain. Slowing the rate of drainage may help minimize the discomfort. After the procedure, patients may experience some discomfort and analgesia should be provided. Mild and moderate pain generally can be controlled with acetaminophen or NSAIDs, with or without a weak opioid. NSAIDs should be avoided in patients who are coagulopathic or have renal impairment. For patients who are reporting pleuritic pain, NSAIDs are the analgesic of choice.

CHEST TUBES

Chest tubes are used whenever there is significant air or fluid in the pleural space or after thoracic surgery. Attention to airway, breathing, and circulation while assessing vital signs and oxygen saturation is critical. Care depends on the hemodynamic stability of the patient. All patients should receive supplemental oxygen to increase oxygen saturation. There are no absolute contraindications to tube thoracostomy, particularly if the patient is in respiratory distress or has a tension pneumothorax.

The associated pain with chest tubes is assumed to be a result from direct irritation of the pleura or periosteum by the chest tube, along with the trauma during insertion. Larger bore chest tubes have been linked with a higher level of discomfort. There are many choices of chest tubes, which may lead to selection of an incorrect size. Chest tube size selection is the flow rate of either the air or the liquid that can be accommodated by the tube (Baumann, 2003; Fysh, Smith, & Lee, 2010). Appropriate chest tube size selection is necessary in order to prevent compromise (Light, 2011; Baumann et al., 2001).

Unless it is an emergency situation, a strong IV opioid analgesic and moderate sedation can be given to reduce patient anxiety and discomfort when a chest tube is being placed. Some clinicians prefer to use local anesthetic alone while others use it in conjunction with moderate sedation. If the patient is hemodynamically stable, use of moderate sedation would be recommended.

Local anesthetic of lidocaine 1% or 2% is used to anesthetize the area of the subcutaneous tissue where the chest tube will be placed. Local anesthetic should be directed along the expected course of the chest tube insertion and into the periosteum, intercostal muscle, and the pleura. While the chest tube is in place the pain is usually mild and generally can be controlled with acetaminophen or NSAIDs (Chapter 6). NSAIDs should be avoided in patients who are coagulopathic or have renal impairment.

The chest tube will remain in place until the original indication for placement is no longer present or the tube becomes nonfunctional. Patients have described chest tube removal as painful in their postoperative recovery and report that the pain is poorly managed (Puntillo & Ley, 2004). There are no standards that exist for analgesia for chest tube removal. Studies are limited and research is needed in this area to see if the efficacy of drugs other than morphine may be effective, including a multi-modal approach. From a study conducted by Puntillo and Ley (2004), they concluded that they were able to maintain excellent pain control during removal of chest tubes using either morphine or ketorolac without adverse side effects if used correctly. Using sufficient doses and performing the procedure at the time that corresponds to the drug's peak effect resulted in good patient outcome.

Treatment

The Eastern Association for the Surgery of Trauma (EAST) made the following evidence-based recommendations for blunt chest wall trauma in their Blunt Thoracic Trauma (BTT) Pain Management guidelines (2004).

The use of epidural analgesia (EA) for pain control after severe blunt injury and nontraumatic surgical thoracic pain significantly reduced patient pain scores, improved pulmonary function tests compared to IV opioids, and is the preferred technique after severe blunt thoracic trauma (Level I).

A combination of an opioid and a local anesthetic (i.e., bupivacaine) provides the most effective EA and the preferred drug combination (Level II). EA is associated with less respiratory depression, somnolence, and gastrointestinal symptoms compared to IV opioids.

Elderly patients 65 years and older with four or more rib fractures should receive EA unless contraindicated (Level II). Patients with cardiopulmonary disease or diabetes are high-risk patients who also would benefit from EA, as these co-morbidities may increase mortality once respiratory complications have occurred (Level II).

ABDOMINAL TRAUMA

Unrecognized abdominal trauma is a major cause of death in trauma patients and the second leading cause of preventable trauma death. Increased incidences of deaths are secondary to hemorrhage, often as a result of a delay in receiving surgical intervention. Abdominal trauma is characteristically categorized as either blunt or penetrating trauma.

Blunt and Penetrating Trauma

Blunt trauma accounts for more than half of all abdominal injuries resulting from motor vehicle accidents, assaults, recreational accidents, or falls. The highest incidence of organ injury after blunt trauma is to the liver and spleen. Intra-abdominal injuries secondary to blunt force are attributed to collisions between the injured person and the external environment and to acceleration or deceleration forces on the person's internal organs. Blunt force injuries to the abdomen can generally be explained by three mechanisms.

Mechanism of Injury

During blunt trauma, the abdominal organs can be injured at three separate times. Initial injury can occur during a rapid change in organ momentum and speed. When organs or adjacent structures suddenly decelerate at different speeds, shearing forces can result in organs tearing at their bases or at the point between two organs. Solid and hollow organs and the vasculature are all at risk for shearing forces.

Organs also can be crushed as a blunt object presses against them, or as organs are compressed against rigid structures in the body. The spleen, kidneys, and liver are all particularly vulnerable to crushing. Lastly, external compression from blunt trauma causes a rise of pressure inside an organ, particularly hollow organs. As a result, hollow organs rupture, spilling their contents into the abdominal cavity.

Penetrating trauma occurs when an object physically enters through the skin and wall of the abdominal cavity. The most common mechanism for penetrating trauma is gunfire, followed by stabbing. As an object enters the abdominal cavity, it injures the organs in two ways. First, the object physically damages organ tissues as it penetrates. While passing through organ tissue, the object sends a wave of pressure in all directions, stretching the organs, which can injure adjacent organs, not just the impacted organ. Organs stretch because of their elastic nature and can cause either a temporary or permanent cavity. The greater the speed of a penetrating object, the more kinetic energy is transmitted to the organs, increasing the chance for ricochet off bony objects and for fragmentation (Collopy & Friese, 2010).

In patients undergoing laparotomy for blunt trauma, most frequently injured organs are the spleen (40%–55%), liver (35%–45%), and small bowel (5%–10%) (ATLS, 2001). Recent studies show an increased number of hepatic injuries, perhaps reflecting increased use of CT scanning and concomitant identification of more injuries.

Assessment

Location of entry and exit sites associated with penetrating trauma must be assessed and documented:

- *Cullen's sign:* A bluish discoloration around the umbilicus; may be present with intraperitoneal bleeding from the liver or the spleen
- *Grey-Turner's sign:* A bluish discoloration of the flank; may indicate retroperitoneal bleeding from the pancreas, duodenum, vena cava, aorta, or kidneys
- Distended abdomen
- Rebound tenderness
- *Kehr's sign:* Left shoulder pain caused by splenic bleeding; it is an acute pain that is a referred pain in the shoulder due to the presence of blood or other irritants in the peritoneal cavity when a person is lying down and the legs are elevated

---

Clinical Pearl	Other signs to consider intra-abdominal bleeding: • Referred shoulder pain • Unexplained hypotension • Multiple traumas present

Diagnosis

■ Diagnostic peritoneal lavage (DPL)
■ Bedside ultrasound: There is insufficient evidence from randomized controlled trials to justify promotion of ultrasonography-based clinical pathways in diagnosing patients with suspected blunt abdominal trauma (Stengel et al., 2005)
■ Chest x-ray
■ CT scan of abdomen

Liver Injury

After the spleen, the liver is the second most commonly injured organ in blunt abdominal trauma. Injury often occurs with fractures of ribs 8–12 on the right side. Injury is common because of the liver's size and location. Severity of injury ranges from a controlled subcapsular hematoma or lacerations of the parenchyma, to hepatic avulsion or a severe injury of the hepatic veins. Injury to the right lobe is far more common than the left, and injury of the posterior segment of the right lobe is more common than the anterior segment. Because liver tissue is very friable and the liver's blood supply and storage capacity are extensive, a patient with liver injuries can hemorrhage profusely and may need surgery to control the bleeding. The mortality rates for blunt hepatic trauma range between 8% and 25%, most commonly associated with hemorrhage (Yoon et al., 2005).

Diagnosis of a liver laceration can be obtained by CT if the patient is stable. If the patient is exhibiting signs of shock or has other critical injuries, a diagnostic peritoneal lavage (DPL) to confirm intra-peritoneal hemorrhage is appropriate. Treatment for large liver lacerations or penetrating wounds may require surgical intervention to either pack or repair the injury. For smaller injuries, close observation and frequent assessment including labs to monitor hemoglobin will be required.

The American Association of Surgery for Trauma (AAST) (1995) developed a grading system to provide a uniform definition of liver injuries.

■ Grade 1: Subcapsular hematoma less than 1 cm, laceration less than 1 cm, isolated periportal blood
■ Grade 2: Parenchymal laceration 1–3 cm deep, parenchymal/subcapsular hematomas 1–3 cm thick
■ Grade 3: Parenchymal laceration more than 3 cm deep and parenchymal or subcapsular hematoma more than 3 cm in diameter
■ Grade 4: Parenchymal/subcapsular hematoma >10 cm in diameter, lobar destruction, or devascularization
■ Grade 5: Global destruction or devascularization of liver
■ Grade 6: Hepatic avulsion

Etiology

The patient with suspected blunt or penetrating liver trauma commonly presents with signs and symptoms of hemorrhage, peritoneal irritation, right upper quadrant pain, and abdominal guarding. There may be rebound tenderness of the abdomen. In the most serious cases, the patient may present with shock, profound hypotension, and decreasing hemoglobin and hematocrit. Patients with blunt liver trauma may develop a liver abscess due to undiagnosed liver damage. These patients will present with signs and symptoms of acute abdominal infections and peritonitis.

Treatment

Non-operative management is currently considered the treatment of choice for the hemodynamically stable patient. Close observation, frequent assessment including labs to monitor hemoglobin will be required. Treatment for large liver lacerations, penetrating wounds, or hemodynamically unstable patients may require surgical intervention to either pack or repair the injury.

Pain is a common complaint in patients with liver trauma. The pain is more generalized and most responsive to opioid treatment. There are many options available for pain control utilizing a multimodal approach on an individual basis including patient's liver function, respiratory and coagulation status, and comorbidities. Ideal postoperative pain control is necessary for early mobilization and improved respiratory function.

The most common opioids used are morphine, hydromorphone, and fentanyl. Side effects of opioid administration include sedation, respiratory depression, nausea, vomiting, constipation, hypotension, and exacerbation of hepatic encephalopathy. Morphine is poorly excreted in patients with renal failure. Hydromorphone and fentanyl elimination is less affected by renal impairment and is a better alternative in patients with liver disease and renal impairment. It is important to closely monitor patients for adverse side effects. For patients who are in critical areas or who are intubated, continuous infusions may be indicated.

- Morphine : 1–4 mg bolus; 1–10 mg/hr infusion
- Fentanyl: 25–100 mcg bolus; 25–200 mcg /hr infusion
- Hydromorphone: 0.2–1 mg bolus; 0.2–2 mg/hr infusion

Epidural anesthesia is also an effective pain management option and can be an adjunct for intravenous opioids. It helps to reduce the pulmonary complications, duration of ileus, and provides better pain control than the use of opioids alone. There are associated risks in patients with an epidural catheter and in patients who are coagulopathic.

There are other drugs that may be useful as adjuncts to opioid management such as intravenous acetaminophen (recommended maximum dose is 2 g/day in patients with hepatic impairment). NSAID use is not recommended post hepatic surgery, in cirrhotic patients, or in patients with renal insufficiency due to the increased risks of bleeding and/or hepatorenal syndrome.

Spleen

The spleen is the most frequently injured abdominal organ in blunt trauma. Fractures of ribs 10–12 on the left should raise suspicion of spleen damage, which ranges from laceration of the capsule or a nonexpanding hematoma, to ruptured subcapsular hematomas or parenchymal laceration. The spleen tends to bleed easily. The capsule around the spleen tends to slow development of shock, although rapid shock occurs when the capsule ruptures. Injury to the spleen can take the form of laceration, intrasplenic hematoma, subcapsular hematoma, or infarction.

The American Association of Surgery for Trauma (AAST) (1994) developed a grading system to provide a uniform definition of splenic injuries.

- I: Subcapsular hematoma <10% of surface; laceration >1 cm deep
- II: Subcapsular hematoma on 10%–50% of surface; laceration 1–3 cm deep
- III: Subcapsular hematoma on >50% of surface or expanding intraparenchymal hematoma >5 cm or expanding
- IV: Laceration of segmental or hilar vessels with major devascularization
- V: Completely shattered spleen or hilar vessel injury with devascularization

Etiology

Clinical findings include the most common—tachycardia, hypotension, and upper left quadrant pain. Rib fractures (9th and 10th) on the left side are also common. If injury to the phrenic nerve is present, the patient may complain of left shoulder/scapular pain as well. Peritoneal signs such as rebounding and guarding will be delayed until the blood causes local irritation to the peritoneum. Other symptoms and signs may include:

- *Ballances' sign*: Dullness to percussion in the left flank left upper quadrant and shifting dullness to percussion in the right flank seen with splenic rupture/hematoma
- *Kehr's sign*: Radiating pain to the left shoulder upon palpation to the left upper quadrant. This highly correlates to the diagnosis
- Rigid abdomen

Treatment

Treatment for a spleen injury may include bed rest, intravenous fluids, opioids and monitoring of lab values. Treatment for large spleen injuries may include a splenectomy or over-sewing to repair the injury. Those that have had a splenectomy are more susceptible to infections. After a splenectomy, vaccinations for pneumococcus, hemophillus, and meningiococcus are usually given.

Pain is a common complaint in patients with splenic trauma. The pain is more generalized and most responsive to opioid treatment. There are many options available for pain control utilizing a multimodal approach based on each individual status and comorbidities. If the patient has postoperative pain, pain control is necessary for early mobilization and improved respiratory function.

The most common opioids used are morphine, hydromorphone, and fentanyl. Side effects of opioid administration include sedation, respiratory depression, nausea, vomiting, constipation, hypotension, and exacerbation of hepatic encephalopathy. Morphine is poorly excreted in patients with renal failure. Hydromorphone and fentanyl elimination is less affected by renal impairment and is a better alternative in patients with liver disease and renal impairment. It is important to closely monitor patients for adverse side effects. NSAIDs are not recommended as the incidence of bleeding is increased.

- Morphine: 1–4 mg bolus; 1–10 mg/hr infusion
- Fentanyl: 25–100 mcg bolus; 25–200 mcg/hr infusion
- Hydromorphone: 0.2–1 mg bolus; 0.2–2 mg/hr infusion

For pain management with either spleen or liver damage, a patient-controlled analgesic (PCA) pump can be used if the patient is able to activate the pump. Using a PCA will help patients breathe easier, move in bed, and become more active as they recover. It also allows the patient to use just the amount of medication needed rather than relying on continuous infusions.

Kidney

The most common kidney injury is a contusion from blunt trauma; suspect this type of injury if the patient has fractures of the posterior ribs or lumbar vertebrae. Other types of renal injuries include lacerations or contusion of the renal parenchyma caused by shearing and compression forces: The deeper a laceration, the more serious the bleeding. Deceleration forces may damage the renal artery; collateral circulation in that area is limited, so any ischemia is serious and may trigger acute tubular necrosis. The American

Association of Surgery for Trauma (AAST) classifies injuries to the kidneys in the following four categories:

- I: Contusions, small corticomedullary lacerations that do not communicate with the collection system
- II: Laceration that communicates with the collection system
- III: Shattered kidney, injury to the vascular pedicle
- IV: UPJ avulsion, laceration of the renal pelvis

Etiology

When there are fractures to the 11th and 12th ribs or complaints of flank pain or tenderness, an injury to one or both kidneys should be suspected. Clinical findings include:

- Complaints of pain on inspiration
- Hematuria
- *Grey-Turner's sign*: Ecchymosis of the flanks caused by the retroperitoneal leak of blood.
- Flank or abdominal tenderness on palpation
- *Cullen's sign*: Peri-umbilical bruising indicative of retroperitoneal hemorrhage

Treatment

The treatment for renal injury has become more conservative over time. Injuries graded I to III can usually be managed with bed rest, intravenous fluids, antibiotics, and observation. Pain medication without antiplatelet drug effects is preferred, especially if hematuria is present.

Lacerations to the kidney can often be managed conservatively and only grades IV and V usually need surgery. Surgical consultation is necessary for a lacerated kidney or kidney injury that shows extravasation of dye during IVP or CT. The goal of injury is to repair the kidney and avoid performing a nephrectomy unless absolutely necessary.

Pancreas

Pancreatic injuries are rare and are accompanied by a high acute vascular mortality due to the location of the pancreas near the aorta, superior mesenteric artery, and the vena cava. Pancreatic injuries are also associated with other injuries. Approximately 50% of pancreatic trauma-related deaths are due to hypovolemic shock from major visceral hemorrhage; therefore, a rapid and accurate diagnosis of pancreatic injury is vital.

The mechanism of injury usually involves compression between the spine and abdominal wall during a forceful blow to this area. Pancreatic injuries generally have very little hemorrhage although leakage of enzymes digests structures in the retroperitoneal space, causing volume loss and potentially, shock. If duct transection is suspected, an emergency endoscopic retrograde cholangiopancreatography (ERCP) or laparotomy may be required.

Etiology

In most cases, pancreatic injury can be symptom free and silent. A contained fracture of the spleen with retroperitoneal hematoma or leak manifests as dull epigastric pain or back pain. The most common scenario for the patient is to exhibit severe peritoneal irritation and a positive abdominal examination that is usually related to injury to other organs. Symptoms of injury to other structures may mask pancreatic injury. It is imperative that excellent assessment skills are utilized to ensure that pancreatic injuries are not missed.

- Epigastric pain, tenderness, guarding
- *Grey-Turner's sign*: Ecchymosis of the flanks caused by the retroperitoneal leak of blood
- Late signs 12 to 36 hours after the injury

Treatment

Diagnosis of pancreatic injury has relied on CT scans, amylase levels, MRI, and ultrasound, with varied levels of success. The optimal management of pancreatic injury once a diagnosis has been made is not well established (EAST, 2009). Non-operative management, suture and repair, non-drainage, or drainage of injury with or without sumps has all been utilized with varying degrees of success. Complications of the pancreatic injury include abscesses, fistulae, pancreatitis, and pseudocysts.

Stomach, Duodenal, Mesentery, and Small Bowel Injury

Hollow viscus trauma is more frequent in the presence of an associated, severe, solid organ injury, particularly to the pancreas. Approximately two-thirds of patients with hollow viscus trauma are injured in motor vehicle collisions.

Injury to the bowel resulting from blunt trauma, although infrequent (<5%), is generally associated with motor vehicle accidents. Injuries can occur as a result of direct compression between the vertebral column and the abdominal wall or a shearing-type injury. Undetected bowel perforation can lead to fatal peritonitis, and a delay of 24 hours without surgical intervention has been shown to increase mortality.

Stab and gunshot wounds account for most patient presentations of penetrating abdominal trauma, with some resulting in apparent peritoneal irritation requiring immediate exploration. The most commonly injured organs associated with penetrating injuries are the small intestine (29%), liver (28%), and colon (23%).

Penetrating injuries below the nipple line and above the symphysis pubis, and between the posterior axillary lines must be treated as injuries to the abdomen and require exploratory laparotomy.

Clinical Pearl	Irritation of the peritoneum is quite painful. In an attempt to relieve the pain, a patient may lie still with the knees pulled into the chest. This position relieves the tension placed on the peritoneum.

Etiology

The classic triad of tenderness, rigidity, and absent bowel sounds only occurs in about 30% of patients. Internal injury and associated internal inflammation to the abdomen may not be evident initially as the symptoms tend to be generalized. Symptoms are produced by intestinal contents, rather than blood loss. Stomach rupture causes rapid onset of burning epigastric pain, followed quickly by rigidity and rebound sensitivity. Small bowel and colon injury may present only with vague generalized pain, with peritonitis developing after a few hours. Duodenal injury may cause back pain. Some of the early signs of hollow viscus injury are as follows:

- Nausea
- Vomiting
- Fever
- Pneumoperitoneum or air or gas in the abdominal cavity
- Disembowelment or evisceration
- Fractured ribs may perforate the abdominal wall causing injury
- Abdominal pain, distension, guarding, rigidity
- Peritoneal signs of inflammation
- Absent bowel signs
- Blood in nasogastric tube
- Shock

Treatment

The majority of patients with penetrating and nonpenetrating abdominal trauma are managed nonoperatively and may be kept for observation for 24 hours in the presence of a reliable abdominal examination and minimal to no abdominal tenderness. Patients who have penetrating abdominal trauma and are hemodynamically unstable or who have diffuse abdominal tenderness should be taken emergently for laparotomy. Those with an unreliable clinical examination as a result of a impaired level of consciousness, spinal cord injury, or need for sedation or intubation should be examined further to determine if there is intraperitoneal injury. Serial examinations should be performed, as a single physical examination is considered unreliable in detecting major injuries to the abdomen.

Consider administering analgesic drugs such as morphine sulfate or fentanyl. Both drugs are safe and effective analgesics. For patients in critical care areas who have severe level pain or are intubated, continuous infusions can be used.

- Morphine : 1–4 mg bolus; 1–10 mg/hr infusion
- Fentanyl: 25–100 mcg bolus; 25–200 mcg /hr infusion

For patients with less severe injuries and pain, or patients who are outside of a critical care area, a patient-controlled analgesic pump (PCA) may be used or intermittent IV injections of pain medications may be sufficient to control pain, For these patients attention will need to be paid to patient complaints of unrelieved pain and opioid dosages adjusted to meet the patient's needs for pain relief.

> *Clinical Pearl*   Blunt abdominal injuries carry a greater risk of morbidity and mortality than penetrating abdominal injuries.

SPINAL CORD INJURY (SCI)

Injuries to the spine commonly result from mechanisms of injury involving high kinetic energy. Mechanisms of injury possibly resulting in spinal injury include falls, motor vehicle accidents, and forceful blows to the head or neck. Any neurovascular impairment and spinal deformity indicate the likelihood of spinal injuries.

With SCI, primary and secondary neurological examinations are performed to assess the severity and location of spinal cord damage. This examination provides information to the practitioner on the level of the SCI, the extent of injury, and the degree of impairment. For the initial assessment where SCI is suspected, a neurological examination should include the following tests:

- Cranial nerve function
- Motor function, or movement, of the major muscle groups
- Reflexes including abdominal, anal, and bulbospongiosus
- Sensation to pinprick, fine touch, and joint position

Each myotome (muscle) and dermatome (region of skin; Figure 17.4) of the body is supplied by an area of the spinal cord and its corresponding spinal nerve. There are 8 cervical nerves, 12 thoracic nerves, 5 lumbar nerves, and 5 sacral nerves. Each of these nerves relays sensation from a particular muscle or region of skin to the brain. By examining the dermatomes and myotomes in this manner, a motor score for level and completeness of a spinal cord injury can be determined.

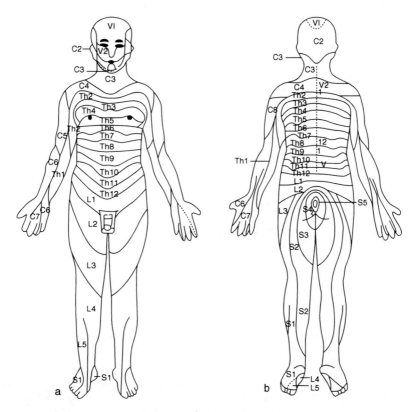

Figure 17.4 ■ Dermatomes.

According to the American Spinal Injury Association (ASIA) standard for neurological classification, the last dermatome or area of skin with intact sensation and normal spinal cord function is considered the level of injury. This may not correspond with the vertebral level of injury, so both neurological and vertebral diagnoses are documented.

Diagnosis

Table 17.1 ■ *Signs and Symptoms of Possible SCI*

• Pain in neck or spine (patient complaint)	• Proprioception deficit
• Painful movement	• Parasympathetic dysfunction in lower sacral nerves: loss of bowel/bladder tone, flaccidity of intra-abdominal muscles, loss of peristalsis
• Spine tenderness/pain/deformity to palpation	
• Paralysis/paresis; abnormal motor exam	• Diaphragmatic breathing
• Paresthesias (upper and/or lower extremities): tingling, numbness, burning	• Neurogenic shock: decreased BP, bradycardia, decreased RR, warm, dry skin with systemic hypothermia
• Abnormal perception/response to pain stimulus (sharp/dull; pinprick)	• Absence of sweating below level of injury
• Ptosis (Horner's syndrome)	
• Position abnormality: head tilt, arms in hold-up or prayer position	

SPINAL CORD SYNDROMES

Incomplete Injuries

Anterior cord syndrome results from injury to the motor and sensory pathways in the anterior parts of the spinal cord.

Mechanism of injury: Occurs with flexion injuries or fractures.

Pathophysiology: Interruption of the anterior spinal artery by occlusion or spasm of the posterior ligaments with subsequent loss of perfusion to the anterior section of the cord. Prognosis for recovery is poor.

Physical findings:
■ Paralysis
■ Loss of pain, temperature, and touch below the lesion
■ Preserves light or crude touch, two-point discrimination, position sense, vibration, and deep pressure

Central Cord Syndrome: Associated with damage to the large nerve fibers that carry information directly from the cerebral cortex to the spinal cord.

Mechanism of injury:

- Hyperextension injury causing damage, hemorrhage, or edema to central cervical segments. Usually no fracture or bony disruption, tears occur to the anterior longitudinal ligament.

- Central cord lesions usually occur following a "smash" or "pinch" type injury of short duration and with a less violent force. The "pinch" results from bony spurs, ligamentous flavum, and intervertebral discs.

- More prevalent in the older population with preexisting conditions such as spondylosis and stenosis due to arthritic changes.

Pathophysiology: Motor fibers in the cord that are most needed (cervical) are central in the cord. Those least critical are distributed toward the surface. In central cord syndrome, the more centrally located (cervical, thoracic) motor and sensory tracts are affected. Lateral fibers to the lower extremities remain intact. Prognosis is usually good; the patient may have some remaining residual loss in the hands.

Physical findings: Patients present with a greater loss of function in the upper extremities than in the lower. There is a variable sensory loss of pain and temperature, and the patient may have bowel and bladder dysfunction.

Brown-Sequard Syndrome: Rare; generally good prognosis

Mechanism of injury: Most common with penetrating trauma and often due to a cervical lesion.

Pathophysiology: Hemi-transection of the cord with complete damage to all spinal tracts on the involved side.

Clinical presentation:

- Injury to corticospinal motor tracts causes an ipsilateral (same-side) motor loss below the lesion.

- Damage to posterior columns that do not cross causes loss of touch, position, pressure, and vibration on the same side below the lesion.

- Injury to ascending spinothalamic (sensory) fibers that cross immediately after entering the cord causes contralateral (opposite side) sensory loss of pain and temperature below the level of the lesion.

Horner's Syndrome: Involves damage to the cervical portion of sympathetic chain. Characterized by ptosis, pupillary constriction (miosis), and anhidrosis (inability to sweat) on the same side as the injury.

Conus medullaris Syndrome: Injury of the sacral cord (conus) and lumbar nerve roots within the neuronal canal, which usually results in areflexic bladder, bowel, and lower limbs.

Cauda equina Syndrome: Injury to the lumbosacral nerve roots within the neural canal resulting in areflexic bladder, bowel, and lower limbs.

PELVIC INJURIES

Fractures of the pelvic ring comprise 2% to 8% of all skeletal injuries and are often associated with high-energy trauma, most commonly motor vehicle accidents and falls from a height. The incidence of pelvic fracture appears to be increasing, secondary to the number of high-speed motor vehicle accidents and the number of patients surviving these accidents due to airbags and safer car designs. Among multiple trauma patients with blunt trauma, almost 20% have pelvic injuries. Mortality rates for patients sustaining pelvic fractures range from 10% to 50% depending, for the most part, on the severity of pelvic fracture bleeding and the presence of associated injuries to the brain, thorax, and abdomen. Death usually occurs from exsanguination or a result of other associated lethal injuries. Management of patients with pelvic fractures and hemodynamic instability remains complex and difficult. The outcomes of patients who present with traumatic pelvic fractures are related to the nature of the fracture, stability of the patient, and institutional resources.

Etiology

The pelvis is made from three bones that are joined together; it supports the upper body and secures the legs to the torso. The pelvis holds organs, nerves, and blood vessels. When the bones of the pelvis are broken, blood vessels, nerves, and organs can be torn, which can result in a large amount of bleeding.

Many organs and blood vessels pass through or near the bones of the pelvis, including the bladder, urethra, end of the large intestine, and internal reproductive organs. Large blood vessels located within the pelvic ring can be the source of severe bleeding and blood from uncontrolled hemorrhage can accumulate in the free space around the pelvis. The bilateral iliac arteries descending from the aorta are located in the pelvis. Blood returns from the lower extremities via the bilateral iliac veins. Major blood vessels also supply the tissue, bones, and organs within the pelvic ring. Blood loss can also originate from bony fracture surfaces and surrounding soft tissue injuries. Uncontrolled bleeding is the leading cause of death for patients with a complex pelvic fracture.

Fracture Types and Classifications

When there is a pelvic injury, there are two common classification systems that are used: the Tile classification and the Young and Burgess classification, both of which are based on the direction of the injury, pelvic stability, and forces involved. Classification helps in identifying associated injuries, the degree of pelvic injury, and is useful in preparing for orthopedic repair. The classification is not essential for early management of patients with pelvic fractures.

Etiology

Signs and symptoms of a pelvic fracture depend on the part of the pelvis that is fractured. General signs and symptoms of pelvic injury:

- Labial, scrotal, and/or perineal swelling/ecchymosis
- Scrotal/labial hematoma
- Neurovascular deficits (numbness or tingling in the genital area or in the upper thighs)
- Discomfort or pain
- Pelvic instability
- Crepitus
- Bloody meatus
- Deformities lower extremities
- Open wounds: rectal
- Sacral nerve root injuries

A broken pelvis is painful, often swollen and bruised. The individual may try to keep the hip or knee bent in a specific position to avoid aggravating the pain. If the fracture is due to trauma, there may also be other injuries to the head, chest, or legs.

- There is usually considerable bleeding, which can lead to shock.
- All pelvic fractures require x-rays, usually from different angles, to show the degree of displacement to the bones. A computed tomography (CT) scan may be ordered to define the extent of other injuries. The physician will also examine the blood vessels and nerves for injury.

Treatment

Stable pelvic fractures are treated with bed rest until the patient's overall condition allows ambulation. Oral analgesics may be prescribed for pain. The patient will have to use crutches or a walker to avoid weight bearing on the hip until the bones heal.

Because mobility may be limited for several months, anticoagulants can be prescribed to reduce the risk of blood clots forming in the legs. Pelvic fractures that result from high-energy traumas are often life-threatening injuries because of the extensive bleeding. In these cases, an external fixator is often used to stabilize the pelvis. This device has long screws that are inserted into the bones on each side and connected to a frame outside the body. An external fixation device remains in place for about 6 to 8 weeks. Pins and insertion sites require frequent cleaning to prevent infection. Unstable fractures may require surgical insertion of plates or screws.

Open fractures are the most devastating and the greatest challenge. The patient is sent immediately to the operating room for exploration, control of bleeding, and repair of soft-tissue injuries. A diverting colostomy may be done at this time to prevent stool contamination of the pelvis and subsequent sepsis. After open fracture repair, daily wound debridement and irrigation done in the operating room is recommended for a few days. Frequent dressing changes in the intensive care unit are important to reduce the risk of sepsis.

Pain management is a high priority during this time, as orthopedic injury is one of the most severe types of pain. Patient controlled analgesia can be used to control pain if the patient is alert and aware enough to push the button. Intermittent IV medication can be used for those patients who cannot push a PCA button. If the patient is in a critical care area, a continuous infusion can be used for the patient with severe level of pain. For these patients in particular a regular bowel regimen is needed to ensure regular bowel movements and avoid constipation.

Complications

When the pelvis is broken there can be many problems including bleeding, bladder rupture, colon injury, infection, lung problems, and liver problems. Other fracture complications include: infection, arthritis, frozen joints, poor healing of the fracture, nonunion, and one leg can be shorter than the other.

Case Study

A 43-year-old female was an unrestrained driver involved in a motor vehicle accident resulting in rollover and ejection from the vehicle. Upon arrival to the ED, the patient was hypotensive, tachycardic, and had left neck subcutaneous emphysema. The patient reported pain 9/10. A chest x-ray revealed multiple bilateral rib fractures, a widened mediastinum, and a left pneumothorax. A left chest tube was placed and had 150 mL of blood return.

Questions to Consider

1. What is the recommended pain modality in patients with multiple rib fractures?
2. What complications is this patient at risk for?
3. Are NSAIDs recommended in chest trauma?

REFERENCES

Alderson, P., & Roberts, I. (2005). Corticosteroids for acute traumatic brain injury. *Cochrane Database of Systematic Reviews*, (1), Art. No. CD000196. doi:10.1002/14651858. CD000196.pub2

Baumann, M. H. (2003). What size chest tube? What drainage system is ideal? And other chest tube management questions. *Current Opinions in Pulmonary Medicine, 9*(4), 276–281.

Baumann, M.H., Strange, C., Heffner, J.E., et al. (February 2001). Management of spontaneous pneumothorax: An American College of Chest Physicians Delphi consensus statement. *Chest, 119*(2), 590–602.

Brain Trauma Foundation, American Association of Neurological Surgeons, Congress of Neurological Surgeons. (2007). Guidelines for the management of severe traumatic brain injury. Hyperosmolar therapy. *Journal of Neurotrauma, 24*(Suppl. 1), S14–S20.

Brims, F. J., Davies, H. E., & Lee, Y. C. (2010). Respiratory chest pain: Diagnosis and treatment. *Medical Clinics of North America, 94*(2), 217–232.

Burgess, A. R., Eastridge, B. J., Young, J. W., Ellison, T. S., Ellison, P. S., Jr., Poka, A., . . . Brumback, R. J. (1990). Pelvic ring disruptions: effective classification system and treatment protocols. *The Journal of Trauma, 30*, 848–856.

Bullock, M. R., Chesnut, R., Ghajar, J., Gordon, D., Hartl, R., Newell, D. W., . . . Surgical Management of Traumatic Brain Injury Author Group. (2006). Surgical management of acute epidural hematomas. *Neurosurgery, 58*, S7.

Centers for Disease Control and Prevention, National Center for Injury Prevention and Control. (2007). *Web-based Injury Statistics Query and Reporting System (WISQARS)*. Retrieved from http://www.cdc.gov/injury/wisqars

Davis, A. E. (2000). Mechanisms of traumatic brain injury: Biomechanical, structural and cellular considerations. *Critical Care Nursing Quarterly, 23,* 1–13.

Finkelstein, E. A., Corso, P. S., Miller, T. R., & Associates. (2006). *Incidence and economic burden of injuries in the United States.* New York, NY: Oxford University Press.

Fysh, E. T., Smith, N. A., & Lee, Y. C. (2010). Optimal chest drain size: The rise of the small-bore pleural catheter. *Seminars in Respiratory and Critical Care Medicine, 31*(6), 760–768.

Goligher, E. C., Leis, J. A., Fowler, R. A., Pinto, R., Adhikari, N. K., & Ferguson, N. D. (2011). Utility and safety of draining pleural effusions in mechanically ventilated patients: A systematic review and meta-analysis. *Critical Care, 15,* R46. Retrieved from http://ccforum.com/content/15/1/R46

Jameel, A. (2010). Torso trauma. In J. B. Hall, G. A. Schmidt, & L. D. H. Wood (Eds.), *Principles of critical care* (3rd ed.). Retrieved from http://www.accesssurgery.com/content.aspx?aID=2298290

Kelly, D. F., Goodale, D. B., Williams, J., Herr, D. L., Chappell, E. T., Rosner, M. J., et al. (1999). Propofol in the treatment of moderate and severe head injury: A randomized, prospective double-blinded pilot trial. *Journal of Neurosurgery, 90,* 1042–1052.

Light, R. W. (2011). Pleural controversy: Optimal chest tube size for drainage. *Respirology, 16*(2), 244–248. doi: 10.1111/j.1440-1843.2010.01913.x

Meyer, M. J., Megyes, J., Meythaler, J., Murie-Fernandez, M., Aubut, J. A., Foley, N., . . . Teasell R. (2010). Acute management of acquired brain injury part II: An evidence-based review of pharmacological interventions. *Brain Injury, 24*(5), 706–721.

Puntillo, K., & Ley, S. J. (2004). Appropriately timed analgesics control pain due to chest tube removal. *American Journal of Critical Care, 13*(4), 292-301; discussion 302; quiz 303–304.

Rupp, T., & Delaney, K. A. (2004). Inadequate analgesia in emergency medicine. *Annals of Emergency Medicine, 43*(4), 494–503.

Savetamal, A., & Livingston, D. H. (2008). Thoracic wall injuries: Ribs, sternal scapular fractures, hemothoraces, and pneumothoraces. In J. A. Asensio & D. D. Trunkey (Eds.), *Current therapy of trauma and surgical critical care* (pp. 252–261). Philadelphia, PA: Mosby.

Stengel, D., Bauwens, K., Sehouli, J., Rademacher, G., Mutze, S., Ekkernkamp, A., & Porzsolt, F. (2005). Emergency ultrasound-based algorithms for diagnosing blunt abdominal trauma. *Cochrane Database Systematic Reviews,* (2), CD004446.

Tintinalli, J. E., Kelen, G. D., & Stapczynski, J. S. (2000). *Emergency medicine a comprehensive study guide* (5th ed.). New York, NY: McGraw Hill.

Wanek, S., & Mayberry, J. C. (2004). Blunt thoracic trauma: Flail chest, pulmonary contusion, and blast injury. *Critical Care Clinics, 20*(1), 71–81.

Xu, J. Q., Kochanek, K. D., Murphy, S. L., & Tejada-Vera, B. (2010). Deaths: Final data for 2007. *National Vital Statistics Reports, 58*(19).

18

Managing Pain in Special Patient Populations

ELDERLY

Pain is common in the older adult but often undertreated because of the concerns for over sedation, decreased drug clearance, and the risk of drug-drug interactions (Jermyn, Janora, & Surve, 2010). These should not be reasons to avoid pain treatment in the older person. It is often the reason that older adults feel that pain is a normal part of the aging process. Older people are more likely to suffer chronic pain from arthritis, orthopedic disorders, back problems, neuralgias, as well as from chronic conditions that typically cause pain.

Adults greater than age 65 years in 2009 were 39.6 million. They represent 12.9% of the U.S. population, about one in every eight Americans. By 2030, there will be about 72.1 million older persons, more than twice the number from 2000 (Administration on Aging, 2010).

Between 25% and 40% of older cancer patients studied had pain on a daily basis. Among these patients, 21% who were between 65 and 74 years of age received no pain medication; of patients who were 75 to 84 years old, 26% received no pain medication; and for those above the age of 84, 30% were left with untreated pain (Kaye, Baluch, & Scott, 2010).

Pain Perception

As we age there are age-related changes that occur in pain perception and the neurophysiology of nociception (Gibson & Farrell, 2005). Gibson and Pickering suggested that pain symptoms and pain presentation may change in the older patient, becoming a less frequent or less severe symptom of a variety of medical conditions most commonly abdominal and chest pain (Gibson & Farrell, 2005, 2003; Gibson, 2006; Pickering & Melding, 2005). They also agreed with findings that the elderly also have an increased pain threshold. The older patient compared with a younger patient may report less pain or atypical pain, report it later, or report no pain at all. Painless disease presentation increases the risk of complications. For example, in older patients, right upper quadrant or epigastric pain associated with cholecystitis may be absent in 85%; 30% of those with peptic ulcer disease and up to 90% with pancreatitis may have no abdominal pain; in those with advanced peritonitis, pain may be a symptom in only 55%; and reports of atypical pain or absence of pain occur in up to 33% of older patients with an acute myocardial infarction and 50% with unstable angina (Pickering & Melding, 2005).

Pain Assessment

The American Geriatrics Society (AGS) (2002, 2009) recognizes and supports that effective pain management occurs when the underlying cause is identified and treated appropriately. A comprehensive examination is necessary to identify whether the pain is from an acute process or an exacerbation of a persistent pain.

Clinical Pearl	Pain is a common symptom among older adults; it often is underdiagnosed and undertreated.

Assessing pain in the older patient takes time and patience. The older patient may be reluctant to report pain for many reasons. These may include fear of becoming a bother, fear of a more serious illness, fear of addiction, or even fear of the costs associated with health care. The older patient may have cognitive or functional impairments that may further delay the pain assessment process.

When assessing the older patient for pain, if possible have the patient sitting upright and with appropriate glasses, hearing aids, or other assistive devices. Ensure appropriate lighting in order for the patient to be able to see. Face the patient when speaking to him or her, get the patient's attention before talking, and speak clearly and loud enough for the patient to understand, allowing enough time for the patient to respond to questions. If the patient cannot communicate verbally because of intubation or a functional impairment, provide alternate means of communication such as pen and paper, nonverbal cues, or a communication board.

When asking patients if they are "experiencing pain" some older patients may say they are not experiencing pain. Using descriptors such as "burning," "discomfort," "aching," or "soreness" may illicit a response as the word pain often has a negative connotation.

The American Society for Pain Management's Nursing Task Force on Pain Assessment in the Nonverbal Patient recommends a comprehensive, hierarchical approach that includes the following five steps: (1) obtain the patient's report of pain, (2) look for potential causes of pain, (3) observe the patient's behavior, (4) obtain surrogate reports of pain or ask others about changes in the patient's behaviors and activities, and (5) attempt an analgesic trial to try to reduce or eliminate pain indicators (Herr et al., 2006, 2011).

Use a standardized tool to assess self-reported pain. A numeric rating scale (NRS) and verbal descriptor scale (VDS) are strong and preferred (Gagliese et al., 2005; Herr et al., 2004, 2007; Jones et al., 2005; Peters et al., 2007; Scherder & van Manen, 2005). The Pain Thermometer and Faces Pain Scale (Wong Baker Faces Scale, Revised-Faces Pain Scale [R-FPS]; Herr et al., 2007; Li et al., 2007; Taylor et al., 2003; Ware et al., 2006) are also strong assessment tools.

Assess pain regularly and frequently—at least every 4 hours. Assess present pain, including intensity, character, frequency, pattern, location, duration, and aggravating and alleviating factors. Monitor pain intensity after giving medications to evaluate effectiveness.

In the patient that is unable to communicate pain, observe for nonverbal and behavioral signs of pain, such as facial grimacing, withdrawal, guarding, rubbing, limping, shifting of position, aggression, agitation, depression, vocalizations, and crying (AGS, 2002, 2010; Herr et al., 2006; Pasero & McCaffery, 2011, 1999). Watch for changes in behavior from the patient's usual patterns (Taylor, Harris, Epps, & Herr, 2005). Gather information from family members about the patient's pain experiences. Ask about the patient's verbal and nonverbal/behavioral expressions of pain, particularly older adults with dementia. A behavioral pain tool is often used in the nonverbal critically ill or the cognitively impaired patient, but in conjunction with a total pain assessment (see Chapter 5).

DELIRIUM

Delirium is an acute confusion disorder characterized by altered mental status, inattention, disorganized thinking, and altered level of consciousness (Schreier, 2010). Delirium is a common complication in elderly patients during hospitalization. In the intensive care unit (ICU), delirium can occur in up to 80% of patients and is an independent risk factor for increased length of stay and 6-month mortality (Truman-Pun, 2007). Causes are diverse, ranging from infection to medications (Table 18.1).

Disorientation, fluctuation, waxing and waning of the above symptoms, and acute or abrupt onset of such disturbances are other critical features of delirium. Delirium is reversible even in the critically ill. Usually, disorientation to time and place and memory loss occur. Perceptual disturbances include auditory, visual, and hallucinations.

Clinical Pearl	Approximately 30–40% cases of delirium are preventable.

It is sometimes difficult to differentiate delirium from dementia because their clinical features such as disorientation and impaired memory, thinking, and judgment are similar. A difference is the onset of symptoms is more chronically progressive and irreversible in dementia than in delirium.

Studies that looked at the relationship of pain and delirium have been generally conducted in surgical hip fracture patients. Morrison et al. (2003) conducted a large prospective cohort study of 541 hip fracture patients in which 16% became delirious. Severe pain was associated with a nine-fold risk of developing delirium.

There are a few different delirium assessment tools: the Intensive Care Delirium Screening Checklist, the Confusion Assessment Method (CAM), and the Confusion Assessment Method for the ICU (CAMICU). The diagnosis of delirium by CAM requires the presence of items 1 and 2 and either 3 or 4 from the following list (Adamis, Treloar, MacDonald, & Martin, 2005):

1. Acute onset and fluctuating course: Evidence of changes in mental status from the patient's baseline that changes in severity during the day.
2. Inattention: Patient has difficulty focusing attention.
3. Disorganized thinking: Patient's thinking is disorganized or incoherent.
4. Altered consciousness: A rating of a patient's level of consciousness as other than alert.

Table 18.1 ▪ *Cause of Delirium*

Elderly	Acidosis	Medication
ETOH abuse	Anemia	Sleep disturbances
Hypertension	Sepsis	Immobilization
Depression	Metabolic	Cognitive impairment
Smoking	Visual/hearing impairment	

The Epworth Sleepiness Scale: Can it be used for sleep apnoea screening among snorers? *Clin Otolaryngol. 24*: 1999; 239–241.

The Society of Critical Care Medicine (SCCM) and the American Psychiatric Association (APA) recommend haldol as the first-line drug of choice in the treatment of delirium. The optimal dosing regimen is not well defined, but starting with 2.5 mg IV and doubling it as required every 20–30 minutes has been recommended. Once the patient is calmer, haldol is prescribed every 4–6 hours, tapering off over a few days. It should be avoided in patients with a prolonged QT interval due to the risk of torsade de pointes. Atypical antipsychotics (i.e., olanzapine, ziprasidone, and haldol) may be helpful in treating delirium in patients unable to tolerate haldol. More research is needed to evaluate these drugs and their effects on patients with delirium.

Hearing loss is a frequently reported risk factor for delirium. Unrelieved pain and hearing loss may have a collaborative effect on cognitive function. Patients with hearing loss are likely to receive lower doses of pain medication and more likely to experience delirium (Robinson, Rich, Weitzel, Vollmer, & Eden, 2008). This finding suggests that lack of effective communication may result in poorer assessment and management of pain in the hearing-impaired older adult.

Researchers have considered the relationship among postoperative pain, pain management, and delirium. Hospitalized adults after hip fracture who received less effective pain management were more likely to experience delirium (Milsen, Lemiengre, Braes, & Foreman, 2005; Morrison et al., 2003). Increased postoperative pain increases the risk of delirium (Vaurio, Sands, Wang, Mullen, & Leung, 2006). Postoperative patients who received greater amounts of pain medication had a delayed onset of delirium (Robinson et al., 2008). When long-term care patients were admitted to an acute care hospital, those who received opioids were more likely to experience mild delirium than moderate to severe delirium (Voyer, McCusker, Cole, St-Jacques, & Khomenko, 2007). These studies suggest that effective pain management reduces the risk for delirium.

Prevention strategies include early involvement of family members in care, optimizing communication through the use of various aids (eyeglasses, hearing aids, etc.), involvement in therapeutic activities, early mobilization, nonpharmacological approaches to sleep and anxiety, adequate nutrition and hydration, and careful and effective prescribing of medication for pain relief. Health care professionals should implement individualized pain management strategies for patients at risk for or experiencing delirium.

Pharmacological Management

Managing the pharmacological interventions in the elderly is complex. There are many physiologic changes that occur and influence pain management. Changes in drug absorption, distribution, metabolism, and elimination may affect the plasma levels and effect of analgesic medications. Drug absorption may be altered as a result of increased gastric pH and decreased gastric motility. Distribution of drugs may change due to a decrease in lean body mass or to a decrease in plasma proteins and albumin from chronic illness and poor nutrition. Hepatic and renal blood flow and glomerular filtration rate are decreased. The glomerular filtration rate also decreases approximately 10% per decade of life, affecting drugs that are cleared via the kidneys. Hepatic metabolism may be decreased and elimination of drugs may change as hepatic clearance decreases. Total body fat increases, while the body's water content and muscle mass decrease. As a result, water-soluble drugs may have a higher initial concentration, while fat-soluble drugs may exhibit a longer half-life due to slow release from fatty tissue.

When beginning pain medications, always start at the lowest dose possible and increase slowly due to the potential toxicity of the therapies. Drug dosages should not be prescribed above the recommended daily dosage including any over-the-counter medications. The 2009 AGS guidelines for pain management are as follows.

Nonopioids

Acetaminophen is and should be considered first in the treatment of persistent pain, unless the patient has a history of liver failure. Use caution in patients with hepatic insufficiency or alcohol dependence. The recommended maximum daily dose is 4,000 mg or 4 g.

Opioids

Opioids should be considered for all patients with moderate to severe pain. When combining opioids with NSAIDs or acetaminophen, caution should be used in not exceeding the maximum dose of NSAID or acetaminophen. Carefully adjust current analgesic regimen so that it is individualized for the patient as "one size does *not* fit all." Utilize multimodal approaches to give lowest effective analgesic doses:

- Acetaminophen, NSAID, anticonvulsant *plus* opioid (Pasero, Rakel, & McCaffery, 2005; Buvanendran & Kroin, 2007)
- Epidural local anesthetic *plus* opioid (Pasero & McCaffery, 2007)
- Perineural local anesthetic *plus* PRN opioid (Pasero & McCaffery, 2007)

Patients should be closely monitored for adverse effects and safe medication use. Reduce the adult starting opioid dose by 50% in the opioid naïve patient (Pasero, Rakel, & McCaffery, 2005). Some patients may require and tolerate regular starting doses (Aubrun et al., 2004). Slow, steady titration of medications will help minimize and prevent adverse effects.

For pain that is continuous, round the clock ordering of analgesics will keep the patient's pain more evenly controlled. Opioid medications have a higher profile for side effects such as hallucinations, delirium, or constipation (D'Arcy, 2009). The older patient who is opioid naïve should be observed for sedation, nausea, mental fogginess, and dizziness, which can increase the risk of falls.

Any older patient who receives opioids should be given a laxative since opioids are constipating. If the patient is nauseated, the health care professional should be aware that the sedating effects of opioids are increased when an antiemetic with sedating effect is added (D'Arcy, 200). Often opioids are to blame for the over-sedation patients may experience, but the link may be associated with concomitant use of opioid, anti-emetic, sleep medication, or antihistamines, which are often used for pruritus.

Adjuvant Drugs

Adjuvant drugs should be considered for patients with pain such as fibromyalgia, back pain, headaches, bone pain, or neuropathic pain. These medications may be used alone or combined with other pain medications. See Chapter 5 for more information on these co-analgesic adjuvant medications.

HIV

Pain associated with disease from HIV is common and multifaceted, with different causes at the different stages of the disease (Cox & Rice, 2008). A frequent cause of pain from the disease is neuropathic pain associated with symmetrical sensory polyneuropathy. These HIV-associated sensory neuropathies (HIVSNs) are attributed to HIV itself and to some of the HIV treatments (Verma, 2001).

Current estimates of global HIV prevalence stand at 33 million, with 2.7 million new infections each year and more patients gaining access to combination antiretroviral therapy (cART; Phillips & Cherry, 2010). With high rates of HIV-associated sensory neuropathies (HIVSNs) reported globally, and up to 90% of affected patients experiencing potentially debilitating neuropathic pain, HIVSN represents a large and potentially worsening source of world morbidity.

Several studies suggest that approximately 25%–30% of ambulatory HIV-infected patients with early HIV disease experience clinically significant pain. A study of pain in hospitalized patients with HIV/AIDS revealed that over 50% of patients required treatment for pain, with pain being the presenting complaint in 30%, second to fever.

> *Clinical*   Pain in HIV/AIDS is often undertreated, especially in women
> *Pearl*   and those with comorbid substance abuse.

Pain is very underreported in this patient population. Factors that influence undertreatment of pain in HIV illness include gender, education, substance abuse history, and a variety of patient-related barriers such as:

- Reluctance to report pain
- Misconceptions regarding addiction
- Wish to limit overall intake of pills
- Wish to use holistic approach to pain management
- Financial concerns

Etiology of Pain in HIV/AIDS

There are various types of pain syndromes that may occur related or unrelated to HIV/AIDS:

- Pain related to HIV infection
- Pain related to immunosuppression or secondary infections/illnesses
- Pain related to HIV/AIDS related therapies such as toxic neuropathies
- Preexisting pain conditions unrelated to HIV

Pain syndromes encountered in HIV illness are varied. The most common pain syndromes reported are painful sensory peripheral neuropathy, Kaposi's sarcoma, headache, oral and pharyngeal pain, abdominal pain, chest pain, arthralgias, and myalgias. Those originating in the nervous system include: headache, painful peripheral neuropathies, radiculopathies, and myelopathies. The HIV virus infects the nerve cells, invading the central and peripheral nervous systems early in the course of the disease. More than 50% of patients with late-stage HIV/AIDS have a neurological complication either directly due to HIV itself or secondary to opportunistic infection, cancer, or medication side effects.

Pain Assessment

The initial step in pain management is a comprehensive pain assessment. The health professional working in the HIV/AIDS setting must have a working knowledge of the etiology and treatment of pain in HIV/AIDS, including an understanding of the different types of HIV/AIDS pain syndromes. A close collaboration of the entire health care team is optimal when attempting to adequately manage pain in the HIV/AIDS patient.

A careful history and physical examination may disclose an identifiable condition such as herpes zoster, bacterial infection, or neuropathy that can be treated in a traditional manner. A pain history may provide valuable clues to the nature of the underlying process and potentially disclose other treatable disorders. Intensity, location, qualities, and radiation of pain should be obtained. Pain descriptors (e.g., burning, shooting, dull, or sharp) will help determine the mechanism of pain (somatic, nociceptive, visceral nociceptive, or neuropathic) and may suggest the appropriate medication treatment. Furthermore, detailed medical, neurological, and psychosocial assessments (including a history of substance use or abuse) must be conducted.

An important element in assessment of pain is the concept that assessment is continuous and ongoing over the course of pain treatment. Continuous assessment includes:

- Pain intensity
- Pain relief
- Pain related function
- Monitoring of effects of intervention

The World Health Organization (WHO, 2002) has devised guidelines for analgesic management of pain that the AHCPR has endorsed for the management of pain related to cancer or HIV/AIDS. This approach advocates selection of analgesics based on severity of pain.

While parenteral administration (IV, IM, SC) will yield a faster onset of pain relief, the duration of analgesia is shorter unless a continuous infusion of opioid is instituted. The use of continuous SC or IV infusions of opioids, with or without patient-controlled analgesia (PCA) devices, has become commonplace in caring for HIV/AIDS patients with escalating pain and in hospice and home settings during late stages of disease.

Pharmacologic Interventions

Pain management in the HIV patient is the same as the oncology patient and the use of the WHO analgesic ladder is recommended (WHO, 2002). Vital to treatment is a comprehensive pain assessment, as the patient will report different types of pain in different locations. This will guide the intervention(s) needed. Symptom management generally requires a multimodal approach to manage pain and the psychological distress.

Nonpharmacologic Interventions

Nonpharmacologic interventions are useful in the management of pain in HIV/AIDS and include a variety of physical and psychological therapies. Physical interventions for pain range from bed rest and exercise programs, to the use of cooling or heat therapies. Other physical or rehabilitative modalities include transcutaneous electrical nerve stimulation (TENS), whirlpool baths, massage, and the application of ultrasound. Acupuncture is now being used frequently in treating HIV/AIDS-related pain. Anesthetic and even neurosurgical procedures (e.g., epidural delivery of analgesics, nerve blocks) are additional options.

Several behavioral interventions that are potentially effective in managing HIV/AIDS-related pain include patient education, hypnosis, relaxation and distraction techniques (e.g., biofeedback and imagery), and cognitive-behavioral techniques.

OBESE PATIENTS

The obesity epidemic consumes a significant portion of health care dollars and the costs continue to skyrocket as the obesity rate continues to climb. In 2008 dollars, medical care costs totaled about $147 billion (Finkelstein, Trogdon, Cohen, & Dietz, 2009). Obesity increases the risk of diabetes, heart disease, and many types of cancer. Prevalence estimates among critically ill patients varies depending on the cohort examined but may be as high as one in four patients. Obesity is defined as a BMI of 30 or higher, morbid or severe obesity is defined as a BMI of 40 or higher, and super-obesity is defined as a BMI in excess of 50.

Prevalence of obesity ranges anywhere from 9% to 26% (Bercault et al., 2004; Ray, Matchett, Baker, Wasser, & Young, 2005) and morbid obesity from 2% to 7% (Ray et al., 2005; Tremblay & Bandi, 2003). In a recent study, Neville et al. reported that 26% of 242 blunt trauma patients requiring ICU care were obese. Bariatric patients requiring surgery may require prolonged ICU care (Neville, Brown, Weng, Demetriades, & Velmahos, 2004).

> **Clinical Pearl** The first postoperative 24 hours seems to be a high-risk period during which more frequent monitoring is indicated. Any dose escalation will prolong the risk.

Pharmacology Challenges

Obstructive Sleep Apnea (OSA)

A major concern that exists when considering opioid medications with obese patients is the risk of adverse events including respiratory arrest, exacerbated or caused by obstructive sleep apnea (OSA). When considering opioid pain medication with obese patients, consider the following:

- Focused history, calculation of BMI and neck circumference in the preoperative evaluation to identify patients at substantial risk or with a history of OSA.
- Sleep apnea study prior to scheduled surgery in patients at risk.
- Use of nonopioid medications (such as NSAIDs) instead of or in combination with careful opioid dosing, and use regional analgesic techniques rather than systemic opioids whenever possible.
- Constant positive airway pressure machines (CPAPs) to alleviate postoperative airway obstruction and decrease major postoperative complications in patients at high risk or those with OSA. Encourage patients with CPAP devices at home to use them while in the hospital, especially if they are receiving opioids.
- Carefully titrate pain medication. Avoid assuming that BMI directly correlates to medication dose.
- Be aware that oral opiates may cause respiratory depression in OSA patients.
- Ensure that everyone involved in the patient's treatment plan is aware of the diagnosis or suspected diagnosis of OSA, particularly in obese patients.
- Train health care professionals providing postoperative monitoring to recognize potential signs of sleep apnea.

Critically ill obese patients must be assessed frequently for anxiolytic, analgesic, and antidepressant needs. Many of these drugs are lipophilic, taken up by adipose tissue and slowly released into the blood. The intravenous and enteral routes are preferred in patients with obesity. Adipose tissue has a decreased blood supply, and drugs given by the subcutaneous route have a delayed onset of action and an unpredictable duration of action. Similarly, transdermal patches are a poor choice for delivery of medications in patients who are obese. Onset of action of transdermal-delivered medications is delayed in patients who are obese, and duration of drug action is erratic and unpredictable.

BURNS

The American Burn Association (2007) estimates that one-half million people with burn injuries receive medical treatment each year, including 40,000 who require hospitalization. Pain is a common experience of all patients with burns; despite the cause, size, or depth of the burn, it can be the worst pain experienced. Patients are not doomed. Over time and with new analgesics, sedatives, and topical agents, burn patients pain can be effectively managed.

The pain associated with burn injury and treatment often is managed poorly. Pain resulting from a burn is one of the most difficult forms of acute pain to treat. The burn injury most likely will produce high levels of pain; as well, burn care of the patient can also intensify whatever pain is present. The therapies can produce pain that is comparable or exceeds the pain experienced by the patient at the time of injury. Therapies may invoke such pain that they may interfere with the care of the patient and thus lengthen the hospital stay. Most burn pain results from tissue damage. Clearly the goal is to avoid the undertreatment of burn pain, although historically patients are undertreated.

The immediate pain that follows a burn injury is due to the stimulation of skin nociceptors. Nerve endings that are completely destroyed will not transmit pain, but those that remain intact will trigger pain throughout the time and course of treatment, as will those still connected to intact afferent fibers.

Researchers have theorized the failure to medicate burn patients adequately is because health care professionals must perform repeated and painful procedures on these patients and have a need for patients to demonstrate pain as a means to create a psychological distance between themselves and the realities of burn care. On the other hand, the fear of creating dependence on opioids may explain the reluctance of some health care professionals to aggressively treat burn pain although there is no evidence to support any higher rates of addiction in burn patients than in other populations requiring opioids for acute pain.

Burn size is measured by percentage of the total body surface area (TBSA) affected by burns, both partial and full thickness. There are several methods of estimating burn size including the rule of nines. The rule of nines divides the body into sections, each corresponding to 9% of the TBSA of an average adult with the perineum and genitalia accounting for the remaining 1%. Accurate burn size estimation is essential in calculating the patient's minimum fluid resuscitation needs within the first 24 hours after using the Parkland formula (4 millimeters X body weight in kilograms X percentage of TBSA burned = the amount of fluid in millimeters).

Superficial (First-Degree) Burns: Reddened, dry unblistered skin with mild edema. The injury is painful and hypersensitive to touch; damage results from momentary contact with a heat source and involves the epidermis and possibly the surface of the dermis. The burned skin blanches with light pressure. Healing usually occurs naturally within a week.

Clinical Pearl The most painful burns are superficial partial-thickness burns because the sensory nerve endings are intact and working but are exposed because of the loss of epidermis.

Partial-Thickness (Second-Degree) Burns: This burn is hypersensitive to touch, air, and temperature; damage to both epidermis and upper dermis results from limited contact with heat source. The burned skin blanches with pressure, but blanching can be slowed in a deep partial-thickness burn. Healing usually occurs naturally in two to three weeks.

Full-Thickness (Third-Degree) Burns: This burn may appear waxy white, tan, or charred, and possibly blistered; injury is lacking feeling, although the area may be surrounded by painful partial thickness burns. Edema and hair loss are always present to some degree. There is complete destruction of both epidermis and dermis resulting from prolonged contact with the heat source. Natural healing of small burns is possible but with risk of infection and scarring. Surgery is usually required.

Deep Full-Thickness (Fourth-Degree) Burns: Charred and hard to the touch, this burn results from the complete destruction of both the epidermis and the dermis, with damage potentially extending into underlying subcutaneous tissue, muscle, and bone. The burned area does not blanch. Surgery is required.

It is important to know that even after the skin is no longer in contact with the heat source that damage to the skin can continue as a result of changes in the structure of the protein molecules. Deep partial thickness burns can develop into full thickness burns within 24 hours of the initial injury.

Pain is not only caused by the direct tissue injury itself but the injury also provokes pain by stimulating both inflammation and hyperalgesia. The inflammatory reaction includes the secretion of histamine, bradykinin, and prostaglandin, irritating substances that stimulate the exposed peripheral nerve endings, producing additional pain (Connor-Ballard, 2009).

Manipulation of the hyperalgesic injury in the course of wound care also exacerbates pain (Stoddard, 2002). At one time it was believed that full thickness burns did not cause pain due to the damage to the nerve endings in the dermis. Burns may have areas of full and partial thickness and there may be areas where the nerves are still functioning, particularly the margins of the wound. An increase in pain in a full-thickness burn around the circumference of a limb may indicate a compartment syndrome–like process, necessitating escharotomy or fasciotomy (Connor-Ballard, 2009). Lastly, full-thickness burns are subjected to repeated painful procedures to prevent infection and promote closure with minimal deformity.

Pain Assessment

Regular, ongoing pain assessment is vital to guide the pain management necessary in order for the patient to not only cope but to heal. Effective detailed pain history and assessment of pain at rest and during movement, breakthrough pain, and procedural pain all warrant individual assessment and documentation throughout the phases of recovery.

- Site or location of pain
- Aggravating and alleviating factors
- Pain descriptors
- Pain rating

It is important to stress the importance of good analgesia to allow patients to participate in their care and potentially have a faster recovery. Assessment scales are useful in assisting the patient in rating their pain, convey a sense of staff empathy, and make the patient's report valid.

- Word descriptors
- Numeric intensity rating scale
- Visual analogue thermometer (Choinere, Auger, & Latarjet, 1994)

Some additional important considerations when assessing for pain:

- Ensure adequate patient education in how to use the pain tool.
- Do not alter the pain score from a self-reporting tool.
- Listen carefully to the patient.
- Assess and reassess frequently, particularly with patients who are in the most acute phase of their injury and treatment.

Pharmacologic Approaches

Burn pain management should be individualized based upon the clinical need for analgesia and limitations imposed by the patient. Health care professionals with a clear understanding of pharmacokinetics and the pathophysiology of the burn patient should be prescribing. During the first 48 hours, decreased organ blood supply will reduce clearance of drugs, but the subsequent hypermetabolic phase (48 hours after injury) is associated with increased clearance (Richardson & Mustard, 2009). Alterations in total body water may affect the volume of distribution. Continued regular and ongoing pain assessment and reassessment is necessary in order to quantify the effect of analgesic agents and thus reduce the impact of these changes.

Opioids

Opioids are the gold standard of pain control in the burn patient. Opioids are very effective and the selection of drugs available provides a range of strengths, routes of administration, and durations of action. Opioids can have clinical significant side effects such as respiratory depression, pruritis, nausea, and vomiting.

IV opioid medications can be given in small incremental doses but the delayed onset of action and long-lasting effects do not allow for adjusting the medications individually. Using a short-term opioid such as fentanyl, alfentanil, or remifentanil is more appropriate; they also have a more rapid onset of action then morphine. These are generally good for procedural pain management due to the short duration of action.

PREGNANCY

Most pregnancies are uneventful so admission to the ICU is rare and thus the existing research is limited. A small percentage of women may experience a life-threatening complication associated with the pregnancy or result from a pre-existing condition. Overall estimates suggest that 1%–3% of pregnant women require critical care services in the United States each year, approximately 40,000–120,000 women (based on 4 million births per year; American College of Gynecologists [ACOG], 2009).

Physiological Changes in Pregnancy

There are a broad range of physiological changes that occur during pregnancy that impact the assessment and management of critical illness. The health care professional must have an understanding of the physiological changes that occur in pregnancy in order to differentiate between what is normal and abnormal in the pregnant patient (Table 18.2). Illnesses that affect the cardiovascular and respiratory systems substantially increase the morbidity and mortality of the mother and/or fetus (Jayasinghe & Blass, 1999).

Maternal Circulation

Treatment of pain during pregnancy and lactation may affect the fetus or nursing child. Analgesics are commonly prescribed during pregnancy. Almost all drugs administered to the mother cross the placenta to the fetus, or are secreted in breast milk.

Maternal circulation and exposure to teratogens influence embryonic and fetal development. Therefore, the health care practitioner must carefully balance all the risks of the treatment on both the pregnant women and her fetus. There are three stages of fetal development:

- Pre-embryonic (first 14 days)
- Embryonic (day 15 through 8 weeks)
- Fetal (8 weeks through 40 weeks/delivery)

Table 18.2 ■ *Maternal Physiological Changes*

Cardiovascular	Respiratory
• Increased heart rate 10–0 beats/min	• Minute volume increased
• SVR, PVR, reduced 20–30%	• Tidal volume increased
• Cardiac output increased elevated 30–50% (25 weeks) (Jayasinghe & Blass, 1999)	• Decreased $PaCO_2$ (Jayasinghe & Blass, 1999)
• Blood volume elevated 40-50% (Price, Germain, Wyncoll, & Nelson-Piercy, 2009)	• Respiratory rate unchanged (although short of breath)
	• Oxygen demand increased
Renal	
• Increase in renal blood flow 30%	
• Increase in glomerular filtration rate 50%	
• Increase creatine clearance	

While most drugs are safe there are particular times of concern, notably the period of organ development (weeks 4 to 10) and just before delivery. When possible the use of nonpharmacological methods should be explored before analgesic medications are initiated.

As stated, certain medications can cross the placenta and have a teratogenic effect on the fetus. Most physicians are extremely cautious with medication use in pregnant patients as it is estimated that at least 10% of birth defects can be attributed to maternal drug exposures. The FDA developed a classification system for medications based on their potential for fetal risk (Table 18.3) to assist health care professionals make an educated choice when determining medications. Medications with recognized harmful effects to a developing fetus are in the categories D and X. Category D medications may provide benefit to the mother in certain medical conditions although the benefit must outweigh the risk to the fetus in order for such drugs to be used. Category X medications are absolutely contraindicated in pregnancy as they are associated with more harm to the fetus than any possible benefit that could be attained.

Pain Medications

Complaints of pain occur in almost all pregnant and lactating women. There is no one superior method to treat pain in the pregnant patient.

Acetaminophen
Acetaminophen is considered as the analgesic of choice during pregnancy.

Table 18.3 ■ *FDA Use-in-Pregnancy Ratings*

FDA Use-in-Pregnancy Ratings	*Medication*
Category-A Controlled studies show no risk: Adequate, well-controlled studies in pregnant women have failed to demonstrate a risk to the fetus in any trimester of pregnancy.	
Category B No evidence of risk in humans: Adequate, well-controlled studies in pregnant women have not shown increased risk of fetal abnormalities despite adverse findings in animals, OR In the absence of adequate human studies, animal studies show no fetal risk. The chance of fetal harm is remote, but remains a possibility.	Acetaminophen NSAIDs (2nd trimester)
Category C Risk cannot be ruled out: Adequate, well-controlled human studies are lacking, and animal studies have shown a risk to the fetus or are lacking as well. There is a chance of fetal harm if the drug is administered during pregnancy; but the potential benefits may outweigh the potential risk.	Fentanyl Morphine Dilaudid Tapentadol Ketoralac Tramadol Gabapentin Pregabalin
Category D Positive evidence of risk: Studies in humans, or investigational or post marketing data, have demonstrated fetal risk. Nevertheless, potential benefits from the use of the drug may outweigh the potential risk. For example, the drug may be acceptable if needed in a life-threatening situation or serious disease for which safer drugs cannot be used or are ineffective.	NSAIDs (3rd trimester)
Category X Contraindicated in pregnancy: Studies in animals or humans, or investigational or post-marketing reports, have demonstrated positive evidence of fetal abnormalities or risk which clearly outweigh any possible benefit to the patient.	

NSAIDs

Use of NSAIDs during pregnancy is associated with increased risk of miscarriage (Li et al., 2003; Nielsen et al., 2004). Considered somewhat safe during early and mid-pregnancy, NSAIDs can produce fetal cardiac and renal complications in late pregnancy, as well as interfere with fetal brain development and production of amniotic fluid; it is recommended to be discontinued in the 32nd gestational week (Ostensen & Skomsvoll, 2004).

Opioids

Most opioids are category C drugs. Short-term use of opioids to treat pain in pregnancy appears safe (Wunsch et al., 2003), but minimizing the use of opioid therapy for chronic pain during pregnancy has been recommended (Chou et al., 2009). Concerns about the effects of opioids on neonates are for those who abuse or those who are in maintenance programs for drug dependence. The developmental effects on the fetus from maternal use can be significant.

Case Study

A 75-year-old women presents to the emergency department. She has been experiencing pain under her right arm. She first noticed it a couple of days ago while getting dressed. Yesterday the pain became worse. She describes "sharp, like lightening" pain near her shoulder blade and traveling under her left arm and breast. It hurts when she raises her arm. Today, the pain is so severe she could not pull her dress over her head. She states she has never had anything like this.

Questions to Consider

1. What is the most likely cause of this patient's pain (differential diagnosis)?
2. What is the physiologic mechanism of pain in this condition?
3. What are your pharmacologic options to improve pain management at this time?

REFERENCES

Adamis, D., Treloar, A., MacDonald, A. J., & Martin, F. C. (2005). Concurrent validity of two instruments (the Confusion Assessment Method and Delirium Rating Scale) in the detection of deliriumamong older medical inpatients. *Age Ageing, 34*, 72.

Administration on Aging. (2010). *A profile of older Americans: 2010.* August 27, 2011. Retrieved from http://www.aoa.gov/AoARoot/Aging_Statistics/Profile/2010/docs/2010profile.pdf

American Burn Association. (2007). *Burn incidence and treatment in the U.S.: 2007 fact sheet.* Retrieved from http://www.ameriburn.org/resources_factsheet.php

American College of Gynecologists. (2009). ACOG practice bulletin No. 100. Critical care in pregnancy. *Obstetrics and Gynecology, 113*(2), 443–450.

Aubrun, F., Bunge, D., Langeron, O., Saillant, G., Coriat, P., & Riou, B. (2004). Postoperative morphine consumption in the elderly patient. *Anesthesiology, 99*, 160–165.

Bercault, N., Boulain, T., Kuteifan, K., Wolf, M., Runge, I., & Fleury, J. C. (2004). Obesity-related excess mortality rates in an adult intensive care unit: A risk-adjusted matched cohort study. *Critical Care Medicine, 32*, 998–1003.

Buvanendran, A., & Kroin, J. S. (2007). Useful adjuvants for postoperative pain management. *Best Practice and Research Clinical Anaesthesiology, 21*(1), 31–49.

Finkelstein, E. A., Trogdon, J. G., Cohen, J. W., & Dietz, W. (2009). Annual medical spending attributable to obesity: Payer- and service-specific estimates. *Health Affairs, 28*(5), w822–w831.

Herr, K., Coyne, P. J., Key, T., Manworren, R., McCaffery, M., Merkel, S., . . . American Society for Pain Management Nursing. (2006). Assessment of pain in nonverbal patients. *Pain Management Nursing, 7*(2), 44–52.

Jayasinghe, C., & Blass, N. H. (1999). Pain management in the critically ill obstetric patient. *Critical Care Clinics, 15*(1), 201–228.

Jermyn, R. T., Janora, D. M., & Surve, S. A. (2010). Assessment and classification of pain in the elderly patient. *Clinical Geriatrics, 18*(08), 16–19.

Kaye, A. D., Amir Baluch, A., & Scott, J. T. (2010). Pain management in the elderly population: A review. *The Ochsner Journal, 10*, 179–187.

Neville, A. L., Brown, C. V., Weng, J., Demetriades, D., & Velmahos, G. C. (2004). Obesity is an independent risk factor of mortality in severely injured blunt trauma patients. *Archives of Surgery, 139*, 983–987.

Pasero, C., & McCaffery, M. (2007). Orthopaedic postoperative pain management. *Journal of PeriAnesthesia Nursing, 22*(3), 160–173.

Pasero, C., Rakel, B., & McCaffery, M. (2005). Postoperative pain management in the older adult. *Pain in Older Persons* (pp. 377–401). Seattle, WA: IASP Press.

Pickering, G., & Melding, P. S. (2005). Foreward. In S. J. Gibson & D. K. Weiner (Eds.), *Pain in older persons* (pp. 67–85). Seattle, WA: IASP Press.

Price, L. C., Germain, S., Wyncoll, D., & Nelson-Piercy, C. (2009). Management of the critically ill obstetric patient. *Obstetrics, Gynaecology, and Reproductive Medicine, 19*, 350–358.

Ray, D. E., Matchett, S. C., Baker, K., Wasser, T., & Young, M. J. (2005). The effect of body mass index on patient outcomes in a medical ICU. *Chest, 127*, 2125–2131.

Robinson, S., Vollmer, C., Jirka, H., Rich, C., Midiri, C., & Bisby, D. (2008). Aging and delirium: Too much or too little pain medication? *Pain Management Nursing,* *9*(2), 66–72.

Taylor, L. J., Harris, J., Epps, C. D., & Herr, K. (2005). Psychometric evaluation of selected pain-intensity scales for use with cognitively impaired and cognitively intact older adults. *Rehabilitation Nursing, 30*, 55–61.

Tremblay, A., & Bandi, V. (2003). Impact of body mass index on outcomes following critical care. *Chest, 123*, 1202–1207.

19

Pain, Addiction, and Opioid Dependency in Critical Care Patients

Pain is a common occurrence in critically ill patients. Although medical and surgical patients who are admitted to critical care may present to the health care team as a post-surgical patient or a critically ill nursing home patient, these patients may have underlying chronic pain conditions that can affect their care. Some may be opioid dependent, using opioids daily for pain control, and require a more comprehensive plan of care for pain management than patients who have not been taking opioids prior to admission. Some patients may be using alcohol regularly or may be addicts using illicit substances such as heroin. No matter how the patient presents to the health care team, pain control will need to be addressed.

Patients who enter the health care system through the emergency department (ED) are at high risk for experiencing pain. Pain is the most common reason for seeking health care in an ED, responsible for more than 70% of all ED visits (Cordell et al., 2002; Todd & Miner, 2010). Unfortunately the pain management in an ED setting is not optimal—in a retrospective study of adults treated in a large metropolitan ED, only 47% received adequate pain relief (Tanabe & Buschman, 1999).

One issue affecting pain management in the ED is the idea of drug seeking. This term is defined as "patient behavior designed to obtain analgesics for pain relief" (McCaffery, Grimm, Pasero, Ferrell, & Uman, 2005). In reality, these patients may be suffering from untreated or undertreated pain. Perhaps the term is better defined as "patients who are seeking relief from unrelieved pain" or "relief seekers." Patients who have pain that is not fully relieved will seek help from those they perceive to have the ability to help manage pain. In a survey of 360 nurses from a variety of practice settings, certain patient behaviors made nurses think the patient was "drug seeking," such as:

- Goes to different EDs to get opioids (84.2%)
- Tells the nurse where to give the drug and how fast (60.4%)
- Tells inconsistent stories about medical history or pain (56%)
- Asks the nurse for a refill because prescription was lost or stolen (58.2%) (McCaffery et al., 2005)

This focus on behaviors rather than the patient's report of pain means the patient may be labeled and left with unrelieved pain. This chapter will discuss the criteria for addiction, opioid dependency, and tolerance, which may help readers examine their own beliefs and thoughts about the use of opioids in the ED and for critically ill patients.

THE PROBLEM OF SUBSTANCE ABUSE

Consider the position of a health care team who is presented with a critically ill patient who needs pain management. One of the biggest problems in the patient's care is the difficult to manage pain. The health care team then considers what the potential causes might be: opioid dependency, a family history of difficult to manage pain, or something unknown. The provider may not have used the best opioid for the patient or the dose may be too low on first consideration, or the patient's genetic make-up for medication metabolism may come into the picture. The issue that may be the hardest to deal with is the patient having a history of substance abuse, which can affect pain. For these patients, there is a heightened sensitivity to pain and diminished response to opioid analgesics.

Unless the patient tells the health care team that he or she has a history of substance abuse or is actively using illicit substances, the health care provider may be caring for a patient who has difficulty with pain control for no detectable reason. These patients can have a simple procedure such as chest tube insertion, yet complain of severe level pain that is not controlled with the usual analgesic medications. Even increasing doses of medication for these patients does not seem to improve the level of pain relief and side effects such as nausea or sedation may start to occur. Although there can be other causes of unrelieved pain, when a patient has a history of substance abuse or is abusing opioids, it tends to remain a problem that reappears when least suspected.

Anyone may be the patient who is an addict or who has a history of addictive disease—trauma patients who are admitted to the hospital, or a homemaker or housewife who became addicted to pain medication after a past surgery. You cannot tell by looking at the patient whether the patient has a history of addictive disease or is addicted to an illicit substance. Not all addicts are young or show behaviors that indicate addiction. They may be an older patient who made a serious mistake with drugs in the past who in later life is still feeling the effects of poor judgment.

PREVALENCE

Addiction is on the rise. It is not only the use of "street drugs" such as heroin but the misuse of prescription medications and teenage abuse of these substances that is increasing. The best estimate on the prevalence of addiction is that 3% to 16% of the 301 million people in the United States have addictive disease (Joranson & Gilson, 2007). The latest government estimate is that prescription drug abuse has increased by 400%. It has become accepted among peer groups and has increased despite public information announcements that highlight the risks of the practice.

The term *psychotherapeutics* is used as a general term for the categories of drugs that include pain relievers, tranquilizers, stimulants, and sedatives (St. Marie, 2010). The most popular drugs abused by teenagers and young adults are:

- Hydrocodone (Vicodin); about 1 in 5 young people
- Oxycodone (Oxycontin); 10%
- Drugs for attention deficit disorder such as methylphenidate (Ritalin) or amphetamine and dextroamphetamine (Adderall); 10% (Generation R_x- Partnership for a Drug Free America).

Where are these young people obtaining their drugs? Most commonly from a medicine chest at home or in a friend's house, from a relative or friend, from a doctor, a drug dealer or stranger, or via the Internet (Substance Abuse and Mental Health Services Administration [SAMHSA], 2006). By 2004, the average American teenager had abused a prescription pain reliever in greater numbers than those who used Ecstasy, cocaine, crack, or LSD (Generation R_x).

Addiction is not only for the young members of our society. It can be found in patients of any age. In the time period of 1992–2003 prescription abuse in the general population increased from 7.8 million to 15.1 million and rose at a rate that is seven times faster than the increase in the United States population (Under the Counter, 2005).

It is unfortunate but health care providers will undoubtedly find they have undetected addicts within their patient groups and even more with a history of addiction. Additionally, many of these patients will have chronic pain or increased pain from acute injuries or surgery.

TERMS

Dealing with patients who have addiction or a history of addiction requires an understanding of the terms addiction, dependency, tolerance, and pseudoaddiction.

Addiction is characterized by the four Cs:
- **C**ontinued use despite harm
- Impaired **c**ontrol over the drug
- **C**raving
- **C**ompulsive use (Savage, Covington, Heit, Hunt, Joranson, & Scholl, 2001)

The formal definition of addiction is a primary chronic, neurobiologic disease influenced by genetic, psychosocial, and environmental factors (Savage et al., 2001). Addicts are driven to look for and find the substance that they favor. They are not concerned with the effect that the drug is having on their lives; they just know that they need it and will go to any lengths to find it and use it. To addicts, the pleasure stimulus that they get from using their drug is worth all that they sacrifice.

Clinical Pearl Opioid dependency is not addiction. However, ALL addicts are dependent on their opioid substance of abuse.

Dependency, on the other hand, is a natural phenomenon that occurs with regular use of a medication. All patients who take opioids for more than 30 days become dependent. It is a state of adaptation manifested by a drug class's specific withdrawal syndrome that can be caused by abrupt cessation, rapid dose reductions, or a decrease in the blood level of the drug by the administration of an antagonist (Savage et al., 2001). Patients who are dependent on opioids for pain relief are *not* addicted. They are simply using the medication to continue with their normal activities of living, working, or pursuing a career. It is not correct to label dependent patients as addicted or drug seeking.

When making chart notes on opioid dependent patients, do not label them as addicts; rather, indicate that they are working toward goals of treatment using the opioids as a part of their treatment plan.

Tolerance is a state of adaptation where an effect of the medication such as pain relief diminishes over time. These patients are the type that have good pain relief for a period of time but then start to complain of increased pain. The new pain may be the result of increased activity relative to their pain control, or just an adaptation mechanism that the patient has no control over. Tolerance does not indicate addiction. It simply means that one or more of the medication effects—nausea, sedation, pain relief—has decreased. Increasing medication doses may reduce the pain level or an opioid rotation as described in the medication section may be needed to restore adequate pain relief.

Pseudoaddiction is the development of patient behaviors that mimic what health care providers would perceive as drug seeking: clock watching, frequent requests for specific pain medications. In reality, this behavior is a result of undertreated pain. Once the pain is treated adequately such behaviors will disappear, unlike addition.

ADDICTION VERSUS ABERRANT DRUG-TAKING BEHAVIORS

Patients whose treatment involves long-term opioid analgesics can develop behaviors that appear to be addictive but in truth are classed as aberrant. Aberrant behaviors are broadly classified as actions that are outside of the agreed upon opioid treatment (Heit & Gourlay, 2010). The development of these behaviors is motivated by a variety of conditions such as past experiences with the health care system or undertreated pain. Some behaviors that are considered aberrant but not addiction include:

- Requesting specific drugs
- Aggressive complaining about the need for higher doses
- Drug hoarding during periods of reduced symptoms
- Unapproved use of the drug to treat another symptom
- Reporting psychic effects not intended by the provider
- Unsanctioned dose escalation once or twice
- Obtaining similar drugs from other medical sources
- Resistance to change in therapy associated with tolerable adverse effects with expressions of anxiety about the return of severe symptoms (Fine & Portnoy, 2007)

When patients develop behaviors that are more predicative of addition, it is a very different situation. The behaviors are more pronounced and severe in nature. They indicate the lack of control the patient has with drugs; often these behaviors manifest very quickly if the health care provider recognizes danger signs and starts to control opioid use. Behaviors that can indicate developing addiction include:

- Injecting or snorting oral formulations for quicker onset
- Forging prescriptions

- Selling or stealing prescription drugs
- Obtaining prescription drugs from nonmedical sources such as drug dealers, other addicts, or over the Internet
- Concurrent use of illicit drugs with the prescribed opioids
- Unsanctioned, continued dose escalations
- Recurrent, frequent prescription losses
- Deterioration in personal life, appearing more unkempt or appearing intoxicated
- Solid resistance to changes in opioid therapy despite demonstrated harm (Fine & Portnoy, 2007)

Once these addictive behaviors start, the health care provider must investigate the source and begin more aggressive urine screening, prescription control, and pill counts, and must mandate compliance with the opioid treatment agreement described in the following sections. Tools for estimating risk with opioid use are also described. These tools can help the health care provider determine which patients may experience difficulty with opioids and start more stringent monitoring earlier in the treatment period.

USING UNIVERSAL PRECAUTIONS

Taking a concept from infectious disease, universal precautions can protect the health care provider who prescribes opioids to patients who may be addicted or have a history of substance abuse, and provide a comprehensive plan for opioid prescribing. This type of assessment process can help identify any additional elements that should be addressed when opioids are being prescribed for long-term pain relief. The basic elements of universal precautions are:

- Diagnosis with the appropriate differential
- Psychological assessment including the risk of addictive disorders
- Informed consent either written or verbal
- Treatment agreement
- Baseline assessment of pain and functionality and post-intervention reassessment
- An appropriate trial of opioid therapy and any co-analgesics as indicated
- Continuing reassessment of pain level and functionality
- Regular reassessment of the four As of pain medicine: Analgesia, Activity, Adverse reaction and Aberrant behaviors
- Periodic review of pain and comorbidity diagnoses
- Documentation (Heit & Gouraly, 2010)

Organizing treatment and office visits using universal precautions can help ensure that all needed information is regularly assessed and documented.

Assessing and Screening

When performing a physical examination on an addicted patient look for signs of current drug use—track marks on the arms, injection sites between toes or in tattoos that can hide the injection marks, or skin popping scars from subcutaneous injections of heroin. Inspect the nares for signs of excoriation or irritation from snorted drugs such as cocaine. Patients who are smoking marijuana or heroin may come in frequently with complaints of cough or shortness of breath. With prolonged heroin abuse with highly contaminated drugs, the patients may have a chest x-ray with tissue damage indicating a "heroin lung," where lung tissues have become blocked with the contaminants. Once obvious signs of drug abuse are identified, a more complete physical work-up including HIV testing and hepatitis tests is indicated. An opioid risk assessment is also clearly indicated.

The patient who has had extended exposure to opioids or has used illicit substances such as heroin will have a decreased response to opioid medications. The patient will also have increased sensitivity to pain. Given these characteristics assessing pain will be difficult. The patient with an addiction history will need more medication but may continue to consistently report high levels of pain.

When discussing the pain complaint, recognize that addicts have often been misidentified, overlabeled, and undertreated. They are less open to discussion about pain management fearing they will again be labeled as addicted and possibly denied treatment with opioids. Dependent patients have had similar experiences where they have been labeled as addicts when in reality they are dependent on opioid medication to relieve their daily pain. Some health care providers see the development of tolerance as a sure sign that the patient is becoming addicted to opioid analgesics. Understanding the difference among the three conditions can help clarify the assessment process.

Using a simple numerical rating scale with 0 to 10 for acute injuries can be all that is needed for pain assessment and for tracking the efficacy of pain management medications and interventions in acute care. Two simple and easy to use screens are the CAGE and TRAUMA screens. They work well for patients who are admitted for care after accidents or are being seen in the ED for acute pain when alcohol abuse or substance abuse is suspected.

To assess a patient using the CAGE screen simply ask the patient these four questions:

- Have you ever tried to <u>c</u>ut down on your alcohol or drug use?
- Have people <u>a</u>nnoyed you by commenting on or critiquing your drinking or drug use?
- Have you ever felt bad or <u>g</u>uilty about your drinking or drug use?
- Have you ever needed an <u>e</u>ye opener first thing in the morning to steady your nerves or get rid of a hangover?

This type of simple screen takes but a few minutes and can give the health care provider an idea about both alcohol and substance abuse. The more positive responses the patient gives, the greater the likelihood that the patient has an alcohol or drug abuse problem (Chou et al., 2009).

To assess a patient using the TRAUMA screen ask the patient the five questions that are related to the patient's injury history.

Since your 18th birthday have you:

- Had any fractures or dislocations to your bones or joints, excluding sports injuries?
- Been injured in a traffic accident?
- Injured your head, excluding sports injuries?
- Been in a fight or assaulted while intoxicated?
- Been injured while intoxicated?

If the patient answers yes to two or more of the questions, there is a high potential for abuse (Chou et al., 2009).

The CAGE and the TRAUMA screens give the health care provider an idea of the potential for substance abuse.

More extensive screens for determining risks associated with opioid prescribing have been developed. These tools are most appropriate for long-term prescribing of opioids but some can identify those patients who will have more problems when opioids are used for analgesia.

- The Opioid Risk Tool (ORT) is used to determine what the risk is when the patient is prescribed opioids for pain. This is a list of simple questions related to family history of substance abuse, personal history of substance abuse, age, history of any preadolescent sexual abuse, any psychological disease, and depression. The patient who scores 0–3 is considered low risk, 4–7 is considered moderate risk, and 8 or greater is considered highly likely to develop aberrant behaviors with opioid use. This tool is designed for determining opioid risk prior to starting opioid therapy (D'Arcy, 2010a; Passik, Krish, & Casper, 2008).
- The Screener and Opioid Assessment for Patients with Pain-Revised (SOAPP-R) is a tool designed to screen patients who are being considered for long-term opioid therapy. It consists of 14 questions related to substance abuse

history, medication-related behaviors, antisocial behaviors, doctor-patient relationships, and personal care and lifestyle issues. A score of 8 or greater indicates a high risk of abuse or misuse (D'Arcy, 2010a; Passik et al., 2008).

■ Diagnosis, Intractability, Risk, and Efficacy (DIRE) score allows a provider to determine if the patient is a good risk for opioid therapy. A score of 14 or higher indicates that the patient is a good candidate for opioid therapy. Patients with lower scores are not good risks for opioid therapy (Passik et al., 2008).

■ Current Opioid Misuse Measure (COMM) is a 17-item self-report tool that is used to identify aberrant behaviors for patients who are currently on opioid therapy. The COMM, as a newer tool, can identify emotional or psychiatric issues, evidence of lying, appointment patterns, medication misuse or noncompliance. This tool is designed for use when aberrant behaviors increase in frequency (Butler et al., 2007; D'Arcy, 2010b).

These tools should always be considered only part of the assessment process and should be used in conjunction with standard pain assessments and consideration of the total patient history. For patients being seen in clinics as outpatients, the numerical rating scale is adequate for assessing and reassessing pain at each visit and tracking the effectiveness of the medications being used. For long-term care, these patients may need more extensive screening and documentation.

The Pain Assessment and Documentation Tool (PADT) is helpful in tracking patients who are on opioid therapy for pain management. It is a tool that is based on the four As:

■ *Analgesia:* Pain ratings during the week, percentage of pain that has been relieved, and whether the amount of pain relief is making a difference in your life?

■ *Activities of Daily Living:* Assessments of physical functioning, relationships, mood, sleep, and overall functioning.

■ *Adverse Events:* Side effects such as nausea, fatigue, itching, constipation, drowsiness, or mental clouding

■ *Aberrant Drug-Related Behavior:* Purposeful over sedation, abuse of alcohol or other illicit drugs, requests frequent early renewals, increases dose without authorization, changes routes of administration, requests prescriptions from other doctors.

Using this tool can indicate that the opioid therapy is producing positive results for the patient or is not providing the expected outcomes. Tracking the patient over time in a consistent format can highlight and be an early indication of change as it occurs, allowing the health care provider to adjust the current medication regimen or taper the patients off the current medications.

DEVELOPING A PLAN OF CARE

Before developing a comprehensive treatment plan for the patient there are some items to consider:

- Do I have enough information to diagnose and formulate a comprehensive plan of care?
- Is a trial of opioids merited and if so what are the risks and benefits?
- Can I treat this patient alone?
- Do I need additional consultants? Who would they be?
- Do I need help to manage the patient?
- Does the patient require care that exceeds my resources (Smith, Fine, & Passik, 2009)?

In most cases the patient who is an addict or has a history of substance abuse will need a team approach. Practitioners skilled in dealing with addiction, psychologists, pain specialists, social workers, psychiatrists, and rehabilitation specialists can all be considered part of the team. Careful planning and teams of specialists can help to ensure that the plan of care includes all that is needed and that it will provide the most benefit with the least amount of risk. The fact that the patient is currently under an opioid agreement from a pain specialist is helpful information for the critical care team to have when considering pain management options.

The community physician prescribing opioids needs to track the patient's progress under the opioid agreement. The use of opioids in the critical care setting may have an impact on the outpatient pain management. If outcomes are not positive, the opioid agreement is broken; if addictive behaviors become pronounced, the patient will need to be tapered off the opioid medications and that part of the care discontinued. The patient can continue to be seen for other health conditions but the opioid therapy will be discontinued. In this case the team can be helpful in making decisions about terminating opioid therapy.

Addicts and patients with a history of substance abuse will need higher doses of medication to control their pain. This is a result of the physiologic changes that take place with substance abuse or long-term opioid use. They also have a heightened sensitivity to pain and a decreased response to opioid medications. Because of these changes, opioid doses will need to be higher than the current standard doses of opioids for chronic pain. For the addicted patient, an estimation of medication will have to be made from the patient's report of substance used on a daily basis.

These questions can be difficult to ask but they will need to be discussed in order to determine what amount of medication will be needed to treat pain and avoid withdrawal syndrome. To develop a plan of care for these patients requires a time commitment to not only the clinical issues, but also to dealing with the psychological coping and additive personality. As outpatients, these patients require close monitoring with frequent urine screens and careful prescription management. In the acute care setting, the focus should be on treating the patient's pain and making appropriate referrals for outpatient services when the patient is discharged. Some patients with a history of substance abuse will be very resistant to using opioids, fearing re-addiction. For these patients a combination of therapies including regional techniques (see Chapter 14), non-opioid medications, and careful opioid use can provide adequate pain control.

It is helpful for the critical care team to understand the scope of the patient's opioid agreement. The treatment plans for patients with addictive disease are very comprehensive. They should be individual and spell out the risk and benefits clearly to both the patients and the health care provider involved in the patient's care. An integral part of the treatment plan for outpatients is a treatment agreement that spells out the terms of opioid use. These agreements are essential for protecting the prescriber from any mis-understandings or legal issues and provide the patient with the necessary information when opioids are being used to treat pain. These agreements define addiction, dependency, and tolerance, and detail what medications are being prescribed, how they should be used, and who should prescribe them. The agreement also details what the penalty will be if illicit drugs are detected in random drug screens and what the options are for the pre-scriber should this occur. Samples of treatment agreements are available at http;//www.painmed.org

Random drug screens or urine drug monitoring (UDM) is an es-sential part of the treatment agreement and these should be random, not scheduled. Starting with a baseline urine screen when opioids are started can be helpful in establishing the procedure for UDM. The response of the health care provider to finding illicit substances not prescribed for the patient in the urine screen should be clearly defined in the treatment agreement.

Urine drug screens can detect the presence of a substance or metabo-lite that indicates that a particular drug is present. Different medications clear the urine more quickly; others like phenobarbital may be present for longer periods of time. The use of urine screens is effective for determining the presence of a particular drug but can also provide a false positive or false negative. Some medications such as antibiotics can cause a false posi-tive. There is usually a 1- to 3-day period of time when drugs are present in the urine and can be detected. Some drugs such as methamphetamine, benzodiazepines, fentanyl, heroin, and most opiates clear the urine within 1 to 5 days, while other drugs such as methadone, phenobarbital, phency-clidine (PCP), and propoxyphene are present for longer periods of time, 7 to 14 days.

Using a urine screen for maintaining an opioid agreement can indicate that the appropriate drug is being taken and no illicit drugs are being used. It can also prove that the prescribed drug is not present in the urine, which may indicate diversion. If there is any concern with the results of a urine screen, a gas chromatography test can further define the findings of the urine screen and give more specific information.

The patient with addictive disease or active addiction is a challenge to treat. Most primary care practices are not prepared for these patients; however, it is inevitable that the addicted patient will surface in most if not all practices. Knowing how to manage these patients and how to assess and treat them will make the experience easier for both the health care provider and the patient.

Case Study

Jessica Jones is a 65-year-old patient admitted to the ICU after a thoracotomy for lung cancer. She reports what seem to be excessive pain intensities—8/10 to 10/10—that cause concern in the critical care team. She is having difficulty maintaining her respiratory status and the team feels if they cannot get the pain relieved, they may have to intubate her. Jessica is using PCA morphine for pain relief. The nurse goes in to speak with Jessica. She asks Jessica about her pain and receives this reply. "It is so bad, I JUST CANNOT GET AHEAD OF IT. I push the PCA button all the time and it just does not work. DO SOMETHING, anything to stop this pain." The nurse reviews the PCA attempts and injections and finds that Jessica has made 154 attempts with 24 injections. She asks the intensivist to increase the PCA settings but when the intensivist speaks with Jessica, she discovers that, for over 6 months, Jessica has been abusing prescription medications purchased on the Internet—hydrocodone, oxycontin, and fentanyl oral tablets—for unrelieved low back pain.

Questions to Consider

1. Just because Jessica looks like an average housewife or professional, should you discount the reason for the unrelieved pain as addiction?
2. Now that you know that Jessica is opioid tolerant, how will you adjust her pain management regimen?
3. How can the nurse help Jessica to manage her pain while understanding that her addiction is causing some of the difficulty with pain management?
4. Should you offer Jessica a referral to an addictionologist or consult one to see her while she is hospitalized?

REFERENCES

American Academy of Pain Medicine, American Pain Society, American Society of Addiction Medicine. Definitions related to the use of opioids for the treatment of pain. *WMJ: Official Publication of the State Medical Society of Wisconsin, 100,* 28–29

American Pain Society. (2008). *Principles of analgesic use in the treatment of acute pain and cancer pain.* Glenview, IL: Author.

Brennan, F., Carr, D. B., & Cousins, M. (2007). Pain management: A fundamental human right. *Anesthesia and Analgesia, 105,* 205–221.

Carlozzi, A., Fornari, F., Siwicki, D., Barkin, R., Nafziger, A., Woodcock, M., et al. (XXX). Anesthesiology News: Pain Medicine News

Chou, R., Fanciullo, G., Fine, P., Adler, J. A., Ballantyne, J. C., Davies, P., …, Miaskowsi, C. (2009). Clinical, guidelines for the use of opioid therapy in chronic noncancer pain. *The Journal of Pain: Official Journal of the American Pain Society, 10*(2), 113–130.

Cordell, W. H., Keene, K. K., Giles, B. K., Jones, J. B., Jones, J. H., & Brizendine, E. J. (2002). The high prevalence of pain in emergency medical care. *The American Journal of Emergency Medicine, 20,* 165–169.

D'Arcy, Y. (2009). Be in the know about pain management. *The Nurse Practitioner, 34*(4), 43–47.

D'Arcy, Y. (2010a). Pain assessment. In ASPMN & B. St. Marie (Eds.), *Core curriculum for pain management nursing.* Indianapolis, IN: Kendall Hunt.

D'Arcy, Y. (2010b). Treating pain in addicted patient: Great challenge, greater reward. *Advance for Nurse Practitioners, 18*(5), 20–25.

Fine, P., & Portnoy, R. (2007). *Opioid Analgesia.* New York, NY: Vendome Group.

Heit, H., & Gourlay, D. (2010). The treatment of chronic pain in patients with history of substance abuse. In S. Fishman, J. Ballantyne, & J. Rathmell (Eds.), *Bonica's management of pain.* Philadelphia, PA: Lippincott Williams & Wilkins.

Joranson, D., & Gilson, A. (2007) A much needed window on opioid diversion. *Pain Medicine, 8*(2), 128–129.

McCaffery, M., Grimm, M., Pasero, C., Ferrell, B., & Uman, G. (2005). On the meaning of "drug seeking." *Pain Management Nursing, 6*(40), 122–136.

Passik, S., Krish, K. L., & Casper, D. (2008). Addiction- related assessment tools and pain management instruments for a screening, treatment planning, and monitoring compliance. *Pain Medicine, 9*(S2), S145–S166.

Passik, S., & Kirsch K. (2009). Pain in the substance abuse population. In H. Smith (Ed.), *Current therapy in pain*. Philadelphia, PA: Elsevier.

Savage, S., Covington, E., Heit, H., Hunt, J., Joranson, D., & Scholl, S. (2001) *Definitions related to the use of opioids for the treatment of pain: A consensus document from the American Academy of Pain medicine, the American Pain Society, and the American Society of Addiction Medicine*. Glenview, IL: AAPM.

Smith, H., Fine, P., & Passik, S. (2009). *Opioid risk management tools and tips*. New York, NY: Oxford University Press.

St. Marie, B. (2010). Coexisting addiction and pain. In ASPMN & B. St. Maria (Eds.), *Core curriculum for pain management nursing*. Indianapolis, IN: Kendall Hunt.

Substance Abuse and Mental Health Services Administration. (2006). Results from the 2005 National Survey on Drug Use and Health: National Findings. Office of Applied Studies, NSDUH Series H-30. DHHS publication No.SMA 06-4194. Rockville, MD. Available at http://oas.samhsa.gov/nsduhLatest.htm

Tanabe, P., & Buschman, M. (1999). A prospective study of ED pain management practices and the patient's perspective. *Journal of Emergency Nursing, 25,* 171–177.

Todd, K. H., & Miner, J. (2010). Pain management in the emergency department. In S. M. Fishman, J. C. Ballantyne, J. P. Rathmell (Eds.), *Bonica's management of pain* (pp. 1576–1587). Philadelphia, PA: Lippincott Wilkins & Williams.

Under the Counter: The Diversion and abuse of controlled prescription drugs in the U.S. (2005). The National Center for Addiction and Substance Abuse at Columbia University. Retrieved November 12, 2012, from www.casacolumbia.org

Webster, L. R., & Dove L. (2007). *Avoiding opioid abuse while managing pain*. North Branch, MN: Sunrise River Press.

Index

A-beta receptors, 13
A-delta fibers, 13
A-delta receptors, 13
A118G single nucleotide polymorphism, 133
A118MOR, 134
AA, 133
AAST. *See* American Association of Surgery for Trauma
ABCDE, 274
Abdominal compartment syndrome (ACS), 215–217
Abdominal exam, components of, 205
Abdominal fluid collections, evacuation of, 217
Abdominal pain
   acute abdomen signs, 205
   etiology, 204–205
   physical examination, 205–206
   treatment, 207
Abdominal trauma
   blunt trauma, 293–295
   hollow viscus trauma, 300
   kidney, 298–299
   liver injury, 295–297
   pancreas, 299–300
   small bowel injury, 300–301
   spleen, 297–298
Abdominal wall compliance, improvement of, 216
Aberrant drug-taking behaviors, 29, 339
   addiction versus, 335–336
Abortive therapy
   cluster headache (CH), 266–267
   migraines, 264–265
Abrasions, 230, 254
Abscesses, 230–237

Acceptable pain relief, 213
Acetaminophen (Tylenol), 65–67, 213, 249–250, 316, 327
   during pregnancy, 326
Acid suppression therapy, 208, 209
Activities of daily living, 339
Acupuncture, 118–119, 320
Acute abdominal pain, assessing and differentiating, 206
Acute aortic dissection, 192
Acute coronary syndrome (ACS), 190
Acute low back pain
   non-pharmacologic therapy for, 249
   red flags, 248
Acute mesenteric ischemia, 210–211
Acute pain, 10, 11, 22, 246
   coanalgesics for, 101–103
   types of, 21
Acute pancreatitis, 212
Acute pericarditis, 194–195
Acute thoracic aortic dissection, symptoms of, 193
Acute upper GI bleeding, 208
Acute versus chronic pain, 11
Addiction
   versus aberrant drug-taking behaviors, 335–336
   and dependency, 334
   formal definition of, 334
   prevalence of, 333
   and pseudoaddiction, 335
   and tolerance, 334–335
Adipose tissue, 321
Adjuvant medications, 63, 105, 317
Adult Nonverbal Pain Scale (ANVPS), 144